TRAUMA-FOCUSED CBT
FOR CHILDREN AND ADOLESCENTS

Also from Judith A. Cohen, Anthony P. Mannarino, and Esther Deblinger

For more information, visit Drs. Cohen and Mannarino's website:
http://pittsburghchildtrauma.net

Effective Treatments for PTSD, Second Edition:
Practice Guidelines from the International Society
for Traumatic Stress Studies
Edited by Edna B. Foa, Terence M. Keane,
Matthew J. Friedman, and Judith A. Cohen

Treating Trauma and Traumatic Grief
in Children and Adolescents
Judith A. Cohen, Anthony P. Mannarino,
and Esther Deblinger

TRAUMA-FOCUSED CBT FOR CHILDREN AND ADOLESCENTS

Treatment Applications

edited by
Judith A. Cohen
Anthony P. Mannarino
Esther Deblinger

THE GUILFORD PRESS
New York   London

Printed in the United States of America

This book is printed on acid-free paper.

Last digit is print number: 9 8 7 6 5 4

The authors have checked with sources believed to be reliable in their efforts to provide information
that is complete and generally in accord with the standards of practice that are accepted at the time
of publication. However, in view of the possibility of human error or changes in behavioral, mental
health, or medical sciences, neither the authors, nor the editors and publisher, nor any other party
who has been involved in the preparation or publication of this work warrants that the information
contained herein is in every respect accurate or complete, and they are not responsible for any errors
or omissions or the results obtained from the use of such information. Readers are encouraged to
confirm the information contained in this book with other sources.

Library of Congress Cataloging-in-Publication Data

Trauma-focused CBT for children and adolescents : treatment applications / edited by
Judith A. Cohen, Anthony P. Mannarino, Esther Deblinger.
    p. cm.
  Includes bibliographical references and index.
  ISBN 978-1-4625-0482-4 (hardback)
  1. Cognitive therapy for children.   2. Cognitive therapy for teenagers.
  3. Post-traumatic stress disorder in children—Treatment.   4. Post-traumatic stress
disorder in adolescence—Treatment.   I. Cohen, Judith A.
II. Mannarino, Anthony P.   III. Deblinger, Esther.
  RJ505.C63T73 2012
  618.92′891425—dc23

                                      2011052458

About the Editors

Judith A. Cohen, MD, a board-certified child and adolescent psychiatrist, is Medical Director of the Center for Traumatic Stress in Children and Adolescents at Allegheny General Hospital, Pittsburgh, Pennsylvania. With Anthony P. Mannarino, she has received funding since 1986 from the National Institute of Mental Health, the Substance Abuse and Mental Health Services Administration, and the U.S. Department of Justice to assess and treat traumatized children. Dr. Cohen is a recipient of the Outstanding Professional Award from the American Professional Society on the Abuse of Children (APSAC) and the Norbert and Charlotte Rieger Psychodynamic Psychotherapy Award from the American Academy of Child and Adolescent Psychiatry.

Anthony P. Mannarino, PhD, is Director of the Center for Traumatic Stress in Children and Adolescents and Vice Chair of the Department of Psychiatry at Allegheny General Hospital. He is also Professor of Psychiatry at Drexel University College of Medicine. Dr. Mannarino has been a leader in the field of child traumatic stress since the 1980s. He has been awarded numerous federal grants from the National Center on Child Abuse and Neglect and the National Institute of Mental Health to investigate the clinical course of traumatic stress symptoms in children and to develop effective treatment approaches for traumatized children and their families. He is a recipient of many honors, including the Betty Elmer Outstanding Professional Award from Family Resources of Pennsylvania, the Most Outstanding Article Award for papers published in the journal *Child Maltreatment* from APSAC, the Model Program Award from the Substance Abuse and Mental Health Services Administration for "Cognitive-Behavioral Therapy for Child Traumatic Stress," and the Legacy Award from the Greater Pittsburgh Psychological Association. Dr. Mannarino is a past president of APSAC and of the Section on Child Maltreatment, Society for Child and Family Policy and Practice (Division 37), American Psychological Association.

Esther Deblinger, PhD, is Co-Founder and Co-Director of the CARES (Child Abuse Research Education and Service) Institute and Professor of Psychiatry at the School of Osteopathic Medicine, University of Medicine and Dentistry of New Jersey (UMDNJ). She has received funding since 1986 from the Foundation of UMDNJ, the National Center on Child Abuse and Neglect, and the National Institute of Mental Health to investigate the impact and treatment of child abuse. Dr. Deblinger has collaborated with Judith A. Cohen and Anthony P. Mannarino over many years on the development, evaluation, and dissemination of trauma-focused cognitive-behavioral therapy, recognized for its efficacy by the U.S. Department of Health and Human Services and the Kaufman Best Practices Task Force. She has coauthored numerous scientific publications and two widely acclaimed professional books on the treatment of child sexual abuse and trauma and traumatic grief, as well as several children's books on body safety. Her work has been recognized with awards from *Woman's Day* magazine and the State of New Jersey's Office of the Child Advocate. In addition, Dr. Deblinger is a recipient of the Outstanding Research Career Achievement Award from APSAC and the Rosenberry Award for Excellence in Teaching, Innovative Research, and Scholarly Vision from the Children's Hospital, Aurora, Colorado.

Contributors

Dolores Subia BigFoot, PhD, Center on Child Abuse and Neglect, University of Oklahoma Health Sciences Center, Oklahoma City, Oklahoma

Angela M. Cavett, PhD, RPT-S, Knowlton, O'Neill and Associates, West Fargo, North Dakota

Judith A. Cohen, MD, Center for Traumatic Stress in Children and Adolescents, Allegheny General Hospital, Pittsburgh, Pennsylvania

Stephen J. Cozza, MD, Center for the Study of Traumatic Stress, Uniformed Services University of the Health Sciences, Bethesda, Maryland

Carla Kmett Danielson, PhD, Department of Psychiatry and Behavioral Sciences, Medical University of South Carolina, Charleston, South Carolina

Michael Andrew de Arellano, PhD, National Crime Victims Treatment and Research Center, Department of Psychiatry and Behavioral Sciences, Medical University of South Carolina, Charleston, South Carolina

Esther Deblinger, PhD, CARES Institute, School of Osteopathic Medicine, University of Medicine and Dentistry of New Jersey, Stratford, New Jersey

Shannon Dorsey, PhD, Department of Psychiatry and Behavioral Sciences, School of Medicine, University of Washington, Seattle, Washington

Athena A. Drewes, PsyD, RPT-S, Astor Services for Children and Families, Rhinebeck, New York

Julia W. Felton, PhD, Department of Psychiatry and Behavioral Sciences, Medical University of South Carolina, Charleston, South Carolina

Christina A. Grosso, LCAT, ATR-BC, BCETS, Center for Trauma Program Innovation, Jewish Board of Family and Children's Services, New York, New York

Matthew Kliethermes, PhD, Children's Advocacy Services of Greater St. Louis, University of Missouri–St. Louis, St. Louis, Missouri

Anthony P. Mannarino, PhD, Center for Traumatic Stress in Children and Adolescents, Allegheny General Hospital, Pittsburgh, Pennsylvania

Laura K. Murray, PhD, Department of International Health, Johns Hopkins University Bloomberg School of Public Health, Baltimore, Maryland

Daniela Navarro, MA, LPC, LCDC, Serving Children and Adolescents in Need, Inc., Laredo, Texas

Susana Rivera, PhD, LPC, Serving Children and Adolescents in Need, Inc., Laredo, Texas

Susan R. Schmidt, PhD, Center on Child Abuse and Neglect, University of Oklahoma Health Sciences Center, Oklahoma City, Oklahoma

Stephanie A. Skavenski, MSW, MPH, Department of International Health, Johns Hopkins University Bloomberg School of Public Health, Baltimore, Maryland

Rachel Wamser, MA, Children's Advocacy Services of Greater St. Louis, University of Missouri–St. Louis, St. Louis, Missouri

Acknowledgments

The growth and dissemination of the trauma-focused cognitive-behavioral therapy (TF-CBT) model as reflected in this book is a direct result of the enormous support we have enjoyed from friends and colleagues too numerous to name. These colleagues include individuals who helped us get started in the field and showed us the ropes and those who supported our efforts along the way, as well as our more recent collaborators. We are particularly indebted to our respective institutions—the CARES Institute at the School of Osteopathic Medicine at the University of Medicine and Dentistry of New Jersey and Allegheny General Hospital/Allegheny–Singer Research Institute—and their leadership for providing the supportive atmospheres in which we have been able to successfully engage in the clinical, research, and training efforts that have made the development, evaluation, and widespread dissemination of TF-CBT possible.

We would like to express our appreciation to our many clinical colleagues, within our institutions as well as those across the United States and the rest of the world. Their creative clinical ideas and insights over the years have greatly contributed to the appeal and flexibility of TF-CBT. In addition, we are very thankful for the commitment and diligence of our research colleagues whose important contributions allowed us to develop the evidence base that sets this treatment model apart and provides clinicians and consumers with confidence that their children can and will overcome the devastating effects of trauma. We are also greatly encouraged by the work of researchers outside of our institutions who are replicating our findings and adding to our understanding of how best to support the healing of children and their families.

We would like to acknowledge the funding agencies that have supported our work for over 25 years. These agencies include the National Center on Child Abuse and Neglect, the National Institute of Mental Health, the National Child Traumatic Stress Network, the Substance Abuse and Mental Health Services Administration, the Foundation of UMDNJ, and the Annie E. Casey Foundation. We would also like to acknowledge the extraordinary collaboration we have enjoyed with our colleagues at the Medical University of South Carolina in developing TF-CBT Web-based training platforms that have contributed so dramatically to TF-CBT dissemination. We thank each of our chapter authors for their critical contributions, as this book would not have been possible without their very impressive knowledge and expertise in applying TF-CBT to special populations in highly diverse settings.

We deeply thank the many parents and children from whom we have learned so much about how families can recover despite extraordinary adversity.

We reserve our greatest appreciation for the love and family in our lives. When editing this book, one of us experienced both the birth of a granddaughter and the death of a parent. This reaffirmed for us that nothing is more important than loving parents and supportive families and friends.

We dedicate this book to all of the parents we have had the privilege to work with and learn from, and to our own parents, whose guidance, support, patience, and love made all the difference: the late Bernard and Anna Foner Cohen; the late Anthony and Marie Mannarino; and Jack and Charlotte Deblinger and Henry and Judy Sosland.

And to Sam and Molly—may you have a lifetime of health, happiness, and love.

Contents

Introduction

ESTHER DEBLINGER
JUDITH A. COHEN
ANTHONY P. MANNARINO

Many individuals experience significant stressors during childhood. These experiences vary considerably in their quality, frequency, intensity, and impact. Some of these stressors are quite common (e.g., peer conflicts, the death of elderly family members), and children usually manage such stressors adequately with no professional intervention. Childhood traumatic events, though less ubiquitous, are also common and are more likely to be psychologically overwhelming because they potentially threaten a child's sense of safety and security and lead to subjective feelings of terror, fear, shame, anger, helplessness, and/or worthlessness. Potentially traumatic childhood events include child sexual or physical abuse, exposure to domestic or community violence, the traumatic loss of a family member whether through death or other means, natural and man-made disasters, war or refugee-related experiences, severe car accidents, fires, and/or medical traumas (Cohen, Mannarino, & Deblinger, 2006).

Many children—perhaps those with stress-resistant temperaments or genetic makeups, naturally effective coping styles, and/or strong support systems—are resilient even to these very traumatic childhood events. However, research has documented that a significant proportion of those who experience childhood trauma develop maladaptive emotional and behavioral reactions that disrupt their psychosocial development and adjustment. Studies examining the significant negative effects of childhood trauma date back many decades. Researchers from the National Institute of Mental Health conducted perhaps the first large-scale study of the impact of trauma on children with their examination of schoolchildren's psychosocial reactions to a tornado striking the movie theater where they were gathered for a matinee (Bloch, Silber, & Perry, 1956). Another seminal investigation of children's reactions to trauma was conducted in the 1970s following a school bus kidnapping in Chowchilla, California. Terr (1985) prospectively examined the unfolding traumatic responses of the kidnapped children compared with a group of nontraumatized children matched on age and sex. Children's post-trauma reactions have continued to be examined by researchers since these early investigations, with studies repeatedly demonstrating strong associations between childhood trauma and an increased risk of developing post-traumatic stress symptoms, depression, conduct problems, psychotic symptoms, substance abuse problems, as well as other emotional and behavioral difficulties (Arseneault et al., 2011; Briere & Elliott, 2003; Kendall-Tackett, Williams, & Finkelhor, 1993; Khoury, Tang, Bradley, Cubells, & Ressler, 2010; Maercker, Michael, Fehm, Becker, & Margraf, 2004; McKay, Lynn, & Bannon, 2005; Putnam, 2003).

In addition, recent research suggests that children who have experienced one traumatic event are highly likely to have experienced traumas of a different nature (Turner, Finkelhor, & Ormrod, 2010). Moreover, the accumulation of traumatic experiences in childhood has been well established to be associated with increasingly severe adverse effects by both retrospective and prospective empirical investigations (Felitti et al., 1998; Finkelhor, Ormrod, & Turner, 2009).

Clinical descriptions of interventions designed to address the effects of childhood trauma date back many decades as well. However, empirical research examining the efficacy of these treatment methods is a more recent development. When we began our efforts to design and evaluate interventions for this population of children, there were no published scientific studies evaluating the efficacy of interventions designed to specifically address childhood posttraumatic stress disorder (PTSD). In essence, trauma-focused cognitive-behavioral therapy (TF-CBT) for children and adolescents was developed and evaluated in response to this clear gap in the scientific literature.

Beginning in the mid-1980s, at separate clinical research sites in Pittsburgh (Judith A. Cohen and Anthony P. Mannarino) and New Jersey (Esther Deblinger), we began conducting independent research studies to identify the specific problems exhibited by children who had experienced trauma, with an initial focus on sexual abuse (Cohen & Mannarino, 1988; Deblinger, McLeer, Atkins, Ralph, & Foa, 1989; Mannarino & Cohen, 1986; Mannarino, Cohen, & Gregor, 1989; Mannarino, Cohen, Smith, & Moore-Motily, 1991; McLeer, Deblinger, Atkins, Foa, & Ralph, 1988) in order to inform the development of evidence-based interventions for this population. We initially implemented and examined the clinical benefits of preliminary treatment protocols (Cohen & Mannarino, 1993; Deblinger, McLeer, & Henry, 1990) and conducted several independent randomized controlled trials of trauma-focused individual (Cohen & Mannarino, 1996, 1998; Deblinger, Lippmann, & Steer, 1996) as well as group therapy (Deblinger, Stauffer, & Steer, 2001) models.

TF-CBT, as described in *Treating Trauma and Traumatic Grief in Children and Adolescents* (Cohen, Mannarino, & Deblinger, 2006), TF-CBTWeb, and this book, reflects the integration of our earlier treatment models (Cohen & Mannarino, 1993; Deblinger & Heflin, 1996) as well as our ongoing collaborative efforts. Our initial large-scale multisite collaboration examined the efficacy of TF-CBT in comparison to child-centered therapy (Cohen, Deblinger, Mannarino, & Steer, 2004). The results demonstrated that, compared with children and caregivers assigned to child-centered therapy, those assigned to TF-CBT exhibited significantly greater improvements with respect to PTSD, depression, behavior problems, feelings of shame, and dysfunctional abuse-related attributions, while their parents reported significantly greater improvements in abuse-specific distress, depression, parenting skills, and parental support. Additionally, these findings were generally maintained over a 1-year follow-up period (Deblinger, Mannarino, Cohen, & Steer, 2006). The findings of our most recent multisite dismantling study documented the overall efficacy of TF-CBT for young children in both 8- and 16-session formats (ages 4–11), while highlighting the benefits of the eight-session trauma narrative condition in most efficiently and efficaciously helping children overcome abuse-related fear and generalized anxiety (Deblinger, Mannarino, Cohen, Runyon, & Steer, 2011). The results also suggested that the skill-building components and the parenting component, in particular, were perhaps most critical in addressing externalizing behavior problems (Deblinger et al., 2011), replicating earlier findings (Deblinger et al., 1996). The efficacy of TF-CBT for children exposed to intimate partner violence (IPV) also has been recently evaluated in a randomized trial conducted in a community setting. The results of this investigation demonstrated that, compared with children assigned to client-centered therapy (usual care), those assigned to eight sessions of TF-CBT exhibited significantly greater reductions in IPV-related PTSD and anxiety (Cohen, Mannarino, & Iyengar, 2011). Recent studies have further documented the benefits of TF-CBT for children who have suffered traumatic grief (Cohen, Mannarino, & Staron, 2006), children traumatized by the events associated with 9/11(CATS Consortium, 2010) as well as Hurricane Katrina (Jaycox et al., 2010), and child populations with high trauma exposure rates, including children in foster care (Dorsey, Cox, Conover, & Berliner, 2011; Lyons, Weiner, & Scheider, 2006) and children exposed to violence and traumatic loss in low-resource countries (Dorsey, Murray, Balusubramanian, & Skavenski, 2011; Murray et al., 2011). While there are many approaches to treating childhood trauma, recent reviews of the empirical literature suggest that TF-CBT has the most extensive empirical support for its efficacy in treating children suffering from PTSD and related emotional and behavioral difficulties (Bisson et al., 2007; Saunders, Berliner, & Hanson, 2004; Silverman et al., 2008). Thus far, there have been 22 scientific investigations examining the efficacy of TF-CBT, including 12 randomized controlled trials. In addition, TF-CBT has received very positive ratings for efficacy, feasibility, and readiness for dissemination based on extensive treatment outcome reviews sponsored by the Department of Justice (Saunders et al., 2004), the California Evidence-Based Clearinghouse for Child Welfare (*www.cebc4cw.org*), and the U.S. Department of Health and Human Services, Substance Abuse and Mental Health Services Administration's National Registry of Evidence-based Programs and Practices (*www.nrepp.samhsa.gov*).

Given the strong evidence supporting its efficacy, it is not surprising that there has been increasing demand for training in this model over the last decade. To date, there have been more than 18 statewide TF-CBT learning collaboratives designed to disseminate training to administrative, supervisory, and direct service providers in mental health agencies across the United States (Sigel & Benton, 2011). We have also created a TF-CBT "Train-the-Trainer" Program to increase the availability of face-to-face clinical trainings. Most notably, we have collaborated with colleagues from the Medical University of South Carolina to create free-of-charge introductory web-based training in TF-CBT (*www.musc.edu/tfcbt*; *www.musc.edu/ctg*) as well as a web-based TF-CBT consult site (*www.musc.edu/tfcbtconsult*) that may be utilized by TF-CBT therapists on an ongoing basis. To date, more than 100,000 therapists from across the United States and around the world have registered for training on the TF-CBT website. These web-based formats also provide data from the field that will continue to inform our efforts to enhance and expand the use of TF-CBT with appropriate populations.

The current book reflects efforts to apply what has been learned in the last two decades from TF-CBT-related research, clinical work, as well as training and dissemination efforts. While cognitive-behavioral principles provided the foundation on which TF-CBT was originally developed, other theories have also informed our efforts to enhance the efficacy of TF-CBT for children who have experienced a wide array of traumas. These theories include humanistic, attachment, family systems, and empowerment models (Cohen, Mannarino, & Deblinger, 2006).

As noted earlier, traumatic experiences have the potential to disrupt the psychosocial development of a child and undermine the well-being of an entire family. Thus, the overarching objective of TF-CBT is to circumvent this process by providing youngsters and their family members with understanding, knowledge, and skills to help them to confront and make meaning of traumatic experiences. At the same time, children and their caregivers learn to optimally manage trauma reminders as well as other stressors and conflicts in the present as they reclaim a sense of enthusiasm and optimism for the future. When children and caregivers successfully complete TF-CBT, they often not only achieve the just-described goals but grow stronger and more resilient as individuals and closer and more cohesive as families.

THERAPEUTIC ENGAGEMENT

Implementing treatment in the aftermath of trauma requires thoughtful consideration of the overall needs of the child and family as well as attention to potential barriers to treatment that may make therapeutic engagement challenging. In the aftermath of many traumas, other pressing issues may take precedence over engaging families in therapy. In the case of child maltreatment, these include child protection and law enforcement investigations, medical examinations, and attention to other safety concerns. Similarly, in the aftermath of widespread disasters, the need for shelter, food, safety, and medical attention usually takes priority over the need for psychological treatment. Recognizing these priorities and providing prompt referrals to needed resources is an important strategy for engaging families in subsequent therapy. After these acute issues have been addressed, the therapist can optimize engagement by discussing potential barriers to treatment such as lack of transportation, scheduling conflicts, or other competing priorities. McKay and others (2004) have demonstrated that both initiation of treatment and session attendance can be improved by utilizing empirically validated engagement strategies such as (1) establishing the need for mental health care, (2) enhancing the caregiver's motivation for treatment, (3) reviewing prior therapy experiences, (4) establishing a collaborative working relationship, and (5) providing assistance in overcoming concrete barriers (e.g., transportation, scheduling). These strategies are highly applicable to engaging families in TF-CBT and have been successfully utilized in prior TF-CBT investigations (i.e., Cohen et al., 2004; Deblinger et al., 1996, 2001; Dorsey & Feldman, 2008). At the outset of treatment, for example, TF-CBT therapists review the assessment findings and acknowledge the impact of the trauma(s) not only on the children but on the parents as well. This process not only establishes the need for trauma-focused therapy, but also normalizes and validates trauma-related feelings and reactions. It is also not uncommon for caregivers and youngsters to report negative prior experiences with mental health therapy and/or social services. Thus, differences between what has been experienced in the past and what can be anticipated in the structure and course of participating in TF-CBT is emphasized. With these expectations carefully outlined, a commitment to participation in an approximate number of sessions is elicited. To further motivate therapy participation and optimism, the scientific research supporting the effectiveness of this treatment approach is highlighted with a focus on the specific benefits of active caregiver participation and collaboration. TF-CBT begins with a focus on the trauma(s) that precipitated the initiation of treatment as well as the clients' related presenting concerns.

CORE VALUES OF TF-CBT

The acronym CRAFTS summarizes the core values of the TF-CBT model. These values apply to all cases regardless of the specific population, community, or setting. This reflects the universality of the human condition in terms of the essential therapy ingredients that contribute to the overall healing of children and their families. The values outlined next highlight that the TF-CBT model is components based; respectful of community, cultural, and religious traditions; adaptable to individualized needs and circumstances; family focused; based on a strong therapeutic relationship; and strongly encouraging of self-efficacy. More specifically, the model is:

Components-based, such that it incorporates knowledge, skills, and processes that build on one another and are integrated in a way that best suits the needs of the particular client and family.

Respectful of individual, family, community, culture, and religious practices, in terms of understanding the impact of the traumatic experience(s) and optimally supporting the child's and family's healing in the context of their family, culture, and community.

Adaptable, as highlighted in this volume by the numerous examples of the importance of the flexible and creative ways that therapists optimally motivate clients and implement the treatment components for diverse populations and settings while maintaining fidelity to the model.

Family focused, in that every effort is made to include supportive family members. Thus, therapists are strongly encouraged to make active efforts to engage parents and/or other caregivers in the treatment process whenever possible. It should be noted that siblings and/or other family members (e.g., a grandparent or a special aunt) are also involved when feasible and clinically appropriate.

Therapeutic relationship centered, such that much attention should be given to creating a therapeutic relationship that allows parents and children to feel safe, accepted, and validated. Such relationships help clients to feel trusting and confident to share their traumatic experiences as well as their most distressing fears, thoughts, and developing beliefs, while also taking the risks necessary to learn and utilize new skills that will produce significant positive change in their lives.

Self-efficacy focused, in that TF-CBT is a short-term, strengths-based model designed to have long-term benefits. In the context of TF-CBT, therapists encourage self-efficacy and feelings of mastery by actively collaborating with clients in planning therapy, motivating clients to follow through on assignments between sessions, acknowledging therapy successes, encouraging and recognizing the ongoing use of TF-CBT skills, and enhancing clients' feelings of preparedness for trauma reminders and other life stressors that they may encounter long after therapy has ended.

ASSESSMENT STRATEGIES

Prior to initiating TF-CBT, it is critical to assess the impact of the traumatic exposures on various domains of functioning. CRAFTS is also used to summarize the potential areas of maladjustment targeted by TF-CBT. These include:

Cognitive problems, such as dysfunctional thought patterns, school learning problems, or concentration difficulties.

Relationship problems, such as increased conflicts at home, in school, or at work and impaired trust or expectations of betrayal in interpersonal interactions.

Affective problems, such as difficulties effectively expressing and/or managing feelings of anxiety, depression, and/or anger.

Family problems, including parenting difficulties, parent–child conflicts, extended family disruptions that may more frequently occur in the context of intrafamilial abuse disclosures, and frequent out-of-home placements (e.g., foster, residential treatment) that arise from early severe interpersonal violence or abuse.

Traumatic behavior problems, including behavioral avoidance of innocuous trauma reminders, sexual behavior problems, aggressive behaviors, and/or noncompliant behaviors.

Somatic problems, including sleeping difficulties, hyperarousal symptoms, headaches, stomachaches, and other physiological reactions to traumatic memories, reminders, and cues.

Assessment of these domains for treatment planning purposes can be accomplished via structured interviews, observations, and standardized measures administered to the children as well as the parents. The use of standardized measures undoubtedly enhances the effective implementation of TF-CBT because they provide objective information that forms the basis for the individual tailoring of the treatment plan for the specific needs of the child and his or her family while also allowing for the assessment of treatment progress.

Given the focus of TF-CBT, the assessment of PTSD and related symptoms is particularly pertinent. A variety of well-validated and reliable PTSD measures are designed for this purpose, including semistructured PTSD interviews such as the Schedule for Affective Disorders and Schizophrenia for School-Age Children—Present and Lifetime Version (Kaufman, Birmaher, & Brent, 1996) and/or child and parent PTSD measures such as the UCLA PTSD Reaction Index (Steinberg, Brymer, Decker, & Pynoos, 2004). Additional measures that may be used to assess other areas of functioning include (1) the Children's Depression Inventory (Kovacs, 1985) to evaluate depression, (2) the Child Behavior Checklist (Achenbach, 1991) or the Strengths and Difficulties Questionnaire (Goodman, 1997) to assess behavior problems, (3) the Multidimensional Anxiety Scale for Children (March, 1997) or the State–Trait Anxiety Inventory for Children (Spielberger, 1973) to assess generalized anxiety, and (4) the Shame Scale (Feiring, Taska, & Lewis, 1996) to measure feelings of shame related to experiences of abuse.

It is critically important to assess parents' overall functioning as well given that they are often directly or indirectly affected by the trauma(s) their children have experienced. This assessment may also help determine the need for a separate therapy referral if the parents' emotional difficulties are of an individual nature, require immediate attention, or are likely to interfere with their ability to participate in treatment on behalf of their child. To assess parental reactions to the child's traumatic exposures, one can utilize measures such as the Impact of Event Scale—Revised (Weiss, 2004) or the Parent Emotional Reaction Questionnaire (Mannarino & Cohen, 1996). Other standardized measures that are useful in terms of assessing parental functioning and planning treatment include the Beck Depression Inventory (Beck, Steer, & Brown, 1996) and the Parenting Practices Questionnaire (Strayhorn & Weidman, 1988) or Alabama Parenting Questionnaire (Frick, 1991) to assess parenting skills.

TF-CBT STRUCTURE
AND TREATMENT COMPONENTS

TF-CBT sessions are structured such that the therapist meets with the child and parent(s) for separate individual sessions, with time increasingly devoted to conjoint sessions over the course of the middle and latter stages of therapy. In cases in which the child is demonstrating behavior problems, however, conjoint sessions may begin early in treatment to allow for the consistent practicing of parenting and coping skills with parents and children together.

The components of TF-CBT are summarized by the acronym PRAC-TICE: Psychoeducation and Parenting; Relaxation; Affective expression and modulation; Cognitive coping; Trauma narrative development and processing; *In vivo* exposure; Conjoint parent–child sessions; and Enhancing safety and future development. These components generally remain the same regardless of trauma types, community environments, or setting differences; however, some additional components are included when working with children suffering traumatic grief reactions. Additionally, if potential trauma exposure is ongoing, some revisions to the order and implementation of these components may be necessary, as described elsewhere (Cohen, Mannarino, & Iyengar 2011; Cohen, Mannarino, & Murray, 2011). It is also worth noting the appropriateness of PRACTICE as an acronym in that the model itself emphasizes the importance of clients *practicing* the TF-CBT skills at home in order to optimize benefits. Moreover, when therapists *practice* what they preach, in relation to using the TF-CBT skills, not only do they more effectively model these skills for their clients, but their experiences using the skills personally may help to inspire their ability to motivate clients to engage in treatment and make the changes necessary to support optimal healing and adjustment.

Theoretical Rationale for Gradual Exposure

As noted earlier, ideas from several theories of psychology have influenced our thinking in terms of the development and refinement of TF-CBT. Cognitive-behavioral principles, however, provide the overarching theoretical rationale for the implementation of this treatment model. TF-CBT includes a variety of strategies that emphasize learning by means of associations, consequences, and observations of others. Based on classical conditioning theory, traumatic events may be conceptualized as unconditioned stimuli that elicit unconditioned or reflexive responses including fear, terror, helplessness, and/or anger. These automatic emotional reactions to trauma are natural and adaptive as they signal the need for protective reactions to real danger such as flight-or-fight response. However, PTSD symptoms may develop when innocuous stimuli (e.g., sounds, sights, smells, images, people, places, or other trauma-related stimuli) present at the time the trauma begin to elicit the same negative unconditioned emotional responses due to their association with the original traumatic threat. Children suffering from PTSD as a result of abuse, for example, may respond to nonabusive people in authority as potential threats as opposed to resources for support. Instrumental conditioning occurs through experience, when children learn

to reduce their anxiety by avoiding innocuous people, places, or things associated with the original trauma(s). Through the process of stimulus generalization, PTSD sufferers avoid a widening circle of innocuous trauma-related
cues that trigger traumatic memories and/or symptoms despite the lack of
real danger.

Observational learning may also play an important role in determining
how children respond to trauma reminders or misperceived threats. Many
children respond to misperceived threats in the environment with progressively more withdrawn, isolative, and/or submissive behaviors. Other children, particularly those exposed to violent traumas, may respond to innocuous reminders or misperceived threats with anger or aggressive behaviors
similar to those exhibited by others in their environment. While aggression and withdrawal are common manifestations of fear in traumatized
children, caregivers may view these behaviors as disobedience and inadvertently respond in ways that exacerbate them. Moreover, as these children
have increasingly problematic interactions with parents as well as others,
unhealthy beliefs about themselves, relationships, and the world develop.
Through these mechanisms of learning, traumatic experiences negatively
impact on children's physiological, emotional, behavioral, and cognitive
functioning. The PRACTICE components of TF-CBT are therefore designed
to enhance coping in each of these domains of functioning.

Gradual exposure (GE) is critical to implementing TF-CBT and is
incorporated into *all* of the TF-CBT components. During each subsequent
PRACTICE component, the therapist carefully calibrates and increases
exposure to trauma reminders while encouraging the child and parent to
use skills learned in previous sessions and praising demonstrated mastery.
In an effort to counter tendencies toward posttraumatic avoidance, gradual
exposure is initiated at the outset of TF-CBT with the direct acknowledgment of the trauma(s) endured and psychoeducation about traumatic stress
reactions. In addition, during psychoeducation, GE might consist of simply
using the words "sexual abuse" rather than referring to "the bad thing that
happened." As the child progresses through the model, the therapist encourages the child and parent to implement the skills with increasing specificity
to reminders of the sexual abuse until, during the trauma narrative, the child
is encouraged to recount his or her traumatic experiences and to share this
with the parent during conjoint sessions when clinically appropriate.

Engaging the child in the trauma narrative and processing component
not only helps to extinguish the intense negative emotions associated with
traumatic memories and reminders, but perhaps more importantly creates new associations such that traumatic memories may elicit feelings of
strength and pride. Moreover, trauma processing and corrective feedback
provided by therapists help children to develop adaptive and contextualized
interpretations of past events such that healthier self, family, and wordviews

may develop. The final skill-building component encourages the development of safety skills. Through discussions and role plays, this component provides additional opportunities for youngsters to differentiate between real dangers in the present and innocuous triggers or reminders. Gradual exposure, as incorporated into each of the practice components outlined below, demonstrates to children and their caregivers that they not only have the strength to confront trauma reminders, but they can also learn and grow by acknowledging and processing traumatic memories.

Psychoeducation

Psychoeducation is provided to the child and parents throughout the course of treatment, but is critical from the start in terms of enhancing therapeutic engagement immediately modeling nonavoidance. After obtaining intake information about the trauma(s) experienced and assessing the child's and parent's trauma reactions, the therapist can offer reassuring educational information that normalizes these trauma responses and outlines the general procedures for treatment. The therapist provides specific feedback regarding the assessment findings as well as the child's strengths and difficulties, particularly in terms of how that information informs the planning of treatment. In addition, the therapist should emphasize the important role of parents in treatment, highlighting how their involvement and support may be the single most important influence on their child's healing. To inspire confidence in the treatment approach and optimism about the child's prognosis, it is important to emphasize the effectiveness of the treatment model both in terms of prior clinical experience as well as the extensive research findings.

General information about the trauma(s) may be provided in a variety of different ways. Even clients who demonstrate extreme avoidance in terms of discussing their personal traumatic experiences are often receptive to general informational discussions about the trauma endured. During the early stages, it is helpful to provide some of the basic facts about the types of traumas experienced in terms of its characteristics, prevalence, impact, common misconceptions, and so on. Educational handouts, books, and games are frequently utilized with children as well as their parents. These activities represent an important early step in the GE process because they undoubtedly trigger memories of the trauma but rarely elicit negative emotions. Rather, during these educational activities, new associations are being created such that trauma memories may begin to be associated with feelings of safety and pride, as knowledge often encourages feelings of empowerment. In general, TF-CBT should not feel like a mysterious process, as clients are educated in a very practical way throughout the treatment concerning the overall therapy objectives and components.

Parenting Skills Training

Parenting skills training is also provided throughout the course of treatment because it is well documented that the parental support and effective parenting skills positively influence trauma recovery in children (Deblinger et al., 1996, 2011; Mannarino & Cohen, 1996). Therapists may initially collaborate with parents in developing family rituals, routines, and structure that will enhance children's feelings of safety and security, while also promoting positive parent–child communication skills such as active listening and the mutual exchange of praise. In order to support the use of effective parenting skills, it is important to conduct functional behavioral analyses, reviewing problematic as well as positive parent–child interactions, on a weekly basis. In the aftermath of trauma, many well-meaning parents inadvertently reinforce problematic behaviors in their children. In the course of conducting functional analyses with respect to parent–child interactions, it is helpful to elicit as much detail as possible, including underlying parental thoughts and feelings that may be driving overindulgent, overprotective, overly harsh, and/or other problematic parenting practices. In the early sessions, the therapist may identify specific problematic child behaviors as well as positive adaptive behaviors that can replace and effectively serve the functions of the problem behaviors (i.e., gaining attention, escaping anxiety, achieving feelings of control). This is particularly important given the natural tendency for parents, in the aftermath of a trauma, to focus on children's difficulties and symptoms, inadvertently reinforcing them. By identifying adaptive behaviors that can replace the maladaptive behaviors, parents can be encouraged to refocus their attention on these positive behaviors by utilizing praise, positive attention, active listening, and tangible rewards when appropriate. Learning to minimize parental attention given to problem behaviors is equally important and often requires very active efforts to dramatically reduce the use of lectures, yelling, and empty threats, which inadvertently increase negative behaviors. Parents and children may also collaborate with the therapist on the development of house rules as well as consequences when the rules are broken. The consequences generally take the form of time-outs, house chores, loss of privileges, and so on, and parents are taught how to optimally administer these consequences in a warm but firm and consistent manner.

Parents are often significantly affected by the traumas their children have personally suffered. GE during the parenting component includes helping parents understand the traumatic impact on both the children and themselves, for example, framing the children's response as due to the trauma that happened to the children rather than the children "being bad." Helping parents to understand that they are their children's most important role models for coping is critical. Thus, parents also are encouraged to learn the coping skills described in the components presented next so that they can both model and reinforce their children's efforts to practice those skills.

Relaxation Training

Relaxation training is introduced early in treatment and provides children and parents with skills they can use to manage daily stressors as well as any distress they may experience in the context of facing traumatic memories in treatment. Focused breathing is a particularly important relaxation skill because it can be mastered easily and used in any context. Other relaxation activities that are commonly utilized in the context of TF-CBT include progressive muscle relaxation exercises and guided imagery, which may be particularly useful with young children. When young children are encouraged to imagine themselves as a tin soldier and then a rag doll, they not only learn the difference between muscular tension and relaxation but, most importantly, learn that they can control muscle tension in their own bodies. Relaxation skills can be particularly valuable for clients with sleeping difficulties and those who experience distress physiologically, such as muscular tension in the form of backaches and headaches.

Mindfulness practices may also be utilized to help TF-CBT clients relax or quiet their minds. This practice encourages the focusing of one's full attention on the present moment through the nonjudgmental observation and acceptance of one's thoughts, feelings, sensations, and surroundings. This disciplined but gentle process of refocusing the mind on moment-to-moment experiences in the present may be very healing for those who have suffered a great deal of trauma in the past and are fearful of the future. Moreover, recent research suggests that this form of meditation not only may decrease feelings of distress but also appears to be instrumental in reducing distractive and ruminative thoughts and behaviors common among PTSD sufferers (Jain et al., 2007). GE during the relaxation component includes encouraging children to implement the techniques just discussed or other relaxation strategies when they experience trauma reminders.

Affective Expression and Modulation Training

Affective expression and modulation training highlights skills that help children and parents communicate and manage feelings more effectively. With young children, this component often begins with exercises designed to identify and review experiences associated with the primary emotions (e.g., happy, sad, mad, scared). Traumatic events often lead to a wide range of other emotions, some of which children may have never experienced before. Thus, it is important to help clients expand their emotional vocabulary beyond the primary emotions just listed to include those frequently associated with trauma (e.g., terror, shame, grief, rage, embarrassment, helplessness). Moreover, by identifying feeling states and labeling them, clients are taking the first steps toward increasing their awareness of their own distressing emotions and managing them more successfully. Part of GE during this component includes helping children and parents to recognize the connection between these negative affective states and children's trauma reminders. In addition, parents and children are encouraged to practice both verbally expressing their own feelings and inquiring about each others' feelings. These skills can help reduce parent–child conflict and are particularly important for children who tend to express negative emotions through aggressive and/or other problematic behaviors. Parents may be encouraged to utilize active listening skills at home when children share their feelings in words as opposed to dysfunctional behaviors. This type of homework greatly contributes to improving parent–child communication and interactions overall.

In the context of TF-CBT, therapists collaborate with clients in identifying coping strategies that will help them tolerate or manage distressing emotions. TF-CBT therapists may review clients' emotional coping repertoire with the objective of reinforcing effective strategies while discouraging the use of less productive coping strategies. Ultimately, parents and children can create a tool kit that includes old and new skills that can be used effectively to manage distressing emotions (e.g. talking to a supportive adult, listening to soothing music, exercising, problem solving); GE is also implemented by helping clients to identify common trauma triggers that lead to distressing emotions so that the coping strategies just presented can be individually tailored to fit the most common circumstances. Thus, for example, when children experience triggers and distress in school, they can be encouraged to engage in coping strategies that allow them to remain in the classroom when possible. Children often find it helpful to create lists or other tools that serve as reminders of what they can do when they are feeling distressed.

Cognitive Coping

Cognitive coping is the component that lays the groundwork for helping children and parents understand the connections between their thoughts, feelings, and behaviors. Even very young children can learn to understand that what they say to themselves (i.e., thoughts) influences how they feel and behave. However, the first step in teaching cognitive coping skills involves helping clients to capture and share internal dialogues that may be fleeting, automatic, and not necessarily in their immediate awareness. Therapists are encouraged to use non-trauma-related examples initially to help clients learn to retrieve everyday thoughts. Asking clients, for example, to share what they said to themselves when they heard their alarm clock ring in the morning is a simple way to begin to elicit internal dialogues. Therapists can introduce a cognitive triangle to demonstrate—using non-trauma-related examples—how different thoughts about the same event can lead to very different feelings and behaviors. Through this process, therapists help children and parents recognize that negative feelings and behaviors are sometimes driven by thoughts that are inaccurate, distorted, or simply unhelpful. Through the process of therapy, clients are encouraged to examine thoughts underlying distressing feelings about everyday events for their accuracy and helpfulness. Ultimately, clients are encouraged to identify inaccurate thoughts that can be corrected and unhelpful thoughts that can be replaced with more helpful, productive thoughts.

Relatively early in treatment, parents are encouraged to share trauma-related feelings and thoughts and, with the help of their therapist, identify inaccurate and dysfunctional thoughts. After devoting some time to eliciting, acknowledging, and simply validating parents' feelings in relation to the trauma, the TF-CBT therapist encourages the examination of thoughts that may be underlying their most distressing feelings. The TF-CBT therapist may then use educational information, Socratic questioning, and role plays to help parents dispute those problematic thoughts. GE is implemented in this manner with parents during the cognitive coping component.

On the other hand, while the TF-CBT therapist may help children examine how their thoughts influence feelings and behaviors on an everyday basis, he or she does not typically challenge the children's trauma-related thoughts until these thoughts and feelings have been expressed, accepted, and validated through the trauma narrative process. When the narrative is almost complete, the therapist can begin to identify problematic thoughts that can be explored and processed, as described next.

Trauma Narrative Development and Processing

Trauma narrative development and processing refers to the middle third of treatment, when therapy focuses increasingly on the specific traumas endured. The trauma narrative is an exposure and processing exercise that typically takes the form of a written book, with an introductory "about me" chapter as well as chapters in which children describe the circumstances of the trauma and associated thoughts, feelings, and sensations experienced. However, some children may prefer to do this work through trauma-specific discussions or other trauma-specific creative work, including poetry, songs, news shows, plays, and art, that reflects the traumatic experiences. The process is designed to help children gradually face increasingly anxiety-provoking trauma-related memories until they can tolerate those memories without significant emotional distress or avoidant responses. In the context of a trusting therapeutic relationship, children learn that recalling and writing about the traumatic experiences does not lead to the overwhelming emotions they suffered at the time of the trauma. This frees children up to share their innermost feelings and thoughts about the traumatic experiences in the context of a validating therapeutic relationship. Moreover, with the help of their therapist, children can begin to process trauma-related thoughts, with a particular focus on identifying and correcting dysfunctional thoughts and developing beliefs. GE is implemented by reviewing the narrative several times during its creation, thus helping the children to gain increasing mastery over these memories. The final narrative chapter often reflects the children's integration of what they have learned and experienced over the course of treatment in terms of its implications for their self-image, relationships with others, worldviews, and expectations for the future. The following are examples of questions therapists often pose to assist children in exploring what they have learned so that they can review and internalize healthy beliefs and incorporate them into the final narrative chapter: What have you learned in therapy? What have you learned about the trauma(s) experienced? What have you learned about yourself, your parents, your family, and/or your world? What are you looking forward to in the future? What are you most proud of? Who could you talk to about past traumatic experiences or other problems faced in the future? What would you tell other children who have had similar traumatic experiences?

In Vivo Exposure

In vivo exposure is a powerful treatment component that is highly effective in helping children overcome problematic avoidant behaviors that develop in the aftermath of trauma. Some trauma-related avoidant behaviors, however, are functional and, therefore, should not be discouraged (e.g., avoiding a sexually abusive individual or a drug-infested street corner where an assault occurred). In contrast, dysfunctional avoidant behaviors develop when the intense negative emotions that were experienced in response to the original trauma generalize to innocuous stimuli associated with it. When this occurs, traumatized individuals work hard to avoid people, places, things, and memories that reflexively elicit these intense negative emotions even though these stimuli in and of themselves may no longer be objectively dangerous. Depending on the circumstances of the trauma, children experiencing PTSD-related avoidance may, for example, begin to object to going to school, sleeping alone, being in dark environments, engaging in social activities, or using certain forms of transportation. The reduced anxiety that children experience when they engage in these behaviors reinforces their avoidance, which can lead to increasingly isolative and withdrawn behaviors. Thus, for these children, the use of the *in vivo* treatment component should be carefully considered in collaboration with parents because it requires a well-developed treatment plan and a full commitment. Certain highly disruptive avoidant behaviors that impact education like school refusal, may be best addressed early in treatment in collaboration with school personnel after a careful assessment of the factors driving the behavior. For many children, missing a great deal of school not only will inadvertently reinforce avoidant behaviors but may significantly undermine their ability to keep up academically, making the return to school increasingly difficult from both an academic and a social perspective. *In vivo* exposure may also be indicated when less disruptive avoidant behaviors do not diminish naturally over the course of the trauma narrative and processing components. In such circumstances, TF-CBT therapists may begin to create *in vivo* plans that gradually encourage participation in anxiety-provoking activities of increasingly greater intensity with simultaneous use of the coping skills learned earlier in treatment to manage the associated distress.

Conjoint Parent–Child Sessions

Conjoint parent–child sessions are designed to help parents and children practice the skills learned and begin to communicate more openly about the traumas experienced. Early in treatment, the TF-CBT therapist spends more time with the children and parents in individual sessions; the amount of time devoted to conjoint sessions over the course of treatment is based on clients' specific needs. When children have significant behavior problems, it is often very useful to begin engaging in brief conjoint parent–child sessions early on to provide opportunities for parents to practice praise, selective attention, and the other coping and behavior management skills they are learning.

The content and timing of initiating the trauma-focused conjoint sessions are based on parents' and children's emotional states and levels of skill development. Ideally, conjoint sessions with respect to trauma-related communication should be initiated when parents have developed sufficient emotional composure to serve as effective coping role models for their children and when children have engaged in enough skills and trauma-focused work to demonstrate pride in sharing their newfound trauma-related knowledge and skills. These conjoint sessions usually begin with more general discussions about the relevant traumas. It is helpful to utilize books and games to create a fun, relaxed atmosphere during the initial trauma-focused conjoint sessions, such as Survivor's Journey (for sexual abuse trauma) (Burke, 1994) or What Do You Know?, a simple question-and-answer game about sexual abuse, physical abuse, and domestic violence (Deblinger, Neubauer, Runyon, & Baker, 2006). These activities help parents and children gain greater confidence and comfort in talking together about the traumas in the abstract prior to reading and discussing the personal trauma narrative.

It is also extremely important to prepare parents for hearing their child read his or her narrative by reviewing the complete narrative with them during individual parent sessions. During individual sessions, parents often greatly benefit from participating in role plays, with the therapist in the role of the child reading the narrative. Role plays help parents become comfortable hearing the narrative while they practice responding to the narrative with active listening, praise, and support for the child. In separate preparation sessions, the therapist may also assist the parents and child individually to identify their trauma-related questions so they can be responded to in therapeutically optimal ways. It should be noted that in a minority of cases it may become apparent early in treatment or during the preparatory individual parent sessions that it is not in the child's best interest to share the narrative because of parental emotional instability or inability to be optimally supportive. The child can still greatly benefit from TF-CBT even if he or she is unable to share the narrative. Often other conjoint activities can take the place of sharing the narrative and can be similarly beneficial (e.g., reviewing general information and/or parents acknowledging how proud they are of their child's work). GE is implemented in this component by sharing the child's narrative together with the parents and/or reviewing trauma-related educational information.

Enhancing Safety and Future Development

Enhancing safety and future development is a component that also may be incorporated into treatment at different stages depending on the traumas being addressed and the family's circumstances (Cohen, Mannarino & Murray, 2011). For children who have experienced domestic or community violence and may have some ongoing exposure despite efforts to minimize such, safety skills may be introduced and practiced early in the course of treatment to enhance safety in high-risk environments and ensure that everyone is in agreement with respect to the safety plan. For children who are less vulnerable to ongoing trauma, it is advisable to delay the focus on safety skills until after much of the narrative is complete. This may minimize children's tendencies to feel compelled to report what they "should" have done in the narrative (as per the safety training) rather than how they actually responded to the trauma. Moreover, focusing on safety skills too early in treatment may inadvertently reinforce feelings of self-blame.

In general, children who have experienced significant trauma are likely to feel an increased sense of vulnerability. Thus, although children cannot and should not be reasssured that they will be completely protected from future traumas—as many parents would like to do—TF-CBT encourages the development of relevant safety skills to enhance children's sense of mastery and self-efficacy when faced with future stressors or traumas. The learning of personal safety skills may be normalized by likening them to other standard safety skills the children may have learned in school or at home (e.g., "stop, drop, and roll" for fire safety; use of seat belts while riding in a car; wearing a helmet while riding a bike). Prior to initiating personal safety skills training, however, it is critical to emphasize to children that the way they responded to the trauma was the best way they could have given their age, knowledge, emotions, and experience at that time. Moreover, children participating in TF-CBT may be reminded that they have already engaged in the most important safety skill—telling a trusted adult about the trauma—and they should be congratulated for doing so given how difficult this step can be. The primary objectives of the safety skills component include (1) assessing children's skills and knowledge regarding potential dangers in their environment; (2) providing and reviewing information about relevant risks, such as child sexual abuse, family violence, community violence, bullying, and Internet danger; (3) developing and practicing communication, assertiveness, problem-solving, body safety, and other safety skills relevant to the trauma endured (e.g., fire safety, pool safety); and (4) involving parents in reviewing the skills and developing safety plans that can be practiced during conjoint and/or family sessions.

Children who have experienced significant losses and traumatic grief may require additional grief-focused components beyond the practice components.

Grief-Focused Components

Grief requires remembering the person who died. Children with traumatic grief avoid thinking about or remembering the deceased person or reminiscing about the deceased person because even happy thoughts segue into traumatic memories about how the person died, and these are too distressing to tolerate. Children with traumatic grief may benefit from additional grief-related treatment components after completing the TF-CBT components as related to the traumatic death. We very briefly summarize them here; interested readers may obtain more detailed information elsewhere in this volume and at *www.musc.edu/ctg*.

> *Grief psychoeducation:* Providing information to the child and parent about the wide range of child grief responses and information about bereavement and mourning. This builds on and supplements earlier psychoeducation provided about death and traumatic symptoms. In so doing, the therapist helps to further establish the importance of maintaining open communication about the traumatic loss of loved ones that for many children and parents might seem easier to avoid.
>
> *Grieving the loss; resolving ambivalent feelings:* Concretizing the death (e.g., through a balloon exercise that describes what the child has lost and what can still be held onto in the relationship with the

deceased); addressing ambivalent feelings toward the deceased helps the child accept the totality of the deceased and address unresolved issues. It is not unusual for lost loved ones to be remembered in only positive terms, as reflected in the widely accepted practice of "speaking no ill of the dead." However, remembering their lost loved one more realistically as a beloved but naturally flawed individual may reduce bereaved children's vulnerability to having unrealistically high expectations for themselves and others. Thus, during this component it is helpful for children to express both what they miss as well as what they don't miss about the lost loved one, while also processing ambivalent feelings and conflicts they may have experienced with that individual in the past.

Preserving positive memories: Encouraging the child and parent to memorialize the deceased and internalize positive aspects of the deceased into self-concept. While the focus on positive and cherished memories of the deceased can be painful, it also provides children with the experience of knowing that they can manage these feelings and need not avoid positive memories. Finding ways to celebrate the lost loved one's life can create new associations such that trauma-related memories may come to be associated with feelings of pride as opposed to intense grief.

Redefining the relationship; committing to present relationships: Accepting that the relationship lives on but is one of memory and the child must commit to relationships with living people. At this stage of therapy, when PTSD symptoms have greatly subsided, with therapeutic support children are typically more able to internalize the love and wisdom shared by lost loved ones in ways that do not interfere with their ability to establish, deepen, and learn from relationships in the present.

Closure issues: Children and parents respond very well to TF-CBT and the related grief components in terms of overcoming highly disruptive PTSD, depression, anxiety, and traumatic grief symptoms (Cohen, Mannarino, & Staron, 2006). However, grieving is a natural process that often extends beyond the end of therapy and thus it is important to prepare parents and children for this in the final phase of treatment. Such preparation may include normalizing the ongoing grieving process; addressing trauma, loss, and change reminders in the future; and encouraging full engagement in life as it is in the present.

Graduating Therapy

Graduating therapy is an important goal that is often discussed at the start of TF-CBT given the time-limited nature of this treatment approach. Establishing the expectation that the children will graduate from TF-CBT encourages confidence and an optimistic view regarding their recovery from the start. For many children and parents, it is reassuring to know that there is a beginning, middle, and end of treatment that they can plan for and look forward to. While confronting and processing trauma experienced in the past is a major objective of treatment, equally important is the focus on the skills learned to be used in the present and the development of optimistic expectations for the future. Thus, setting high expectations for what clients will accomplish and complete over the course of therapy is consistent with the core value of encouraging client self-efficacy in the context of TF-CBT.

TF-CBT is often provided to children who have experienced numerous unexpected traumas and losses. Therefore, as treatment termination nears, a reminder of the number of sessions remaining is especially helpful to children and their parents. In the final phase of treatment, it is also important to readminister standardized measures to review progress and confirm the appropriateness of the clients' therapy graduation. Children who are receiving longer term care at agencies or institutions may graduate from the TF-CBT portion of their treatment and continue on with other forms of treatment (e.g., supportive counseling, mentoring, skill building). Still, these children can benefit from taking time to celebrate their TF-CBT graduation. On the basis of assessment, the therapist may make referrals, if appropriate, for other services and provide guidelines for reconnecting if booster sessions are needed in the future. This is an important time to acknowledge the feelings of loss that termination may elicit while simultaneously highlighting the positive factors associated with the ending of the weekly therapy sessions. For example, therapy graduation reflects the children's success in treatment, the parents' ability to provide the support needed, and the opportunity to utilize this time for other positive activities (e.g., after-school activities, clubs, and sports).

After completing the trauma-focused conjoint sessions, the final individual sessions provide clients opportunities to share their thoughts and feelings about those sessions, while also reviewing overall progress and what they have learned in terms of their self-view, their relationships with others, as well as their worldview. These ideas may already be incorporated into the final chapter of their trauma narrative and thus may be read and/or reviewed one last time. In addition, it is important to discuss and plan for future trauma reminders and steps that can be taken to prevent emotional and behavioral relapses. The therapist should collaborate with clients to create a relaxed, fun celebration, incorporating, when possible, the clients' favorite activities and/or graduation mementos, such as certificates, graduation hats, balloons, and cake. This celebration provides another opportunity to reinforce feelings of strength, pride, and family togetherness in the aftermath of the trauma rather than the distressing trauma-related thoughts and feelings that originally brought the family to treatment.

CONCLUSION

The concept for this book grew out of the dramatic growth in the utilization of TF-CBT with children of all ages and from diverse cultures and settings. While this introduction outlines the basic principles, values, and treatment components associated with TF-CBT, the chapters that follow highlight the individual tailoring of TF-CBT to optimally serve children's and adolescents' specialized needs. Outstanding authors were invited to contribute chapters based on their extensive experience utilizing TF-CBT in the special contexts described. Thus, the chapters to follow offer specific recommendations for maintaining overall fidelity to the model while simultaneously creatively applying TF-CBT to optimally address applications across different settings, developmental issues, and special populations. Two chapters highlight the value of play in creatively engaging children of different ages in the educational, skill-building, as well as exposure and processing components. Other chapters demonstrate how to adjust TF-CBT to overcome the barriers to treatment or accommodate the special circumstances in which traumatized children are receiving treatment (e.g., residential settings, foster placements, low-resource countries). A unifying theme throughout this book is the importance of building and maintaining a positive, trusting, and collaborative therapeutic relationship. The chapters and the many case examples bring to life the unique aspects of utilizing TF-CBT with children at different developmental stages, from different cultural backgrounds, and in diverse settings in the United States and around the world. Although we recognize that there is still much to be learned to enhance the resiliency of children and families, we hope that the ideas offered here support the many professionals around the world working to help children and their families build more hopeful futures.

REFERENCES

Achenbach, T. M. (1991). *Manual for the Child Behavior Checklist and Revised Child Behavior Profile*. Burlington: University of Vermont.

Arseneault, L., Cannon, M., Fisher, H. I., Polanczyk, G., Moffitt, T. E., & Caspi, A. (2011). Childhood trauma and children's emerging psychotic symptoms: A genetically sensitive longitudinal cohort study. *American Journal of Psychiatry, 168*, 65–72.

Beck, A. T., Steer, R. A., & Brown, G. K. (1996). *Manual for the Beck Depression Inventory (2nd ed.)*. San Antonio, TX: Psychological Corporation.

Bisson, J. L., Ehlers, A., Matthews, R., Pilling, S., Richards, E., & Turner, S. (2007). Psychological treatments for chronic post-traumatic stress disorder: Systematic review and meta-analysis. *British Journal of Psychiatry, 190*, 97–104.

Bloch, D. Silber, E., & Perry, S. E. (1956). Some factors in the emotional reaction of children to disaster. *American Journal of Psychiatry, 113,* 416–422.

Briere, J., & Elliott, D. M. (2003). Prevalence and psychological sequelae of self-reported childhood physical and sexual abuse in a general population sample of men and women. *Child Abuse and Neglect, 27,* 1205–1222.

Burke, R. B. (1994). *Survivor's journey: A therapeutic game for working with survivors of sexual abuse.* Charlotte, NC: KidsRights.

CATS Consortium. (2010). Implementation of CBT for youth affected by the World Trade Center disaster: Matching need to treatment intensity and reducing trauma symptoms. *Journal of Traumatic Stress, 23,* 699–707.

Cohen, J. A., Deblinger, E., Mannarino, A. P., & Steer, R. (2004). A multi-site, randomized, controlled trial for children with sex abuse-related PTSD symptoms. *Journal of the American Academy of Child and Adolescent Psychiatry, 43,* 393–402.

Cohen, J. A., & Mannarino, A. P. (1988). Psychological symptoms in sexually abused girls. *Child Abuse and Neglect, 12,* 571–577.

Cohen J. A., & Mannarino, A. P. (1993). A treatment model for sexually abused preschoolers. *Journal of Interpersonal Violence, 8*(1), 115–131.

Cohen, J. A., & Mannarino, A. P. (1996). Factors that mediate treatment outcome of sexually abused preschool children. *Journal of the American Academy of Child and Adolescent Psychiatry, 34*(10), 1402–1410.

Cohen, J. A., & Mannarino, A. P. (1998). Interventions for sexually abused children: Initial treatment outcome findings. *Child Maltreatment, 3,* 17–26.

Cohen, J. A., Mannarino, A. P., & Deblinger, E. (2006). *Treating trauma and traumatic grief in children and adolescents.* New York: Guilford Press.

Cohen, J. A., Mannarino, A. P., & Iyengar, S. (2011). Community treatment of IPV related PTSD. *Adolescent Medicine, 165,* 16–21.

Cohen, J. A., Mannarino, A. P., & Murray, L. K. (2011). Trauma-focused CBT for youth who experience ongoing traumas. *Child Abuse and Neglect, 35*(8), 637–646.

Cohen, J. A., Mannarino, A. P., & Staron, V. R. (2006). A pilot study of modified cognitive-behavioral therapy for childhood traumatic grief (CBT-CTG). *Journal of the American Academy of Child and Adolescent Psychiatry, 45,* 1465–1473.

Deblinger, E., & Heflin, A. H. (1996). *Treating sexually abused children and their non-offending parents: A cognitive behavioral approach.* Thousand Oaks, CA: Sage.

Deblinger, E., Lippmann, J., & Steer, R. (1996). Sexually abused children suffering posttraumatic stress symptoms: Initial treatment outcome findings. *Child Maltreatment, 1,* 310–321.

Deblinger, E., Mannarino, A. P., Cohen, J. A., Runyon, M. K., & Steer, R. A. (2011). Trauma-focused cognitive behavioral therapy for children: Impact of the trauma narrative and treatment length. *Depression and Anxiety, 28,* 67–75.

Deblinger, E., Mannarino, A. P., Cohen, J. A., & Steer, R. A. (2006). Follow-up study of a multisite, randomized, controlled trial for children with sexual abuse-related PTSD symptoms: Examining predictors of treatment response.

Journal of the American Academy of Child and Adolescent Psychiatry, 45, 1474–1484.

Deblinger, E., McLeer, S. V., Atkins, M., Ralph, D., & Foa, E. (1989). Post-traumatic stress in sexually abused children: Physically abused and non-abused children. *International Journal of Child Abuse and Neglect, 13,* 403–408.

Deblinger, E., McLeer, S. V., & Henry, D. E. (1990). Cognitive/behavioral treatment for sexually abused children suffering post-traumatic stress: Preliminary findings. *Journal of the American Academy of Child and Adolescent Psychiatry, 29,* 747–752.

Deblinger, E., Neubauer, F., Runyon, M., & Baker, D. (2006). *What do you know?: A therapeutic card game about child sexual and physical abuse and domestic violence.* Stratford, NJ: CARES Institute.

Deblinger, E., Stauffer, L. B., & Steer, R. (2001). Comparative efficacies of supportive and cognitive-behavioral group therapies for young children who have been sexually abused and their non-offending mothers. *Child Maltreatment, 6,* 332–343.

Dorsey, S., Cox, J. R., Conover, K. L., & Berliner, L. (2011, Summer). Trauma-focused cognitive behavioral therapy for children and adolescents in foster care. *Children, Youth, and Family News.* Available at *www.apa.org/pi/families/ resources/newsletter/index.aspx.*

Dorsey S., Murray, L. K., Balusubramanian, K., & Skavenski, S. (2011, January). *Trauma-focused cognitive behavioral therapy: International training and implementation.* Paper presented at the 25th Annual San Diego International Conference on Child and Family Maltreatment, San Diego, CA.

Feiring, C., Taska, L. S., & Lewis, M. (1996). A process model for understanding adaptation to sexual abuse: The role of shame in defining stigmatization. *Child Abuse and Neglect, 20,* 767–782.

Felitti, V. J., Anda, R. F., Nordenberg, D., Williamson, D. F., Spitz, A. M., Edwards, V., et al. (1998). Relationship of childhood abuse and household dysfunction to many of the leading causes of death in adults: The Adverse Childhood Experiences (ACE) Study. *American Journal of Preventive Medicine, 14,* 245–258.

Finkelhor, D., Ormrod, R. K., & Turner, H. A. (2009). Lifetime assessment of polyvictimization in a national sample of children and youth. *Child Abuse and Neglect, 33*(7), 403–411.

Frick, P. J. (1991). *The Alabama Parenting Questionnaire.* Unpublished rating scale, University of Alabama.

Goodman, R. (1997). The Strengths and Difficulties Questionnaire: A research note. *Journal of Child Psychology, Psychiatry, and Allied Disciplines, 38*(5), 581–586.

Jain, S., Shapiro, S. L., Swanick, S., Roesch, S. C., Mills, P. J., Bell, I., et al. (2007). A randomized controlled trial of mindfulness meditation vs. relaxation training: Effects on distress, positive states of mind, rumination and distraction. *Annals of Behavioral Medicine, 33*(1), 11–21.

Jaycox, L. H., Cohen, J. A., Mannarino, A. P., Walker, D. W., Langley, A. K., Gegenheimer, K. L., et al. (2010). Children's mental health care following Hurricane Katrina: A field trial of trauma-focused psychotherapies. *Journal of Traumatic Stress, 23,* 223–231.

Kaufman, J., Birmaher, B., & Brent, D. (1996). Schedule for Affective Disorders and Schizophrenia for School-Age Children—Present and Lifetime Version (K-SADS-PL): Initial reliability and validity data. *Journal of the American Academy of Child and Adolescent Psychiatry, 36,* 980–988.

Kendall-Tackett, K. A., Williams, L. M., & Finkelhor, D. (1993). Impact of sexual abuse on children: A review and synthesis of recent empirical studies. *Psychological Bulletin, 113,* 164–180.

Khoury, L. K., Tang, Y. L., Bradley, B., Cubells, J. E., & Ressler, K. J. (2010). Substance use, childhood traumatic experience, and post-traumatic stress disorder in an urban civilian population. *Depression and Anxiety, 27,* 1077–1086.

Kovacs, M. (1985). The Children's Depression Inventory (CDI). *Psychopharmacology Bulletin, 21,* 995–998.

Lyons, J. S., Weiner, D. A., & Scheider, A. (2006). *A field trial of three evidence-based practices for trauma with children in state custody* (Report to the Illinois Department of Children and Family Services). Evanston, IL: Mental Health Resources Services and Policy Program, Northwestern University.

Maercker, A., Michael, T., Fehm, L., Becker, E. S., & Margraf, J. (2004). Age of traumatisation as a predictor of post-traumatic stress disorder or major depression in young women. *British Journal of Psychiatry, 184,* 482–487.

Mannarino, A. P., & Cohen, J. A. (1986). A clinical-demographic study of sexually abused children. *Child Abuse and Neglect, 10,* 17–28.

Mannarino, A. P., Cohen, J. A., & Gregor, M. (1989). Emotional and behavioral difficulties in sexually abused girls. *Journal of Interpersonal Violence, 4,* 437–451.

Mannarino, A. P., Cohen, J. A., Smith, J. A., & Moore-Motily, S. (1991). Six- and twelve-month follow-up of sexually abused girls. *Journal of Interpersonal Violence, 6,* 484–511.

March, J. S. (1997). *Multidimensional Anxiety Scale for Children: Technical manual.* New York: Pearson.

Mannarino, A. P., & Cohen, J. A., (1996). Family-related variables and psychological symptom formation in sexually abused girls. *Journal of Child Sexual Abuse, V 5*(1), 105–120.

McKay, M. M., Hibbert, R., Hoagwood, K., Rodriguez, J., Murray, L., Legerski, J., et al., (2004). Integrating evidence-based engagement strategies into "real world" child mental health settings. *Community Medicine, 4*(2), 177–186.

McKay, M. M., Lynn, C. J., & Bannon, W. M. (2005). Understanding inner city child mental health need and trauma exposure: Implications for preparing urban service providers. *American Journal of Orthospsychiatry, 75*(2), 201–210.

McLeer, S. V., Deblinger, E., Atkins, M., Foa, E., & Ralph, D. (1988). Post-traumatic stress disorder in sexually abused children: A prospective study. *Journal of the American Academy of Child and Adolescent Psychiatry, 27*(5), 650–654.

Murray, L. K., Skavenski, S., Jere, J., Kasoma, M., Dorsey, S., Imasiku, M., et al. (2011). *An international training and implementation model: Trauma-focused cognitive behavioral therapy for children in Zambia.* Manuscript submitted for publication.

Putnam, F. W. (2003). Ten-year research update review: Child sexual abuse. *Journal of the American Academy of Child and Adolescent Psychiatry, 42,* 269–278.

Saunders, B. E., Berliner, L., & Hanson, R. F. (Eds). (2004). *Child physical and sexual abuse: Guidelines for treatment* (Revised report). Charleston, SC: National Crime Victims Research and Treatment Center. Available at *www.musc.edu/cvc*.

Sigel, B., & Benton, A. (2011, July 14). *Findings for statewide dissemination programs using trauma-focused cognitive behavioral therapy (TF-CBT) with children and adolescents*. Paper presented at the 19th annual colloquium of the American Professional Society on the Abuse of Children, Philadelphia.

Silverman, W. K., Ortiz, C. D., Viswesvaran, C., Burns, B. J., Kolko, D. J., Putnam, F. W., et al. (2008). Evidence-based psychosocial treatments for children and adolescents exposed to traumatic events. *Journal of Clinical Child and Adolescent Psychology, 37*(1), 156–183.

Spielberger, C., D. (1973). *Manual for the State–Trait Anxiety Inventory for Children*. Palo Alto, CA: Consulting Psychologists Press.

Steinberg, A. M., Brymer, M. J., Decker, K. B., & Pynoos, R. S. (2004). The University of California, Los Angeles Post-traumatic Stress Disorder Reaction Index. *Current Psychiatry Report, 6*, 96–100.

Strayhorn, J. M., & Weidman, C. S. (1988). A parent practices scale and its relation to parent and child mental health. *Journal of American Academy of Child and Adolescent Psychiatry, 27*, 613–618.

Terr, L. (1985). Psychic trauma in children and adolescents. *Psychiatric Clinics of North America, 8*(12), 815–835.

Turner, H. A., Finkelhor, D., & Ormrod, R. (2010). Poly-victimization in a national sample of children and youth. *American Journal of Preventive Medicine, 38*(3), 323–330.

Weiss, D. S. (2004). The Impact of Event Scale—Revised. In J. P. Wilson & T. M. Keane (Eds.), *Assessing psychological trauma and PTSD* (2nd ed., pp. 168–189). New York: Guilford Press.

PART I

TF–CBT SETTING APPLICATIONS

1

Schools

SUSANA RIVERA

RATIONALE FOR TF–CBT
APPLICATIONS IN SCHOOLS

There are a significant number of school-age children who have been exposed to trauma and are in need of mental health treatment. However, there is a gap between the number of children in need of mental health services and those actually receiving treatment. Service access may be compromised for various reasons, including lack of knowledge of available services and how to access them, cost, lack of transportation, lack of child care for younger siblings, parental stress, work obligations, scheduling conflicts, logistics, and the stigma still often attached to receiving mental health services. Reaching out to trauma-exposed children and ensuring that they receive needed services thus becomes a priority.

All children are required to attend school and this is where they spend the majority of their time, making schools a logical avenue through which children can access services. School counselors and teachers are often the first to identify children in need of services for two primary reasons. First, trauma-exposed youth may experience a wide range of emotional and behavioral problems, including academic difficulties. It is these behavioral and academic concerns that usually bring children to the attention of school staff, most likely for disciplinary action. Second, school faculty is often aware of which children and families are experiencing certain difficulties and may benefit from intervention. Unfortunately, for reasons previously mentioned, not all families referred for services will follow through on their referrals and actually access services. This makes the accessibility of school-based services all the more beneficial for children and their parents. By providing services on campus, children have immediate access to treatment that they may not otherwise receive.

For the successful implementation of school-based services, school faculty, including administrators, counselors, and teachers, must be actively involved in the service delivery process. Therapists interested in providing school-based services must begin by working closely with school administrators to address the impact of trauma on all areas of children's functioning and the benefits of making school-based services available. Administrators who are supportive of providing treatment on campus will help pave the way for therapists to gain access to the children and may also make school resources more readily available. Once children begin receiving services, teachers and counselors will be able to provide therapists with critical information regarding changes in school performance, mood, and behavior. Teachers and counselors may also help to reinforce the skills being taught to the children if they are engaged in the treatment process. Although counseling may not be considered to be within the academic mission of the school, and there may be administrative concerns regarding interruption of children's class time, therapists can stress the benefits of providing services on campus: Children will receive services they may not otherwise receive, will learn the skills necessary to cope with their trauma, and will likely experience improvements in posttraumatic stress symptoms as well as emotional, behavioral, and academic functioning. Focusing on improvements in children's academic performance may serve to encourage school cooperation, since administrators are held accountable for their students' academic performance.

Therapists stress to school faculty that past traumatic experiences may interfere with children's academic success. Trauma symptoms may cause children to experience difficulties in concentrating, completing tasks, learning new concepts, and even engaging with classmates. Moreover, children may exhibit behavioral, emotional, and physical reactions to trauma reminders as well as trauma reenactment behavior problems, which may greatly interfere with their functioning in school. School faculty are provided with psychoeducation so that they learn to recognize trauma responses and to respond appropriately rather than in a manner that might inadvertently further dysregulate the children. School faculty are also taught basic relaxation and coping skills that they can implement in the classroom if the children become triggered and behaviorally or emotionally dysregulated. Therapists also stress the importance of not automatically attributing all behavioral problems to trauma. It is important that the trauma not define the children or be used as an excuse for all unacceptable behaviors. Rather, an enhanced understanding of the traumatic etiology of behavior problems may help school personnel proactively identify ways to minimize the occurrence of trauma-related behavior problems, while simultaneously encouraging more positive coping behaviors through their use of praise, attention, and other school-based rewards. In addition, teachers and other personnel can be supported in firmly, consistently, and sensitively enforcing school rules and consequences to discourage problematic behavior of any origin. By including teachers and other school personnel in the treatment team, school-based therapists are likely to have more success in helping children overcome behavior problems and heal in the aftermath of trauma.

CASE EXAMPLE

One middle school teacher often complained about Jose, a 12-year-old boy with a history of exposure to domestic violence that had only ended upon his father's recent incarceration. The teacher described Jose as being very hyperactive, never sitting still, being disruptive in class, and rarely completing class assignments. Prior to referring Jose to school-based trauma-focused treatment, the teacher managed his behavior, at the recommendation of his mother, by not allowing Jose to consume sugar during the day, believing that sugar was triggering his hyperactivity and inattentiveness. However, Jose would hoard his lunch money and visit the snack bar, where he would purchase soda and candy. The teacher quickly realized that attempts at limiting Jose's sugar intake were ineffective and his disruptive behavior continued. Jose was referred to treatment not because of his exposure to domestic violence but rather because of his disruptive classroom behavior. The teacher was engaged in treatment and learned about trauma reactions and relaxation techniques. When Jose became dysregulated in class, the teacher reminded him of his relaxation techniques, and he soon began exhibiting calmer behavior. By the end of treatment, Jose was being less disruptive and more attentive and was completing more tasks. His sugar consumption was also no longer an issue.

School-based services are delivered in both individual and group sessions, although there are advantages to providing the majority of services in group sessions. First, groups are more cost-effective. They allow the therapist to see multiple children simultaneously, resulting in a larger number of children being served. Second, in the peer group children learn from—and can practice their newly learned skills with—each other. Third, groups promote peer support, which is important considering how isolated many trauma-exposed children feel. Despite the advantages of group sessions, there are components of trauma-focused cognitive-behavioral therapy (TF-CBT) that will be critical to implement in individual sessions.

There are advantages and disadvantages to providing school-based services. Therapists providing school-based services have access to children's academic information, including grades, classroom behavior, and interactions with peers and teachers, critical data that they may not be able to access otherwise. When providing outpatient services, this type of information has to be elicited from parents, who may not be able to provide it, and the therapist may not have access to the children's teachers. School-based therapists also have regular access to the children and are able to provide them with a "safe place" within the school. For many children, school is the only place where they are exposed to positive adult support. School-based services also allow the children opportunities to practice their newly learned skills in a generalized, real-world setting. Considering the stigma often still attached to accessing mental health treatment, providing services in a familiar setting such as a school may allow families to view treatment as more acceptable "school guidance counseling" and may encourage participation.

Disadvantages arise from the fact that schools do not typically offer therapeutic services and may not be equipped to do so. Space is often limited, and therapists may find themselves forced to provide services in areas of the building that are less than ideal. It is important to communicate with school personnel and stress the importance of privacy and confidentiality when trying to access space. Problems also arise when children are involved in treatment and are abruptly withdrawn and transferred to another school, where therapists may not be granted access to them in order to continue treatment. Also, if children are consistently absent or truant, continuity and treatment progress may be compromised. In these cases, therapists can make arrangements with parents to complete treatment either in the clinic or at home, depending on the needs of the family. It is also an opportunity for the therapists to learn more about additional traumas that may be preventing the children from attending school regularly. Gaps in treatment also occur during school holidays or testing periods, and the therapists may not see the children for up to 2 or 3 consecutive weeks. However, these occurrences are usually scheduled in advance and thus can be planned for accordingly. On rare occasions, therapists have reported disruptions during sessions because of unanticipated lockdowns or drills, which unfortunately cannot be planned for and must simply be adjusted to. Another challenge to providing school-based services is the limited access that clinicians may have to the families and other home-based information beyond the intake process. Every effort is made throughout the course of treatment to engage parents continually.

This chapter focuses on TF-CBT applications in school settings, including methods for addressing some of the obstacles just described as well as creative methods for implementing TF-CBT model components in school-based environments.

IDENTIFYING WHO WILL RECEIVE SERVICES

Potential clients are referred by teachers and schools counselors, who are generally well informed regarding their students' trauma history. However, not all children in need of services will be identified. School faculty tend to be more aware of "public" traumas such as grief, exposure to natural disasters, and medical crises and less aware of personal traumas such as physical abuse, sexual abuse, and exposure to domestic violence. Children also tend to be most often referred by school faculty for behavioral or academic problems as opposed to trauma exposure. Because treatment is presented as trauma focused, this may result in some children not being appropriately referred if the teacher or counselor is either unaware of a trauma history or does not perceive the child's history as being traumatic. Referrals are still encouraged if trauma exposures are suspected even if no index trauma can be immediately identified. Once a child is referred to treatment and an assessment is conducted, a trauma history may be identified and the appropriateness of TF-CBT can then be determined. The assessment process is completed by gathering information from the child during individual intake sessions and from the primary caregiver during parent sessions.

When a child is first referred for services, the therapist is provided with caregiver contact information. Written information describing services is sent home, along with a consent form for the child to participate in treatment. If the parental consent form is signed and returned, the child receives an explanation of services and is also asked to sign a consent form to participate before being screened for service eligibility. Eligibility to receive trauma-focused treatment first depends on whether there is an identifiable trauma. If the child is deemed an appropriate candidate for services, the therapist contacts the caregiver and further explains the assessment process, course of treatment, and expectations for child and caregiver participation. This second contact may occur by phone, although a home visit is preferable. Evidence-based engagement strategies (McKay et al., 2004) may be utilized to enhance caregiver commitment and participation (see Deblinger, Cohen, & Mannarino, Introduction, this volume).

After consent forms are signed and a child has been deemed eligible to receive services, the formal assessment process begins. The therapist meets with the child individually and administers standardized trauma assessment measures. Commonly used measures are the UCLA PTSD Reaction Index and the Trauma Symptom Checklist for Children. Baseline intake forms are also completed at this time. On the basis of these assessments, some children may be determined to require services beyond that which can be provided in a school setting. For example, children exhibiting psychotic symptoms or severe behavioral problems, reporting active substance use, engaging in self-injury behaviors, or endorsing numerous severe trauma symptoms may be referred to clinic-based or other services as appropriate. During this process, therapists may also find themselves having to report suspected cases of abuse depending on state reporting laws.

The most challenging aspect of assessment in a school-based setting is the possibility that children may become behaviorally or emotionally dysregulated during the session, particularly if this is the first time they have spoken of the trauma. In this case, it is difficult to simply end a session and send the children back to class, where they will have to continue to deal with their trauma reminders without any support. In anticipation of this possibility, extra time is devoted to the assessment process, and arrangements are made to excuse children from class for a prolonged period and provide crisis intervention if necessary.

The screening and assessment process occurs at the start of each school semester, and groups are formed within the first 2 weeks of class. Groups are composed of children from the same grade level and never have more than 10 members. Whenever possible, children are grouped according to trauma type, although most often there are a mix of traumas represented in each group because the majority of children have identified multiple traumas. Groups may meet once a week but no more than twice within the same week. Exceptions to weekly sessions are made, and no sessions are conducted during school holidays or when students are taking state-mandated standardized tests. Although the majority of services are being delivered in group sessions, individual sessions are also conducted when the therapist determines that a child requires more individual attention or if a child expresses significant unease at participating in a group session. Children are monitored so that those who are having difficulty working within a group format to the point that they are not benefitting (e.g., a child who is extremely withdrawn because of shame or significant depression and who may need additional help) will be seen in individual sessions. All sessions are conducted during school hours and last for one class period at a time that has been mutually agreed upon by the therapist, teachers, and school counselors. Every effort is made to ensure that the children's classroom time is disrupted as minimally as possible, and most sessions are conducted during an elective or study period. Children who are absent and miss a group session meet with the therapist individually prior to the next session for a makeup session so that they can catch up with the rest of the group. Sessions are generally held for approximately 16 weeks, and the end of treatment is meant to coincide with the end of the semester. However, children requiring long-term treatment are accommodated as necessary.

When implementing TF-CBT in a school setting, all of the components of the model are implemented just as in a clinical setting, with the primary difference being that skill-building components may be delivered in a group format.

PARENTAL INVOLVEMENT IN TREATMENT

Parental involvement in school-based treatment is often difficult, and therapists may find themselves having to use creative engagement strategies to achieve this. Aside from the common barriers to accessing services mentioned previously, some parents may be uncomfortable in a school setting because they may associate school calls and visits with their children being in "trouble." Many children are living in chaotic homes characterized by domestic violence, parental substance abuse or mental illness, parental incarceration, involvement in the child welfare system, custody disputes, and unstable caregiver presence. These issues often interfere with supportive parental involvement and are addressed prior to engaging parents in treatment. In these cases, the therapists will gather as much information as possible from school faculty and will conduct home visits in an effort to gather additional information and determine the extent of the children's needs. If possible, and if consent is obtained, the therapists may also gather additional information by talking to extended family members. If there are ongoing safety concerns or if the situation is deemed highly unstable, the therapists will likely make the decision not to initiate TF-CBT until these more pressing issues are addressed.

Parents often have to be oriented to what trauma is and the importance of addressing it in treatment. Children receiving school-based services are typically referred to treatment by school faculty, not parents, which may result in parents not being as committed to treatment. Parents also may not be aware that a trauma has occurred, may not identify a particular event as having been traumatic for their children, or may not acknowledge the importance of treatment. Cultural influences should be explored because these may play a role in terms of these issues as well as the parents' overall receptivity to treatment for their children (Cohen, Deblinger, Mannarino, & de Arellano, 2001). Many cultures discourage mental health treatment, preferring to keep personal issues within the family and to deal with them privately. Assessing for and incorporating cultural beliefs into treatment may help families to overcome their reluctance. Integrating cultural beliefs into treatment may also result in greater treatment attendance and completion as well as better outcomes.

Many children are referred to treatment by school faculty because of specific behavioral problems and a suspicion of a trauma history. Upon assessment, therapists often learn that the children do indeed have a trauma history, one that has possibly never been disclosed. Children may not disclose trauma for various reasons, including fear of retaliation by a perpetrator, fear of removal from the home, and concerns over upsetting their parents. Psychoeducation becomes especially important in these cases so that the children are able to disclose the trauma to parents and can begin to move forward with treatment. In these cases therapists must address reporting concerns within a specified time frame; thus, it is important for school-based therapists to be knowledgeable of their state's child protection reporting requirements and community resources that will be helpful to the family.

Caregivers and children who have been exposed to repeated domestic violence may be desensitized to it, and parents may not thus perceive it as traumatic for the children. As a result, they may not understand the effects of trauma exposure on their children or may not attribute the children's emotional or behavioral problems to the trauma. Rather, they may view the children's actions as acting-out behaviors as opposed to trauma reactions. When this is addressed, feelings of guilt over being a "bad" parent may arise, which will have to be a focus of treatment. It is important to validate parents' feelings of inadequacy, guilt, or self-blame and acknowledge how overwhelmed they may have been under the circumstances. It is also important to address the role of the parents in the children's treatment and help them see themselves as part of their children's recovery, not part of the problem. Not uncommonly, when parents learn of their children's trauma, they may reveal that they themselves were victimized as children but never disclosed it. In these cases, parents may adopt an attitude of "I got through it on my own, so why does my child need counseling?" The therapist must then acknowledge the parents' strength in the face of adversity and explain individual differences in coping with trauma. It should also be stressed to parents that their children's response to the trauma is not a reflection on their parenting abilities.

The first step in engaging parents is to initiate positive contact through a phone call, letter, or home visit. Prior to providing services, while attempting to acquire consent, therapists have the opportunity not only to promote the proposed services but also to stress how crucial parental involvement is in the child's treatment. Parents can be encouraged to attend sessions at the school if that setting will put them at ease, or home visits can be provided, depending on their preferences and logistical needs. It is also important to define "family" broadly and not limit caregiver involvement to parents only. Any adult who plays a significant role in the child's life may be encouraged to participate with proper parental consent.

Parent sessions parallel to child sessions are scheduled weekly at a time and location convenient for the primary caregiver. School-based parent groups sometimes prove difficult to coordinate for various reasons, including conflicting work schedules, lack of transportation, lack of child care for preschool-age children, and discomfort in the school setting. Thus, home-based parent sessions have proved to be most effective. Occasionally, some parents will request clinic-based services and should be accommodated accordingly. Potential barriers to accessing services are important to identify prior to treatment so that any obstacles can be overcome without interrupting or compromising treatment.

Every semester therapists encounter parents who, although they consent to their child receiving services, indicate that they prefer not to participate in parent sessions. In these rare cases, the therapists meet with the parents in an effort to determine why they are hesitant to participate, answer any questions they may have about treatment, address their concerns, and overcome their reluctance if possible. If the parents continue to refuse to participate, efforts are made to identify another adult who may, with parental consent, engage in the parent sessions and provide support for the child. If an alternate adult cannot be identified, services are still provided to the child, and parents are kept informed of treatment progress. Regardless of whether parents choose to engage in parent sessions, they are still encouraged to participate in the assessment process and complete their own standardized assessment measures related to their child's trauma history and symptoms. This will allow the therapist to form a comprehensive picture of the child's needs. The measures most commonly used with parents are the UCLA PTSD Reaction Index (Steinberg, Brymer, Decker, & Pynoos, 2004) and the Child Behavior Checklist (Achenbach, 1991).

Parent sessions are initially conducted individually, with a focus on psychoeducation and the skills the child is learning as well as parenting skills. The PRAC components of TF-CBT are introduced, and parents are assigned homework that will encourage communication and reinforce these skills at home. As the child nears the trauma narrative component of TF-CBT, the therapist continues to meet with parents individually and prepares them to hear their child's narrative. Conjoint sessions will follow as the child shares the completed narrative. These conjoint sessions are usually held at the home after school hours. After the narrative has been shared, individual sessions may resume as the therapist prepares the parents for the end of treatment.

The goal is for children and parents to take the skills that are being taught and apply them not only to trauma-related but also to real-life scenarios, including those that play out at home. Parents generally want to focus on managing behavioral problems, and are taught that parenting techniques can be applied with all children in the household, not just the identified client. As treatment progresses, parents also typically report decreases in their own depression and anxiety associated with their child's trauma.

APPLICATION OF TF-CBT
COMPONENTS IN SCHOOL SETTINGS

Considerations for implementing TF-CBT in school settings include modifications for delivery in group sessions, length of treatment, and delivery in a nonclinical setting.

Psychoeducation

Psychoeducation is meant to provide trauma information and normalize a child's reactions to trauma. In a school setting, psychoeducation is typically delivered in group format at the beginning of treatment. This component actually begins during the assessment phase as the child is oriented to trauma and a rationale is provided for the initiation of the trauma-focused assessment and treatment. Psychoeducation groups focus on providing general trauma information and normalizing a child's behavioral and emotional reactions to trauma. Because each child in the group has a unique trauma history, it is difficult to focus on any one specific trauma type when providing psychoeducation. Therapists will instead provide general trauma information by addressing all trauma types and common affective and behavioral reactions to trauma. Since the therapists know each child's trauma history, they provide more detailed psychoeducation about specific trauma types that are relevant to group participants, but will do so without singling out any child as having experienced a particular trauma unless the child identifies him- or herself as having experienced a particular trauma. Typically, the first group session will be the only "official" psychoeducation session, although this component will be revisited during each subsequent session as the children continue to learn about trauma and trauma reactions and how the trauma relates to them.

Case Example

Twelve-year-old Juan was referred to treatment following the death of his father. At assessment, Juan did not identify the loss of his father as a trauma. In fact, he did not endorse any trauma at all. He did, however, endorse trauma symptoms that he had been experiencing recently but did not relate them to the loss of his father. Although Juan questioned why he was referred to treatment, the fact that some of his friends would also be participating encouraged him to consent to participate. His mother readily consented to treatment because of her concerns over how he was coping with his father's death; she noted that Juan had become quiet and withdrawn, had given up his favorite extracurricular activities, and was experiencing a drop in his grades. Despite the fact that Juan did not identify any trauma, the therapist still decided to engage him in treatment considering the information his mother provided. During the first psychoeducation session, the therapist introduced different types of traumas that children experience, including the loss of a loved one. With Juan's loss in mind, the therapist even shared how, as a child, she had lost somebody who she loved, and she spoke about how confusing that had been. Following this discussion, the therapist asked if anybody in the group had ever lost somebody they loved. After a few quiet moments, Juan spoke up: "That's like what happened with my dad." Prior to this, he had never openly acknowledged the loss of his father. After this session, he gradually began talking about his memories of his father and his feelings about his loss.

Parenting Skills

Parenting skills—specifically how to manage behavioral problems—is the one topic that parents generally want to focus on. Because most children are referred for behavioral problems they are exhibiting in school, the therapist is in an ideal position to work closely with both parents and teachers to support positive behavior and reduce behavioral problems. Although behavior management skills and contingency reinforcement programs are routinely discussed during individual parent sessions, they may also be addressed during conjoint sessions among parents, teachers, and school counselors. If behavioral problems are a significant concern, the therapist may schedule a conjoint session between parents and teachers to identify the problematic behaviors, as well as previous successful and unsuccessful techniques for addressing them, and to develop a behavior management plan emphasizing the importance of reinforcing positive behaviors. The children may also be involved in the development of this plan so that they understand the expectations in terms of specific desirable and undesirable behaviors being exhibited and the rewards and consequences for ensuing behaviors both at home and at school. Of course, behavioral interventions will always be tailored to the developmental level and needs of the child.

Relaxation and Stress Management Techniques

Relaxation and stress management techniques are meant to help reduce the physiological manifestation of stress and posttraumatic stress disorder and are also taught in a group format. Once the rationale for these techniques is introduced and clients have learned about the physiological manifestations of stress, the therapist introduces basic relaxation techniques such as deep breathing, progressive muscle relaxation, and the use of imagery. The group also collectively identifies and discusses other activities they find relaxing, such as art, music, and sports. Together, the group practices some of these activities. In the past, therapists have provided children with "mood pencils," which change color when held. Surprisingly, these pencils became a source of relaxation: The children found that rolling the pencils in their hands in order to change the color had a calming effect on them.

Teachers and school counselors frequently report that children exhibit trauma symptoms in class, causing disruptions in the class routine. In consideration of how trauma reactions can affect children at school, therapists address stress reactions and relaxation techniques as they apply to the school environment. In addition, therapists address not only trauma-related but also school-related stressors and how relaxation techniques can be effective under these circumstances as well. The goal is for children to see that the skills they are learning can be generalized and applied to real-life situations regardless of whether they are trauma related. Similarly to the psychoeducation component, relaxation and stress management techniques are continuously addressed during subsequent sessions after they are first introduced.

Case Example

Thirteen-year-old Lisa was referred to treatment because of immigration-related trauma, the kidnapping of her father, and traumatic grief. Her most overwhelming trauma symptom was anxiety, which was affecting her functioning in every aspect of her life. Her anxiety made it difficult for her to concentrate in school or to focus on basic tasks at home. As a result of her trouble concentrating at school, she had never been able to earn a passing score on state-mandated standardized tests. Her mother pressured her about the importance of doing well in school, which increased Lisa's anxiety when taking any test. After learning about relaxation techniques and how they can be applied in school, Lisa practiced deep breathing before her next test and at the following group session reported that she had calmed down enough to focus on the questions and answer them correctly. She continued to practice deep breathing before tests and eventually earned a passing score on her next state-mandated standardized test. The following school year the therapist was informed that not only had Lisa earned a passing score on that year's state test, but she had earned "Commended Recognition," the highest level of achievement recognition.

Affective Expression and Modulation Skills

Affective expression and modulation skills are meant to help children manage and express their feelings in a healthy manner and are also addressed in a group format when implemented in a school setting. It is not unusual for children to experience difficulty in identifying emotions. In a group setting, children may be reluctant to discuss trauma-related feelings in the presence of peers, many of whom may not know each other well. There may be concerns about showing vulnerability or being ridiculed. Therefore, emotions are initially introduced in a general manner. Group members identify common positive and negative emotions that children may routinely experience and also identify situations that may elicit those emotions. Another approach is to discuss common situations that children encounter daily and identify positive and negative emotions that those situations may elicit. Once the group members become at ease discussing emotions in general, the focus turns to identifying and normalizing emotions elicited by trauma and trauma reminders. These trauma-related emotions are also discussed in general terms (i.e., what might a person who witnessed domestic violence feel). Once this becomes a comfortable topic, the focus then turns to specific trauma-related emotions that the group members have experienced. This component may take several sessions to move through as children become comfortable with owning and expressing their emotions.

CASE EXAMPLE

Miguel is a 14-year-old boy who was referred to treatment for traumatic grief. Miguel's father stabbed his mother to death while under the influence of drugs when Miguel was 6 years old and is currently incarcerated for the crime. Miguel is being raised by his maternal grandmother and other maternal relatives, and has no contact with his father or any paternal relatives. As a result of these circumstances, Miguel has grown up angry and has directed his anger at his father. He has been expressing his anger through aggressive outbursts, impulsive acts, and risky behaviors. His teacher and school counselor reported that he became especially angry whenever anybody talked about parents in his presence. Miguel reported having some memories of his mother, but felt he mostly knew her through the many positive stories he had been told about her by his family. In regard to his father and the stabbing, Miguel had only vague memories and told the therapist that much of what he knew was probably from details that his older brother had shared with him. When discussing emotions in his group, Miguel would not identify or acknowledge any feeling other than anger, always referring to his father taking his mother away from him. He also reported that he knew his father had never loved him or his mother and expressed anger over that as well. The therapist made several attempts at helping Miguel acknowledge other feelings that may be underlying his anger, but Miguel would not endorse any. The therapist then provided psychoeducation on the role that drugs can play in the occurrence of violence, thereby indirectly addressing the fact that Miguel's father was under the influence at the time. The goal was not to excuse his father's actions but rather to help Miguel realize that his father may have not acted rationally and did not intentionally take his mother from him because he did not love them. Miguel recalled an incident at a family gathering when a relative became intoxicated and acted in a manner uncharacteristic of her. Later in treatment, during individual processing sessions, Miguel began to consider the possibility that his father had not fully comprehended what he was doing when he stabbed his mother because he was high on drugs. The therapist had previously worked on a responsibility pie with Miguel, where he had placed 100% of the blame for the murder on his father. Following the discussion about the effects of drugs and alcohol, Miguel worked on another responsibility pie and attributed part of the blame to the drugs, although the majority of the blame was still allocated to his father for making the decision to use drugs in the first place. After this Miguel was encouraged to speak with a family member and ask questions about his mother, her relationship with his father, and his early childhood. Miguel soon came to realize that his parents had actually loved each other and that his father had loved him. As he came to terms with this new information and his newly acquired insight into his father's state of mind on the day of the murder, Miguel was able to begin acknowledging different emotions regarding his father, his mother, his family, and especially himself. By the end of treatment, Miguel was still endorsing anger, but he was also acknowledging sadness and positive emotions as well.

Cognitive Coping Skills

Cognitive coping skills are meant to help children identify the difference between thoughts and behaviors and learn how their thoughts and feelings influence their behaviors. These skills primarily focus on helping children change their feelings and behaviors by recognizing and changing their unhealthy or inaccurate thoughts. This component is also delivered in a group format, where members learn to take the feelings they identified during the affective expression and modulation component and begin to identify thoughts that may trigger distressing feelings. As they master identifying thoughts that underlie positive and negative feelings, examination of resulting behavioral reactions is introduced. As with the affective expression and modulation component, the skills are taught in a general fashion before focusing on specific trauma-related thoughts. The therapist then moves to having the children differentiate unhelpful thoughts, inaccurate thoughts, and accurate thoughts. Interestingly, it is the group members who are able to help others identify inaccurate thoughts, pointing out their cognitive distortions for them. This has allowed the children to focus closely on their behaviors, particularly at school, and how they have been motivated by irrational thoughts. They have then been able to shift their focus to their behaviors at home and the thoughts and feelings behind those behaviors. As they learn how their behaviors are influenced by their trauma-related thoughts and feelings, they begin to learn ways of changing their thoughts. This also occurs in part through the influence of their group peers. Group members are often adept at recognizing their peers' unhealthy thoughts and behaviors more easily than their own. In addition, they also offer each other support and encouragement as they work on changing their thoughts.

CASE EXAMPLE

Two children were influenced not to join in gang activities as a result of the cognitive coping skills they learned in treatment. Maria, a 14-year-old girl living with her elderly maternal grandmother, was referred to treatment for bullying and aggressive behaviors toward classmates as well as a suspicion of her own physical abuse. During the assessment, Maria confirmed not only physical abuse by her mother (who was currently incarcerated for drugs) but also sexual abuse by a male relative when she was between the ages of 3 and 12 years. Maria did not have feel as if she had anyone who served as a strong source of support for her and she seemed to be looking to belong. Throughout treatment Maria revealed that she was contemplating joining a gang and that the aggressive behavior she had been exhibiting toward her classmates had actually been part of a gang initiation ritual she had been forced to engage in. She reported that she was considering joining a gang because she needed a "family" that would "have her back" and keep her safe from harm by anyone. Maria had no sense of safety from her family after the years of physical and sexual abuse and was looking for it from an alternate family. She was quick to recite the reasons why she should join a gang and how it would be beneficial to her in terms of belonging and a perceived sense of physical safety and was unable to identify any negative consequences. While working through the cognitive coping component, she slowly began to reevaluate her reasons for wanting to join a gang and by the end of treatment had decided against it. Maria revealed to the therapist that she had used the cognitive triangle to make her final decision about joining the gang and had changed her mind after she closely considered how she felt and the possible consequences of being a gang member. She had realized that being involved in a gang might actually cause her further physical harm, and that was one of the deciding factors against joining. The therapist suspected that the conjoint sessions may have also helped Maria to feel more connected to her grandmother as a source of support versus gang involvement.

Kevin, a 12-year-old boy who was already in a gang, was referred to treatment after both having witnessed and having been a victim of gang violence. Kevin's father was absent from his life, and Kevin reported missing this relationship. Kevin revealed that he often felt isolated and lonely and joined a gang because he wanted to belong. He was completely involved in all aspects of gang life and, since joining, had perpetrated violent acts against others, had been physically beaten by rival gang members, and had also begun experimenting with drugs and alcohol. Although he appreciated the fact that he finally belonged and had a "family" in the form of his fellow gang members, Kevin began to question his actions and how he felt about them as he worked through the cognitive coping component. He also began to think about himself and the other gang members differently. At the end of treatment, he was still a member of the gang but was reevaluating his membership and what it meant for him. The following school year, Kevin approached his therapist on campus and reported to her that he left the gang and now belonged to an organized sports team instead. The therapist acknowledged how difficult it must have been to make that decision and praised him for leaving the gang. Kevin replied that it was the cognitive triangle that had made him think about what he was doing and had also made him realize that he didn't like the way he thought of himself when he was engaging in certain gang-related activities. This made him rethink his reasons for joining and convinced him to leave. He added that he still appreciated the sense of belonging he felt, but now the sports team gave him a more positive impression of himself because he was "acting better."

Trauma Narrative

The trauma narrative is an exposure and processing intervention that encourages children to share details of their traumas and become desensitized to trauma reminders by unpairing thoughts and reminders of the trauma from overwhelming negative emotions. When the group reaches this point in treatment, group sessions are temporarily suspended so that trauma narrative sessions can be conducted individually. This allows each child the privacy and time needed to develop and complete the trauma narrative. These individual sessions are still conducted on campus, although therapists try to conduct them later in the school day to avoid possible distraction from schoolwork. Many sensitive details come up during the development of the trauma narrative and, although they have already mastered their PRAC skills, sometimes the children become dysregulated during these sessions. It is difficult for the therapist to have them share these sensitive details and then send them back to their classroom, where they might have difficulty concentrating because their mind is still on the narrative session. Relaxation techniques are revisited and practiced prior to ending each session in an effort to address this. As in clinic-based treatment, the children are allowed flexibility and creativity in how the trauma narrative will be developed.

Prior to this interruption of group sessions, the therapist explains to the children what will come next. The therapist has already explained the value of facing traumatic memories, and the children are now reminded of this, with examples of how a trauma narrative or other similar activities will help them achieve that goal. The therapist decides how many weeks the group sessions will be suspended for based on his or her clinical evaluation of how the members are progressing individually. Members are informed of the date that group sessions will resume so that they are prepared. Children who have not completed their trauma narrative by this date are still allowed to rejoin the group, but continue to meet with the therapist individually to complete their trauma narratives.

Case Example

Twelve-year-old Sam was referred to treatment for traumatic grief. When Sam was 8 years old his father died, murdered during a drug deal that went wrong. However, Sam was unaware of the circumstances of his father's death because his mother withheld the truth in order to protect him. During the skill-building group sessions, Sam had diligently worked on group activities but never related any of what he was learning to the loss of his father. He was also silent during most of the discussions. When the therapist addressed his silence, Sam numbly replied that "it wasn't time to talk about it yet." When the time came to begin work on his trauma narrative, at Sam's request, the decision was made to develop the narrative during conjoint sessions with Sam and his mother. Sam learned about his father through stories, pictures, and videos that his mother shared with him during the development of the narrative. Most of what Sam learned was information that was new to him, as were the pictures and videos. During this time, Sam also learned the true circumstances of his father's murder. Initially, he was very angry with his mother for having kept these details from him, but came to accept that she lied in order to protect his feelings and to help him maintain a positive image of his father. As Sam continued to communicate with his mother and learn more about his father, he came to acknowledge how he had been affected by his father's death. In his trauma narrative, Sam included his memories and related thoughts and feelings about his father, the murder, his relationship with his mother, and how he had coped with it all. Although trauma narratives are not typically developed in conjoint sessions, in Sam's case it proved beneficial because it was the catalyst for him feeling that "it was time to talk about it now," and his mother provided him with the information that he needed to develop his narrative, which helped him to more fully grieve the loss of his father.

Cognitive Processing

Cognitive processing follows the completion of the trauma narrative and allows for the identification and correction of the child's trauma-related cognitive errors. When TF-CBT is delivered in a school-based setting, this component is also provided in individual sessions held on campus. There have been no notable differences in how the processing of the narrative occurs in a school setting compared with a clinical setting.

In Vivo Exposure

In vivo exposure is meant to gradually and repeatedly bring a child in closer contact with a feared stimulus. This component is difficult to implement in a school setting, particularly if the feared stimulus is not school related. In order to successfully work through this component when providing school-based services, a plan is developed early in the treatment process between the therapist and parent after the therapist has worked with the child and has identified the stimulus that the child is struggling with. The gradual exposure plan is reviewed and progress and setbacks are discussed during weekly parent sessions. The therapist works with the parent on following through with the plan (i.e., getting the child to sleep alone in his own bed all night) and provides the necessary support to ensure success. This may also be addressed during individual sessions with the child if the therapist considers it necessary. Gradual exposure, of course, also occurs throughout the course of treatment as the child is exposed to trauma reminders and trauma-related thoughts and feelings.

Often, the feared stimulus is not necessarily school related but may manifest itself at school. For example, a child who has been sexually abused may be uncomfortable changing clothes for gym class because of feelings of shame. In this case, these feelings and the child's response to them would be addressed during the affective expression and modulation component as well as during the cognitive coping component. In regard to *in vivo* exposure, the therapist may, for example, engage both the child and the gym teacher in developing an exposure plan that will allow the child to gradually become more comfortable changing clothes in the locker room.

Conjoint Sessions

Conjoint sessions are meant to promote effective communication between the child and the caregivers regarding trauma and the child's reaction to it. These sessions are not always feasible when providing school-based services because the child is seen on campus and parents are typically seen off campus. Conjoint sessions tend to occur most often when sharing the trauma narrative. However, the therapist does have the option of conducting conjoint sessions whenever necessary. These conjoint sessions may be delivered on campus or in the home, depending on what is most convenient for the parent. Conjoint sessions may be used to review the PRAC skills, to review homework, or to share new and important information. Many times these conjoint sessions occur early in the treatment process when a child discloses a trauma and reports that the parent is unaware of it or when the therapist learns from the parent critical details about the trauma that the child is unaware of but needs to know in order to effectively work through treatment. Most often, these are details regarding the circumstances surrounding a death that the parent is trying to protect the child from. Conjoint sessions occur as often as the therapist deems necessary throughout treatment (e.g., if there are significant behavior problems) and are coordinated accordingly with the parent.

Enhancing Safety and Future Development

Enhancing safety and future development is meant to identify potential safety concerns and help the child develop skills necessary to stay safe in the future. Although it is the final PRACTICE component, it may be delivered earlier in treatment if safety concerns are a priority. However, if implemented before the narrative, it is particularly important to emphasize to the child that he or she would not have been expected to utilize these skills at the time of the traumas given his or her young age, emotional distress, and/ or lack of knowledge. If the therapist determines that the child is at risk or simply does not feel safe, the therapist may work with the child individually or conjointly with both the child and parent to develop an appropriate safety plan. Even if safety is addressed early in treatment, safety planning will still be reviewed prior to ending treatment in order to reinforce safety skills. This is typically done in individual and/or conjoint sessions, although safety skills may also be addressed in a group session.

Group sessions resume after the children have completed, processed, and shared their trauma narratives. By this time, the end of the semester is near and treatment will begin to wind down. Final group sessions focus on reviewing the skills learned and enhancing safety and problem-solving skills.

TERMINATING TREATMENT

Children who receive school-based services are generally able to work through the components in 12 to 16 sessions. Treatment ends with a group graduation after the final session, during which children are presented with "diplomas" acknowledging successful completion of treatment. Prior to receiving their diplomas, however, the therapist has the children create their own personal message for future TF-CBT participants, in which they share why they were involved in treatment, their thoughts and feelings at the start of treatment, what they learned, and what they would tell another child going through a similar experience. Their message is anonymous and is signed with only their initials, age, and gender. Their written message may also be personalized with a paint-dipped handprint in their favorite color. These messages are compiled into a scrapbook and shared with future participants as psychoeducation and inspiration.

Those children who require more intensive intervention should be referred for such after the end of the group sessions. The end of treatment is also the time for therapists to evaluate each child's progress and facilitate referrals for additional services if needed.

CONCLUSION

For various reasons, not all trauma-exposed children in need of mental health treatment are able to access clinic-based services. However, because all children are required to attend school, the school setting is a logical place to reach children in need of treatment and bring the services to them. Trauma-focused treatment, although typically delivered in a clinical setting through individual sessions, has been effectively implemented in group format as well (Deblinger, Stauffer, & Steer, 2001; Stauffer & Deblinger, 1996) and more recently in school-based group programs, with positive outcomes. By delivering school-based services and using a group format, more children can be reached and can reap the benefits of TF-CBT.

REFERENCES

Achenbach, T. M. (1991). *Manual for the Child Behavior Checklist and Revised Child Behavior Profile*. Burlington: University of Vermont.

Cohen, J. A., Deblinger, E., Mannarino, A. P., & de Arellano, M. A. (2001). The importance of culture in treating abused and neglected children: An empirical review. *Child Maltreatment, 6*(2), 148–157.

Deblinger, E., Stauffer, L. B., & Steer, R. (2001). Comparative efficacies of supportive and cognitive-behavioral group therapies for young children who have been sexually abused and their non-offending mothers. *Child Maltreatment, 6,* 332–343.

McKay, M., Hibbert, R., Hoagwood, K., Rodriguez, J., Murray, L., Legerski, J., et al. (2004). Integrating evidence based engagement strategies into "real world" child mental health settings. *Community Medicine, 4*(2), 177–186.

Stauffer, L., & Deblinger, E. (1996). Cognitive behavioral groups for nonoffending mothers and their young sexually abused children: A preliminary treatment outcome study. *Child Maltreatment, 1*(1), 65–76.

Steinberg, A. M., Brymer, M. J., Decker, K. B., & Pynoos, R. S. (2004). The University of California, Los Angeles Post-traumatic Stress Disorder Reaction Index. *Current Psychiatry Report, 6,* 96–100.

2

Children in Foster Care

SHANNON DORSEY
ESTHER DEBLINGER

UNIQUE ASPECTS
OF THE FOSTER CARE POPULATION

Children in foster care have significantly higher rates of trauma exposure and trauma-related symptoms than the general population as well as high rates of behavioral problems (Kolko et al., 2010; Pecora et al., 2003). These clinical concerns make trauma-focused cognitive-behavioral therapy (TF-CBT), which includes both specific trauma treatment components as well as a parenting component, a particularly relevant treatment approach for the foster care population. However, there are a few unique features and considerations that often raise questions for clinicians in terms of how to implement TF-CBT with both children and adolescents in foster care and with their foster and biological parents. These include:

- Multiple, chronic, trauma exposure histories
- Significant behavioral problems
- High levels of emotional dysregulation
- Multiple presenting problems and diagnoses
- Difficulty engaging the primary caregiver (foster parent)
- Complexities regarding the involvement of biological parents

Our goals in this chapter are to address these concerns and to offer practical clinical suggestions and resources. In most ways, providing TF-CBT to children in foster care is not significantly different from providing TF-CBT to other children; however, in some cases, children and adolescents in foster care who present for treatment have multiple diagnoses and presenting problems, have prior experience with therapy, may be on multiple medications, and may have attachment difficulties. This combination of factors can be daunting to clinicians and can result in hesitancy in providing TF-CBT. Cognitive-behavioral therapy (CBT), generally, has been found to be effective for diverse cultural and ethnic groups (Huey & Polo, 2008) and is considered a frontline treatment for depression and anxiety as well as behavioral problems, when the emphasis is on the "B" in CBT (i.e., behavioral, parenting skills). Even when children have significant attachment difficulties, which many in foster care do as part of a normal reaction to inconsistent caregiving and disrupted placements, the best tools for treatment include CBT, a targeted focus on skills that can be beneficial across a number of areas (e.g., posttraumatic stress disorder [PTSD], depression, anxiety, behavior problems), consistent foster parent involvement, and concentration on reinforcing the child's and foster parent's use of skills at home and in the community. In a review of more than 70 studies of interventions designed to improve attachment security in children (Bakermans-Kranenburg, van IJzendoorn, & Juffer, 2003), the more effective interventions had common characteristics, including being shorter term, goal oriented, and focused (like TF-CBT) versus more extensive and broader in focus.

EVIDENCE FOR TF-CBT WITH CHILDREN AND ADOLESCENTS IN FOSTER CARE

In addition to the general evidence for CBT and targeted, structured approaches detailed previously, TF-CBT, specifically, has been found to be effective with children in foster care. All TF-CBT studies have included some children and adolescents in foster care, and two studies—one published and one underway—have found that TF-CBT has been effective specifically with this population (Dorsey, Cox, Conover, & Berliner, 2011; Lyons, Weiner, & Schneider, 2006; Weiner, Schneider, & Lyons, 2009). In the Weiner and colleagues (2009) study, ethnically diverse children in foster care who received TF-CBT, when compared with those who had received treatment as usual through the systems of care, reported significantly greater reductions in trauma symptoms and significantly fewer placement changes and runaway attempts (Lyons et al., 2006). In an ongoing randomized controlled trial of standard delivery of TF-CBT compared with TF-CBT plus evidence-based engagement strategies with youth in foster care, TF-CBT was found to be effective in both conditions for significantly reducing PTSD symptoms, based on both child and foster parent report (Dorsey et al., 2011). The TF-

CBT plus evidence-based engagement strategies resulted in fewer dropouts during treatment, suggesting the importance of focused engagement strategies for this population.

These findings should be generalizable to community-based practice: Both of these studies were effectiveness trials that included few study exclusionary criteria and included ethnically and culturally diverse children and adolescents. Clinicians were predominantly masters'-level clinicians, all of whom were employed in community mental health settings. Additionally, despite the fact that children were in foster care, the average number of sessions provided by community-based mental health clinicians in the Dorsey, Cox, and colleagues (2011) trial was 16 to 17, which is in the suggested range (i.e., 8–20 sessions), noteworthy also because most clinicians were providing 50- to 60-minute sessions (vs. 90-minute sessions).

COLLABORATION WITH CHILD WELFARE

Child welfare social workers play an important role in the lives of children in foster care and thus can be a critical source of support for the TF-CBT therapist. These workers are important collaborators who can provide information about the children's history, reunification, or permanency plans and updates, and can offer support and encouragement for both child and foster parent participation in treatment. In our work with youth in foster care, connecting with the child welfare workers has been critical for staying informed about any upcoming court dates, visitation plan changes, and placement changes and for incentivizing foster parents to participate in treatment. Child welfare workers who are supportive of evidence-based practices have been able to creatively encourage foster parents to be more involved in treatment, sometimes providing incentives such as mileage reimbursement, licensure hours for therapy participation, and reinforcement of treatment participation during home and safety visits (Dorsey, Kerns, Trupin, Conover, & Berliner, 2011).

As part of this collaborative effort, the child welfare workers, who are typically the state "representative guardians," should also be generally informed about their clients' progress in treatment (as should foster parents, who are the day-to-day caregivers). In our experience, when clinicians provide regular, brief treatment updates (e.g., once a month) about child and foster parent attendance and treatment progress (e.g., on trauma narrative), caseworkers greatly appreciate the effort and can then support the therapy in any decisions related to the children's care. When child welfare workers are not involved, they may inadvertently make recommendations or other referrals that are counter to the CBT approach to treating trauma (e.g., avoiding vs. facing trauma reminders).

Another important role of social workers is in helping clinicians determine whether, when, and how to involve biological parents in treatment (see additional discussion later in this chapter). Although the children may be in foster care, clinicians should consider the role of the biological parents up front—most children continue to see their parents either formally (court-ordered visits) or informally (in the community), and a substantial number will reunify. Social workers can help clinicians understand the parents' current role, and their involvement with the children—information that is key in determining the biological parents' level of involvement in treatment. In some cases, a meeting early in the process between clinician and biological parent—and not necessarily including the child (see later discussion for guidelines for conjoint sessions)—can do much to reduce resistance to treatment and defensiveness later when it is clear that parent and child will reunify and that biological parent involvement will, therefore, be essential.

FOSTER PARENT INVOLVEMENT

One primary challenge often mentioned by clinicians when providing TF-CBT to children and adolescents in foster care involves engaging foster parents. In TF-CBT, the day-to-day caregivers are ideally involved in treatment to support the children's acquisition and practice of skills and to offer emotional support throughout the therapy process. Caregiver involvement is particularly important when the children have significant behavioral problems, as is the case with many children and adolescents in foster care, as behavioral problems are predominantly addressed through behavior management strategies covered in the parenting component of TF-CBT.

Research on predictors of engagement indicates that perceptual barriers to engagement appear to be just as significant as concrete barriers, if not more so (McKay, Pennington, Lynn, & McCadam, 2001). For many foster parents, primary barriers to engaging in therapy are related to past negative experiences and to perceptions that mental health therapy will not be helpful. McKay, Stoewe, McCadam, and Gonzales (1998) have developed specific evidence-based engagement strategies that were applied to TF-CBT with youth in foster care, resulting in greater retention in treatment (Dorsey et al., 2011). These strategies, described briefly here and in more detail in McKay and Bannon (2004), focus on addressing prior negative experiences with mental health, increasing expectations that therapy can be helpful, identifying foster parents' perception of why children might need treatment, and beginning active treatment in the initial telephone contact and in the first in-person meeting (vs. focusing solely on appointment scheduling and completing intake paperwork).

In TF-CBT, an important part of building expectations that therapy can be helpful involves describing the model, the research on its effectiveness, how treatment will be structured, and expectations about treatment (e.g., attend sessions weekly, practice skills in session and at home), while also soliciting questions, concerns, and hesitations about participation so that these can be discussed in session. In our qualitative work, some foster parents have indicated that it is important as well to clarify that the therapy involves providing support to the foster parent.

In some cases, clinicians are hesitant to involve foster parents because of their own past negative experiences with foster parents not wanting to be involved or being unsupportive. However, foster parents are the day-to-day, 24-hour caregivers for the children in their homes, are often inadequately prepared by foster parent training programs to handle behavioral and emotional problems (Dorsey et al., 2008), and to respond supportively to trauma-related discussions and symptoms.

In cases in which a foster parent cannot be engaged, identifying and engaging another adult who is important in the child's life (e.g., aunt, mentor, fictive kin) is an option. When working with foster families, one should be aware of differences in the experiences of nonrelative and kinship foster parents. For example, when foster parents are relative caregivers, they may be much more likely to be emotionally affected by the child's trauma. Kinship caregivers may have experienced additional stress related to taking the child into the home (e.g., strained extended family relationships, disruption in their immediate family). As one kinship caregiver reported, after taking her cousin's children into her home, "You get a call late at night, and you can either take in these children or they go into the system. You don't get to take a class or make a decision that you want to be a foster parent. You don't get to prepare your own children. Your family changes overnight." Kinship caregivers may greatly benefit from the cognitive coping and processing techniques that are part of TF-CBT in order to cope with their own thoughts and feelings regarding the child's trauma, often inflicted by their own family member.

ENGAGING CHILDREN
AND ADOLESCENTS IN FOSTER CARE

Foster children, having often grown up in disorganized, chaotic, and/or violent family environments, benefit a great deal (as do all children) from structure and predictability in the therapy environment. Thus, beginning and ending session in consistent ways and creating very clear session rules and end-of-session rewards can effectively encourage active session participation while also helping to reduce avoidance and noncompliance. Therapists can identify session rewards that are particularly meaningful to their clients, such as a favorite song, game, or activity (e.g., basketball). Clinicians can also encourage foster parents to praise the children for participation in therapy and to identify small rewards that can be used to incentivize participation.

COMPONENT-SPECIFIC ADDITIONS/ CONSIDERATIONS FOR TF–CBT WITH CHILDREN IN FOSTER CARE

In addition to the considerations already discussed, there are other applications, specific to children in foster care, for some of the TF–CBT components, discussed next.

Psychoeducation

Depending on the child's situation, it can be beneficial to supplement the psychoeducation provided as part of TF–CBT with psychoeducation on the foster care system. For some older children, it is important to clarify the role of child welfare workers, clinicians, and the court in terms of making decisions about their reunification or adoption as well as visits with parents and siblings. Two resources that clinicians have found helpful are *Maybe Days: A Book for Children in Foster Care* (Wilgocki & Wright, 2002), which provides general information about foster care, and *Murphy's Three Homes: A Story for Children in Foster Care* (Gilman & O'Malley, 2008), which focuses on multiple placements and related feelings and thoughts. Although not specific to foster care, another book that has been helpful for understanding and treating children's reactions to traumatic events and that was used frequently in one of the foster care studies is *A Terrible Thing Happened* (Holmes & Mudlaff, 2000).

Additionally, because many children enter foster care subsequent to neglect and abuse related to parental substance use, it can be helpful to provide some education on substance use and how and why substance use makes it challenging for parents to care for and parent children appropriately. In addition to often having been hurt by a parent through abuse and neglect, as have many children who receive TF–CBT, foster children also struggle with understanding why their parents were unable or chose not to do whatever was necessary to retain custody of them. Explaining substance use—addictive qualities (e.g., hard to resist and refuse) complicates parental ability to make appropriate decisions—can assist children in understanding and coping cognitively with why parents were, or still are, unable to meet expectations in order to gain custody (e.g., "My mom loves me, but she can't make good decisions when she is using drugs").

Some additional areas of psychoeducation with foster parents that may be important to cover include (1) the child's trauma exposure history; (2) the child's relationship and attachment to biological parents and siblings; and (3) normalizing some behaviors (e.g., normative sexual behaviors) and explaining other seemingly "odd" behaviors that result from abuse and neglect experiences (e.g., hoarding food, stealing, clinginess, low expressed need for emotional support). We have repeatedly heard from foster parents that they are unaware or have limited knowledge of the trauma history for the foster child in their home (Dorsey, Burns, et al., in press). The TF-CBT therapist can help the foster parent understand the child's experiences from their assessment of the child's trauma exposures and symptom presentations and from collaborative contacts with the child's welfare worker. This education is an important first step that continues through the narrative and processing phase so that the foster parent can understand and support the child more effectively, particularly with respect to the trauma history and related difficulties. Moreover, a greater understanding of the traumatic experiences suffered by the child in their care often helps foster parents to empathize with and respond to the child's emotional and behavioral reactions with greater consistency, sensitivity, and compassion.

Despite the fact that biological family members may have caused emotional or physical pain, most children still love their family and hope for a relationship. Some foster parents struggle to understand this, given the hurt they perceive the family has caused the child. It can often be helpful to normalize this experience—both that the child may remain attached to, and defensive of, his or her parents and their actions and that foster parents may find it hard to understand. In foster care, as in cases of divorce, it is best that the foster parents not talk negatively about the child's biological family. However, the therapist can validate the foster parents' feelings of anger and frustration, particularly when biological family members miss visits, act inappropriately in visits, or talk negatively about the foster parents. TF-CBT includes skills for emotion regulation and cognitive coping, and clinicians can encourage the foster parents to use these skills to cope with their own feelings and thoughts about the biological parents. It can also be important to provide some psychoeducation to foster parents about family visits with parents and siblings—how these visits are often important for maintaining family contact, despite some difficulties surrounding them, including family no-shows, child distress, and behavior problems before and after visits.

Parenting

Children in foster care have high rates of behavioral problems that often reach clinical levels and warrant intervention. Behavioral problems of children and adolescents are responsible for 20% of unplanned placement changes

(James, 2004; James, Landsverk, & Slymen, 2004). Behavior problems both lead to and are exacerbated by placement changes. For these reasons, when children in foster care who are receiving TF-CBT have behavioral difficulties, it is even more critical that clinicians engage foster parents and include a significant and targeted focus on parenting skills early in treatment. Focusing on parenting can address behavioral problems and, in turn, stabilize the placement. In TF-CBT, the early parenting focus is on positive parenting strategies—using praise, attention, and rewards to reinforce positive behavior or the opposite of the behavioral problem (e.g., listening when given a direction; presenting oneself to unknown adults by saying "hello" vs. jumping into their lap and hugging them immediately). Given their inconsistent or negative past parenting experiences, an initial focus on positive parenting skills is particularly important for children in foster care.

For example, one TF-CBT therapist worked with a 7-year-old boy who threw repeated temper tantrums approximately three times a day. In his first foster placement, the foster mother repeatedly questioned the boy about why he had tantrums and would give him a lot of attention when the tantrums occurred, offering candy, hugs, video games, or anything she thought might stop the tantrum. The foster mother could not be engaged in using positive parenting skills, ignoring, and offering praise for times when he stayed calm and did not throw tantrums. She eventually requested that the child be removed from her home because the behavior did not improve. The child's next foster parents were highly receptive to the clinician's suggestion of offering praise and rewards for times when he stayed calm and did not throw tantrums and ignoring him when he did throw tantrums. With a focus on positive parenting, the tantrums decreased to only three to four times per week.

Often, foster parents may not be interested in trying specific parenting strategies, having successfully raised their own children. To overcome foster parents' resistance to trying positive parenting and behavior management strategies, it is helpful to explain that, unlike children parented since birth or early adoption, children in foster care may have had inconsistent or negative parenting experiences, which may require the addition of particular tools to their existing parenting skill toolbox. We have also used the common CBT technique of asking foster parents to experiment with the positive parenting strategies, even if they are unsure whether they will be effective. In addition, it is often necessary to help foster parents understand how to apply the same behavior management strategies to behaviors related to neglect or abuse (i.e., hoarding, stealing, lying, sexualized behavior). Positive parenting strategies are also effective for behaviors that result from insecure attachments. Although there are many approaches to addressing behaviors that are consistent with insecure or disorganized attachment, the American Professional Society for the Abuse of Children recommends

CBT treatments that teach positive parenting strategies, like TF-CBT, as the frontline approach (Chaffin et al., 2006).

A resource that has been found to be particularly helpful for parenting children in foster care is *Off Road Parenting* (Pacifici, Chamberlain, & White, 2002), a book and DVD package that includes short chapters and cartoons describing basic behavior management strategies. In the video vignettes, parenting strategies are acted out, with demonstrations of the child responding positively and negatively to the various techniques and how the parent or foster parent handles each scenario. For foster parents interested in additional training in behavior management strategies, specifically for some of these challenging behaviors, the same group that published *Off Road Parenting* has developed an online program, *Foster Parent College* (*www.fosterparentcollege.com*), that offers training in addressing these particular behaviors ($10 per course). Some research (nonexperimental design) supports the effectiveness of the Foster Parent College courses in improving foster parent behavior management skills (Pacifici, Delaney, White, Nelson, & Cummings, 2006).

Parenting of children in foster care may also require additional reassurance and safety rituals, given that the children have had repeated trauma exposure and continue to live in a state of uncertainty ("Will I go home to my mom?", "What will happen in my next visit with my dad? If he even comes, he'll probably only play with my brother"). Some of the challenging behaviors exhibited by youth in foster care may be related to anxiety (e.g., bedtime refusal, school refusal), and may not only be noncompliance. Clinicians will need to work with foster parents to conduct a thorough functional analysis of problematic behaviors in order to understand the factors that trigger them. This information is critical in identifying appropriate positive behaviors (to replace the problem behaviors), behavior management skills that would support an increase in those positive replacement behaviors, and/or appropriate coping skills (e.g., relaxation, affective regulation, problem solving).

Relaxation and Affective Expression and Modulation

Given the repetitive and chronic nature of their trauma exposure, some youth in foster care may need additional time focused on learning and practicing skills in order to regulate their emotions. However, as mentioned earlier in the chapter, in a number of cases, duration of treatment was no longer than that for children living with their biological or adoptive families. Decisions to spend more time on relaxation and affective modulation should be made based on clinical assessment and on the children's ability to use skills (e.g., deep breathing, listening to music) to cope with difficult or distressing emotions or tension in session and between sessions.

It can be important also to work with both the child and the foster parent on using their skills at foster care–specific times that are distressing: for example, preparing for and coming home from visits with parents, siblings, and other family or upcoming parent court dates and placement decisions (when children are aware of them and are experiencing distress). Many foster parents report that children are emotionally distressed or that behavioral problems are exacerbated before and after visits. Clinicians can work with children and foster parents to develop a coping and transition plan that includes relaxation and affective modulation strategies, which can be used consistently to build a coping routine before and after the visit. For some children, developing a safety plan for visits is one way to reduce distress before, during, and after the visits. Cognitive coping strategies can also be beneficial as part of this plan, and are addressed in the "Cognitive Coping" section. Some children like to carry a "favorite coping strategies" card that they created to refer to when they are feeling distressed and to have with them on their visits as a reminder. TF-CBT therapists can laminate these coping cards to make them sturdy and durable.

As for any youth receiving TF-CBT, during the session it is beneficial to demonstrate that using relaxation and affective modulation strategies work, and that the child can change his or her feelings and their intensity. One activity implemented with success involves having the child write down or draw current feelings, rate their intensity, and then watch a funny video on YouTube (e.g., twin babies talking) or play a fun game for a few minutes. Following this, the child re-rates the feelings and writes or draws any new feelings. This type of activity provides an excellent springboard for demonstrating the child's efficacy in changing feelings and/or their intensity.

Case Example

A 9-year-old girl in foster care was missing her biological father, who she witness being stabbed by her mother. She had frequent nightmares about the stabbing. In conducting the affective modulation component, the first strategy the child identified that would help when she had nightmares was having her biological father sing to her, which was not possible because she was in foster care. The clinician validated and normalized this desire and then asked if there was anyone in her foster home who could sing to her. She identified her foster mom as someone who could sing her a song and, working with the foster mother, a plan was created whereby she could knock on her foster mother's door and listen to a short song when she was having nightmares. The foster mother also implemented a calming routine with the child before bedtime. After singing a gentle song, the foster mother also would give the child a hug and help her do some cognitive coping ("I am safe. My dad is OK"). After a period of time, the nightmares decreased.

Cognitive Coping

Cognitive coping is an incredibly helpful strategy for all children in learning that, although we cannot always control what happens or happened, we can control how we think about it. This often decreases children's feelings of helplessness and empowers them to feel some control over the impact of particular events or situations. For children in foster care, there are a number of important events and decisions that are often out of their control, including past traumatic experiences and inconsistent caregiving, where and with whom they live in the short term (e.g., placement changes and disruptions) and in the long term (reunification vs. long-term foster care or adoption), as well as visits with family. When parents or siblings do not show for or cancel family visits, additional distress and/or fear can result (e.g., "Something bad must have happened to my mom"; "My dad doesn't love me enough to come"). Helping children identify different ways to think about missed visits that help them feel better, blame themselves less, and worry less can be important (e.g., "My mom sometimes misses visits, and she has always been OK. She takes care of herself pretty well"; "My dad misses visits sometimes because he's drinking and forgets, but he doesn't miss them because of me").

These children can also apply cognitive coping skills to handle difficult thoughts and feelings related to their relationship with their biological parents. In one case, a 17-year-old girl was experiencing a lot of anger and was engaging in physically aggressive behavior in her foster home and at school. The clinician was working with the foster mother on behavioral management strategies, and at the same time was conducting cognitive triangle exercises (i.e., helping her to connect thoughts, feelings, and behavior) with the client to identify what was going through her mind at times when she was angry and most likely to be aggressive. The client reported that she was often thinking about her mom and how angry she was that her mom had become "addicted to drugs" after injuries from a car accident. Since the accident, her mother had not cared for her and her sister, which resulted in their placement in two different foster care homes. In the cognitive coping activity, the clinician worked with the client to identify a more helpful thought for when she would think about her mom and become angry (see Figure 2.1). This activity was immediately helpful for the client in recognizing the role her thoughts played in her aggressive behavior and her feelings of anger.

Trauma Narrative Development and Processing

One important component of TF-CBT with children in foster care is helping them identify which of the typically many traumatic events should be discussed as part of the trauma narrative (TN). For all children, the TN

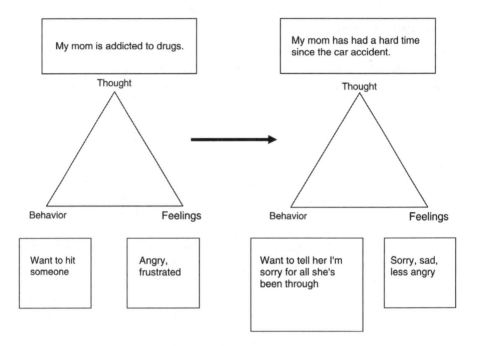

FIGURE 2.1. Cognitive triangle exercise.

can include multiple traumatic events of different types (e.g., sexual abuse, neglect, witnessing domestic violence), but it does not need to be, and should not be, entirely comprehensive (because of the time this would necessarily involve). Instead, the goal is for the children to talk about and become desensitized to some of their worst and the most distressful memories. The children should also be allowed the option of beginning the TN with a less difficult memory, and working toward the more difficult ones, so that the TN is gradual in nature.

For some children, the process of entering foster care and/or particularly troublesome placement changes may be included in the more difficult memories. For children in foster care trauma exposure is typically chronic in nature, and they often have had multiple different foster and kinship placements and sometimes disrupted reunification or failed adoption. To help children organize their experiences and decide what to include in the TN, many clinicians have found a table of contents or timeline to be a helpful strategy. Evidence suggests that individuals who have more organized and coherent trauma memories are less prone to developing PTSD.

One helpful resource that can be used earlier in psychoeducation but also may help to prepare children to develop their TN is Levy's *Finding the*

Right Spot (2004). This book is a useful tool for children who have experienced significant distress dealing with foster care or with parents who do not follow through with visitation or contact. Reading books about foster care not only helps children bring up their own thoughts and feelings about similar experiences (thereby supporting the goal of gradual exposure), but also provides a model for how they might write a book about their own experiences.

Cognitive Processing

Helping children to make meaning of and contextualize their trauma exposure is one of the most important aspects of TF-CBT, especially for those in foster care who have not yet had resolution for their experiences (e.g., as a result of trauma exposure, lack of permanent placement). Clinicians should address children's thoughts as recommended in TF-CBT and be on the lookout for thoughts related to self-worth, ability to be loved, and perspective on the future. Children in foster care often have had repeated negative experiences with caregivers and abuse or stability-related experiences (e.g., failed placements) and, therefore, are prone to developing negative beliefs about themselves. In TF-CBT, identifying negative self-beliefs and helping the children develop a more positive or less self-blame-oriented perspective about their past experiences and future is important. Unfortunately, some experiences in foster care can seem to confirm children's negative beliefs (e.g., "See? I'm not a kid people like. I told you what happened with my parents, and the last two foster families I had didn't want me for more than a few weeks"). The goal, as much as possible, is to help children avoid self-fulfilling prophecies, such as "I won't be loved" or "It doesn't matter if I try to act right or fit in. Nobody wants me around for long."

Additionally, thoughts related to beliefs about their parents' love for the child can be particularly distressing when parents have given up custody voluntarily or have repeatedly missed visits or when the children are old enough to recognize that their parents are not complying with expectations to regain custody. It may be challenging for even the clinician to find a more helpful, positive perspective. In one case, an 11-year-old boy who was sexually and physically abused and neglected by his father and then placed in foster care had difficulty making sense of why his father had given up his parental rights voluntarily and was not pursuing custody of his children. The client struggled with understanding why his father did not want to try to get custody of him and his younger brother and how he could have hurt them. During cognitive reprocessing, the therapist used logical/Socratic questioning to help the child reflect on the psychoeducation regarding neglect provided earlier in treatment (e.g., What is a parent's job? What should parents do for children? Do parents know the rules about sexual abuse and physical abuse?) and helped him think about the situation in a different way: that, by giving up custody, the father was also involved in making sure the children would be cared for by someone who, unlike himself, *would* fulfill parental expectations—feed the children, clothe them appropriately, and be home for them. This new thought (e.g., "My dad knows it's best for other adults to take care of us") helped the client focus on some of the more positive aspects of the situation, although he still, as would be expected, reported sadness about not having a dad who wanted to "do a parent's job" and keep his children at his home. The foster father was involved and in conjoint sessions was instrumental in reinforcing that this child was loved, that nothing that happened was his fault, and that the dad just did not have the ability to care for his children himself.

Conjoint Parent–Child Sessions

As with other children who receive TF-CBT, ideally a caregiver is involved in each session and is prepared to be involved in conjoint sessions, including a conjoint TN sharing session. In some cases, these conjoint TN sessions are similar to any other conjoint TN session. Ideally children share all of their TN but can choose whether or not they want to discuss certain aspects (e.g., because of a low sense of emotional closeness to the foster parent, privacy reasons). Our goal is to assess *why* the child does not want to share the TN to ensure that reasons are not related to self-blame, shame, or other unhelpful cognitions ("If my aunt hears this part, where I talk about how I went over to his house even though my mom repeatedly told me not to, she will be angry and think part of it was my fault").

In some cases, when either a caregiver has not been involved or the child does not want to share with the caregiver for appropriate reasons (e.g., the foster parent has not been emotionally supportive of the child's traumatic experiences), the clinician can help the child think creatively about someone with whom it would be appropriate to share the TN and who could offer ongoing emotional support. We have had some children share with an adult sibling, a teacher, a mentor, or a former foster parent. In all situations, the therapist took the same time as one would with a caregiver to provide psychoeducation about trauma exposure and common reactions and to allow the individual time to hear and desensitize to the TN prior to the conjoint TN sharing session.

INVOLVING BIOLOGICAL/ADOPTIVE PARENTS FROM WHOM CHILDREN HAVE BEEN REMOVED

Clinicians often ask about how and when to involve biological parents in treatment. In our experience, this varies case by case and special consideration should be given to (1) reunification plans, status, and timing (e.g., is this child going to be reunified with his/her parents and when?); (2) parent's role in the abuse (was the parent the perpetrator?); (3) abuse type (sexual abuse vs. other types); and (4) parental receipt of and response to their own treatment. In considering parental involvement, consultation with the child welfare social worker is important. When a child will reunify with parents, we often involve the parents in learning the PRAC components of TF-CBT so that they know the skills the child has learned and can reinforce these skills in the home when the child returns. We also often work with the biological parents on safety. We recommend that decisions about sharing the child's TN with the parent, even when the child wants to do so, include careful consideration of the factors just presented. In some situations, when the parent was the perpetrator or contributed to the abuse (e.g., did not monitor other adults in the home because of his or her own substance use) but has received treatment, has taken responsibility for the abuse, and developed a plan for safety in the future, the parent can be involved in conjoint sessions for the TN. Two CBT treatments are available that incorporate or build on TF-CBT skills that specifically include the physically abusive parent: alternatives for families CBT (Kolko, 1996; Kolko & Swenson, 2002) and combined parent–child CBT (Runyon, Deblinger, & Steer, 2010). If the parent was involved in perpetration but has not yet received treatment and has not taken responsibility for the abuse, sharing the TN is not advised because of concerns that the parent may reinforce child blame or deflect responsibility and may be unable to provide emotional support to the child.

In cases in which the parent has received treatment and participated in TF-CBT, children can share their TN with both their foster parents and their biological parents—the share does not have to happen only once with one caregiver. We had one client who first shared her TN with her grandmother (her kinship caregiver who participated in TF-CBT each week). Then, after two to three conjoint sessions in which the therapist met with the client's biological mother as well as her therapist, during which the mother was oriented to TF-CBT and prepared for the share, the client was also able to share her TN with her biological mother, who had been the victim of the domestic violence to which this client was exposed. The share was very effective in reestablishing the mother's ability to offer support to her daughter, but only after it was clear she could be emotionally supportive during the TN share.

CLINICAL CASE DESCRIPTION

Ten-year-old Thomas was placed in foster care for the third time after his 26-year-old biological mother was hospitalized following a violent domestic dispute with Thomas's biological father, whose whereabouts were unknown.

In his two prior foster placements, Thomas exhibited significant acting out and attempted to run away numerous times, once successfully, getting as far as 5 miles.

Because of his trauma history, suspected PTSD, and acting-out behaviors, Thomas was referred for TF-CBT at a local outpatient clinic. Thomas and his foster mother, Ms. Bell, participated in the initial assessment, which consisted of interviews, observations, and the completion of standardized measures. Although Thomas was cooperative in completing the measures, he was highly reticent to talk about any of the violence to which he was exposed, including the physical abuse by his father, which had been substantiated by the child protection agency on two occasions. He was more willing, however, to talk about the drug use by his parents that he witnessed and his negative experiences in prior foster placements, including being bullied by a foster teenager in his last home.

On the basis of the assessment, Thomas was rated in the clinical range on the Externalizing and Internalizing scales of the Child Behavior Checklist, and he met *Diagnostic and Statistical Manual of Mental Disorders* (fourth edition, text revision) criteria for oppositional defiant disorder as well as for PTSD. Thomas also reported some symptoms of depression and feelings of shame.

During the initial treatment session, Ms. Bell was provided with information from the assessment about Thomas's trauma exposure as well as his emotional and behavioral functioning. Ms. Bell was surprised to learn the extent of the violence Thomas experienced and reported that it helped her understand some of his behavioral reactions and discomfort being around her husband. She further indicated that she had not been asked to participate in therapy with her prior foster child and would be willing to do so with Thomas if it would help him. She acknowledged that she had requested that her prior foster daughter be removed from her home because she could not manage the teenager's behaviors, and she was worried that she might not be able to tolerate Thomas's behaviors much longer if something did not change. The therapist validated Ms. Bell's feelings of regret concerning her prior foster child and the challenges involved in being a foster parent, and praised her efforts on behalf of Thomas. The therapist also reviewed the proposed treatment plan, pointing out that she would be meeting with Ms. Bell each week in addition to meeting with Thomas and that there would also be conjoint sessions. The therapist explained that this approach was highly effective and would greatly assist Ms. Bell in understanding and managing Thomas's emotional and behavioral difficulties, and that they would start immediately on developing a plan to improve Thomas's behavior, particularly his refusal to listen to her directions. In addition, the therapist discussed the nature, characteristics, prevalence, and common effects of family violence on children, including the increased aggression that Thomas had been demonstrating, as well as the stressors associated with placement in foster care.

Thomas engaged readily in casual conversation with the therapist from the start and easily shared a detailed, positive narrative about a recent adventure in the park with his friends in the new neighborhood. However, when asked to share what had brought him to Ms. Bell's home, he responded with "Read my file." The therapist indicated that she could do that but preferred to hear his thoughts on why he was placed with Ms. Bell or maybe what his first day at Ms. Bell's home was like for him, just like he had told her about his adventure exploring the new neighborhood. Thomas insisted that he did not know why he was "taken from" his mom, but he briefly shared his first day with Ms. Bell, with minimal details and emotions compared with his earlier narrative. Thomas explained, "My worker picked me up and brought me to a big red house. Ms. Bell came to the door and said 'Hi.' I said nothing 'cause I was mad. Then she showed me my room and it was green—I don't like green, but I did like the car picture on the wall. Then I tried to sleep because it was late, but I couldn't for a long time." The therapist reflected back a summary of what Thomas shared, and validated his feelings, praising him for helping her understand what that day was like for him. During the sessions that followed, the therapist taught Thomas relaxation skills to help him relax in the evening before bed, a time when Thomas worried a lot about his mom. The therapist inquired about a place Thomas considered most relaxing. Using his favorite place, the beach, the therapist engaged in a guided imagery exercise incorporating ocean and beach images and sounds.

During the weekly individual sessions with Thomas and his foster mother, the therapist introduced affective expression and modulation and cognitive coping skills. It was particularly important to help Thomas expand his identified emotions beyond "mad" and "angry" to include, for example, "scared," "sad," and "ashamed." In the course of considering all the different feelings kids might have when placed in foster care or if they experience any kind of violence within their families or in their community, Thomas was able to create a long list of emotion words. When asked simply to circle any feelings he had experienced himself, after initially only circling *mad* and *angry*, he acknowledged that he had also felt sad and scared. Still, he insisted that most often he felt angry and sometimes he did not even know why. The therapist explained that she could help Thomas to understand better what might be causing him to get angry so frequently and to manage those feelings better to avoid getting in trouble. Thomas showed some interest, but reminded the therapist that he had not been in trouble for almost a week, so he had figured that out himself. This provided a starting point to help Thomas identify how he had kept himself out of trouble in the past week and led to the identification of some useful impulse-control and affect regulation skills, such as ignoring those who teased him and problem-solving alternatives to fighting, including making friends with the nicer kids who would protect him. He also insisted that he had the right to be mad about being away from his mom, and the therapist agreed and suggested that there were many ways he could express those feelings—in drawings, poems, or even by writing rap, like many celebrities have done about things in their lives that were difficult. The rap song idea appealed to Thomas, who wondered if any celebrity had ever been in foster care "because of his stupid dad."

Conjoint sessions began early in treatment in order to assist Ms. Bell with the parenting and behavior management skills she was learning. Ms. Bell complained that Thomas did not cooperate with her the way her sons did when they were young. The therapist explained that Thomas had not learned to cooperate with his parents; rather, in order to survive in his family environment he learned to be aggressive toward others, but he could unlearn these behaviors with her help. In the conjoint therapy sessions, Ms. Bell had an opportunity to practice the behavior management skills to increase Thomas's compliance, starting with sessions in which she would praise Thomas for cooperative behaviors. Thomas was also encouraged to prepare specific praise to share with Ms. Bell during conjoint sessions (e.g., he thanked for picking him up everyday after school). This ritual of ending sessions with a mutual exchange of praise became a highlight of the sessions that led to an important daily ritual that Ms. Bell insisted she would continue after therapy had ended because she enjoyed hearing praise from Thomas so much.

In parent-only sessions, the therapist and Ms. Bell role-played how to praise Thomas each time he listened or cooperated and how to minimize the attention she gave him when he talked back to her. As sessions progressed, the therapist and Ms. Bell developed a rewards plan for Thomas to reinforce his listening to her instructions the first time or with a subsequent warning. Each week, Ms. Bell practiced these skills with Thomas and reported back to the therapist about how the skills had worked or not worked, allowing modification of the behavior management plan. Ignoring Thomas's talking back was challenging for Ms. Bell, who viewed it as disrespectful. In the first week that Ms. Bell had planned to ignore the talking back, she reported to the therapist that she had not followed through with this practice, and that it was particularly challenging to ignore the disrespect—respect for adults was an important principle in her home. The therapist and Ms. Bell worked to reframe her thoughts about his talking back—that it was a way Thomas had learned to get attention, both in his previous placements and with her. Working with Ms. Bell to view the talking back through this lens (e.g., attention seeking) allowed her to feel less frustrated by Thomas's behavior and better able to use active ignoring and praise for respectful behavior. The more she ignored the talking back, the less Thomas engaged in this behavior and showed more respect.

At times, Ms. Bell reported that practicing the parenting skills, although helpful, was a lot of work. When the therapist asked about the amount of time Ms. Bell felt she had spent trying to manage Thomas's noncompliance and her former foster daughter's noncompliance, Ms. Bell reported that it had taken all of her energy. The therapist validated how challenging it can be to use the new behavior management skills consistently, but that the investment of time now should decrease the energy she would have to spend managing Thomas's noncompliance in the future.

After about six sessions and some success with using the parenting skills for managing noncompliance, Ms. Bell reported that, although Thomas seemed happier and more comfortable in her home and was listening better, he had missed several days at school in the past week, refusing to go because of headaches and stomachaches. Moreover, he insisted that his biological mom frequently allowed him to stay home from school. Ms. Bell reported that the mornings were extremely frustrating, so she sometimes lost her patience and would simply give in and send Thomas back to bed, but eventually would allow Thomas to watch TV in the family room. The therapist explored with Ms. Bell possible reasons why certain days might be particularly anxiety provoking at school, and she indicated that Thomas seemed to hate gym and complained most about going to school on those days.

Initially, the therapist did not let on with Thomas that she was aware of his avoidance of school, but simply taught Thomas about the cognitive triangle and how thoughts influence feelings and behaviors. The therapist indicated that when we wake up in the morning we often have a thought before we say anything out loud. She asked Thomas what thought popped into his head when his alarm went off in the morning. Surprisingly, seemingly caught off guard, Thomas indicated that this morning he thought, "I hate school and I feel sick. So I'm not going." The therapist validated his feelings, acknowledging that many kids hate school and inquiring what he hated most about school. Thomas immediately reported that gym was what he hated most. After asking many open-ended questions about school, Thomas eventually acknowledged that he hated gym the most because in his class the boys might see the scars on his legs and would "know I was beat by my Dad for being a bad kid." The therapist helped Thomas process his feelings and his thoughts. The therapist showed Thomas pictures from medical books of people with scars on their legs—some worse than Thomas's. She asked Thomas to guess what caused the scars. Even before guessing, Thomas seemed to understand that he had "no idea" what happened but guessed anyway and was wrong each time. Although he was still concerned that the other boys might tease him, Thomas felt better knowing that if he did not tell the children, they would likely not know how he got his scars.

During the conjoint session, the therapist and Ms. Bell acknowledged that it took a lot of courage for Thomas to go to new schools so often and to make new friends. Ms. Bell praised Thomas for his assertiveness skills, and also explained that each day that he went to school cooperatively in the morning, she would let him play video games on Mr. Bell's computer in the evening after homework.

Thomas continued to be reticent about discussing anything relating to his parents, although he seemed more than happy to talk about Mr. and Ms. Bell and his previous foster parents. When the therapist asked Thomas if he would like to read a book about kids in foster care, Thomas was interested. After reading *Maybe Days*, the therapist suggested that Thomas could write a similar book about his experiences. Thomas said that he would like to draw pictures for the book but did not like writing. When the therapist offered to type his story and create a fancy book based on his experiences, Thomas seemed cautious but willing. First, Thomas was asked to create a timeline of events he might like to include in his book in the form of chapters titles. The initial chapters included:

1. "Thomas and My Maybe Days"
2 "My First Time in Foster Care"
3 "My Second Time in Foster Care and the Teenage Bully"
4 "My Third Time in Foster Care"
5 "The End"

After some coaxing to include additional experiences that might help other kids understand why kids have to be in foster care sometimes, Thomas included a chapter about his parents using drugs and a chapter about the "scary" night before he went to Ms. Bell's house.

When the narrative was almost complete, the therapist praised Thomas for being so brave and writing about many things that were confusing and scary for kids. She explained when kids and adults talk and write about things like he did, it not only helps them but also helps to stop the secrets that keep violence in families going. She encouraged him to write one or two more chapters about anything else that happened to him that he thought he would never want to talk about before he got so brave. The therapist waited out a long silence until Thomas said he wanted to write one chapter about the beatings he got from his dad. After completing that chapter, Thomas and his therapist reread his entire book, highlighting the many accurate and important feelings he expressed while also identifying and correcting dysfunctional thoughts, including the cognitive distortion that he was placed in foster care because of his misbehavior in school. With these lessons learned in mind as well as with encouragement and guidance from his therapist, Thomas wrote his final chapter:

I am 11 years old now and I still live with Ms. Bell. I used to be mad at her and everyone all the time. I don't get mad that much anymore. When I get mad, I take a few deep breaths and say to myself "Chillax" and it works most of the time. I used to think if I could take care of my mom she would not do drugs, but now I know kids can't stop people from doing drugs—only doctors, therapists, and maybe hospitals can help my mom with this. My mom and dad had problems with drugs, anger, and violence. I don't know why they were so angry, but sometimes people don't know why, they just need help to stop fighting. When my father was angry, he hurt me and said very mean things to me—probably this was because he was on drugs, because other times he was nice. I don't see my Dad anymore because no one knows where he is. I hope he is OK, but I'm glad he can't hurt me or my mom anymore. My mom is working hard to get better and she loves me. We don't want any more violence. Ms. Bell is my mom too and I really like Mr. Bell too. I want to be a teacher and a dad like Mr. Bell. He doesn't hit, just says "1, 2, 3" and he tries to make me laugh with his funny voices. Maybe I will stay with Ms. Bell and maybe I will not, but I will always be in her heart. If you ever have to go to foster care—don't worry it won't be that bad, especially if you get the Bells.

The therapist prepared Ms. Bell for a conjoint session in which Thomas would present his narrative by sharing sections of Thomas's narrative with her as he was developing it. This sharing enhanced Ms. Bell's compassion for Thomas's circumstances and experiences that were markedly different from her own children's. She reported that this helped her to have greater patience and willingness to persevere with Thomas. This seemed to be particularly important when Thomas's behavior problems worsened temporarily because of an extinction burst when Ms. Bell was beginning to implement behavior management (i.e., praise and active ignoring) and Thomas was really testing the limits in the Bell home. Toward the end of treatment, Thomas spontaneously asked if he could share his entire narrative with his foster mom, and Ms. Bell seemed very well prepared emotionally and pleased that Thomas was excited to share it with her. In preparing for this conjoint session, the therapist encouraged Ms. Bell to practice her active listening and praise skills in a role play during an individual parent session in which the therapist played the role of Thomas reading the narrative. The therapist also explained that Thomas had some questions that he wanted to ask her after sharing his narrative, including, "Do you think my dad wouldn't have hit me so much if I had listened better?"; "Will I always get to stay with you if I want to?"; "Do you think my dad thinks about me sometimes?" With the help of the therapist, Ms. Bell carefully prepared answers to these questions that were honest but also therapeutic for Thomas. Finally, during this session, the therapist encouraged Thomas and his foster mom to think about how they would like to celebrate their therapy graduation.

Ms. Bell expressed that she was pleased that they did not have to continue in therapy endlessly, but would really miss the support and guidance she had been receiving and hoped she could call from time to time or drop in. The therapist encouraged her to call not only for an occasional booster session but also with good news about Thomas's progress as well. This seemed to relieve Ms. Bell's anxiety about termination and allowed her to look forward to and plan an elaborate (i.e., graduation cap, balloons, music, and special "Bell classic" double chocolate cake) graduation celebration with greater enthusiasm.

CONCLUSION

As noted earlier, children placed in foster care have high rates of trauma exposures and related emotional and behavioral difficulties (Kolko et al., 2010; Pecora et al., 2003). The escalation of such difficulties often leads to placement disruptions that are highly predictive of additional adjustment problems in adolescence and adulthood. Thus, it is imperative that foster children receive mental health services that are efficient and effective in addressing their unique and individualized needs. This chapter describes the implementation of TF-CBT, which has been demonstrated to be effective with this population, with special attention to their unique concerns and circumstances. In addition, methods for enhancing the active engagement of foster parents in treatment are highlighted, along with suggestions and factors to consider concerning the involvement of biological/adoptive parents from whom children were removed. TF-CBT has shown great promise in serving the needs of foster children; however, much still needs to be learned through collaborative clinical and research efforts to ensure that we are optimally caring for the comprehensive needs of these children.

REFERENCES

Bakermans-Kranenburg, M. J., van IJzendoorn, M. H., & Juffer, F. (2003). Less is more: Meta-analysis of sensitivity and attachment interventions in early childhood. *Psychological Bulletin, 129,* 195–215.
Chaffin, M., Hanson, R., Saunders, B., Nicols, T., Barnett, D., Zeanah, C., et al. (2006). Report of the APSAC/APA Division 37 Task Force on attachment therapy, reactive attachment disorder and attachment problems. *Child Maltreatment, 11,* 76–98.
Dorsey, S., Burns, B. J., Southerland, D., Cox, J. R., Wagner, R., & Farmer, E. M. Z. (in press). Prior trauma exposure for youth in treatment foster care. *Journal of Child and Family Studies.*
Dorsey, S., Cox, J. R., Conover, K. A., & Berliner, L. (2011, Summer). Trauma-

focused cognitive behavioral therapy for children and adolescents in foster care. *CYF News.*

Dorsey, S., Farmer, E. M. Z., Barth, R. P., Greene, K. M., Reid, J., & Landsverk, J. (2008). Current status and evidence base of training for foster and treatment foster parents. *Children and Youth Services Review, 30,* 1403–1416.

Dorsey, S., Kerns, S. E., Trupin, E., Conover, K. A., & Berliner, L. (in press). Child welfare workers as service brokers for youth in foster care: Findings from Project Focus. *Child Maltreatment.*

Gilman, J. L., & O'Malley, K. (2008). *Murphy's three homes: A story for children in foster care.* Washington, DC: American Psychological Association.

Holmes, M. M., & Mudlaff, S. J. (2000). *A terrible thing happened: A story for children who have witnessed violence or trauma.* Washington, DC: Magination Press.

Huey, S. J., Jr., & Polo, A. J. (2008). Evidence-based psychosocial treatments for ethnic minority youth. *Journal of Clinical Child and Adolescent Psychology, 37,* 262–301.

James, S. (2004). Why do foster care placements disrupt? An investigation of reasons for placement change in foster care. *Social Service Review, 78*(4), 601–627.

James, S., Landsverk, J., & Slymen, D. J. (2004). Placement movement in out-of-home care: Patterns and predictors. *Children and Youth Services Review, 26*(2), 185–206.

Kolko, D. (1996). Individual cognitive behavioral treatment and family therapy for physically abused children and their offending parents: A comparison of clinical outcomes. *Child Maltreatment, 1*(4), 322–342.

Kolko, D. J., & Swenson, C. C. (2002). *Assessing and treating physically abused children and their families: A cognitive behavioral approach.* Thousand Oaks, CA: Sage.

Kolko, D. J., Hurlburt, M. S., Zhang, J., Barth, R. P., Leslie, L. K., & Burns, B. J. (2010). Posttraumatic stress symptoms in children and adolescents referred for child welfare investigation: A national sample of in-home and out-of-home care. *Child Maltreatment, 15,* 48–62.

Levy, J. (2004). *Finding the right spot: When kids can't live with their parents.* Washington, DC: Magination Press.

Lyons, J. S., Weiner, D. A., & Schneider, A. (2006). *A field trial of three evidence-based practices for trauma with children in state custody* (Report to the Illinois Department of Children and Family Services) Evanston, IL: Mental Health Resources Services and Policy Program, Northwestern University.

McKay, M. M., & Bannon, W. M., Jr. (2004). Engaging families in child mental health services. *Child and Adolescent Psychiatric Clinics of North America, 13*(4), 905–921.

McKay, M. M., Pennington, J., Lynn, C. J., & McCadam, K. (2001). Understanding urban child mental health service use: Two studies of child, family, and environmental correlates. *Journal of Behavioral Health Services and Research, 28*(4), 475–483.

McKay, M., Stoewe, J., McCadam, K., & Gonzales, J. (1998). Increasing access to child mental health services for urban children and their care givers. *Health and Social Work, 23,* 9–15.

Pacifici, C., Chamberlain, P., & White, L. (2002). *Off road parenting: Practical solutions for difficult behavior.* Eugene, OR: Northwest Media.

Pacifici, C., Delaney, R., White, L., Nelson, C., & Cummings, K. (2006).Web-based training for foster, adoptive, and kinship parents. *Children and Youth Services Review, 28,* 1329?1343.

Pecora, P. J., Williams, J., Kessler, R. C., Downs, A. C., O'Brien, K., & Hiripi, E. (2003). *Assessing the effects of foster care: Early results from the Casey National Alumni Study.* Seattle, WA: Casey Family Programs.

Runyon, M. K., Deblinger, D., & Steer, R. (2010). Comparison of combined parent-child and parent-only cognitive-behavioral treatments for offending parents and children in cases of child physical abuse. *Child and Family Behavior Therapy, 32,* 196–218.

Weiner, D. A., Schneider, A., & Lyons, J. S. (2009). Evidence-based treatments for trauma among culturally diverse foster care youth: Treatment retention and outcomes. *Children and Youth Services Review, 31,* 1199–1205.

Wilgocki, J., & Wright, M. K. (2002). *Maybe days: A book for children in foster care.* Washington, DC: Magination Press.

3

Residential Treatment

Judith A. Cohen
Anthony P. Mannarino
Daniela Navarro

UNIQUE FEATURES OF RESIDENTIAL TREATMENT THAT REQUIRE TF-CBT APPLICATIONS

More than 100,000 children[1] in the United States currently receive mental health treatment in residential settings. These children ("residents") typically spend from 4 months to 2 years in residential treatment facilities (RTF). This chapter focuses on trauma-focused cognitive-behavioral therapy (TF-CBT) applications in RTF, but these applications may also apply to children receiving treatment in group homes or long-term inpatient treatment programs.

Two distinguishing features of RTF require unique TF-CBT applications: (1) The primary reason for RTF placement is to address severe externalizing behavior problems; and (2) RTF direct care milieu staff members are responsible for managing children's problems in the RTF milieu setting.

RTF settings exist for children with serious externalizing behavior problems that have not responded to interventions in less restrictive settings. Although RTF programs are increasingly recognizing that trauma contributes to these problems, trauma-focused treatment will likely only be viewed positively in RTF to the extent that it contributes to behavioral

---

[1] Many RTF only serve older youth. Please note that throughout this chapter the terms "child" or "children" is used to refer to both children and adolescents.

improvement, shorter length of stay, or other RTF-relevant outcomes. Thus, TF-CBT treatment must not only resolve trauma symptoms but contribute to resolution of the behavioral problems for which the child was sent to RTF. Therapists should clarify for residents, RTF staff, administrators, and parents how TF-CBT treatment will contribute to residents' behavioral regulation.

Parental involvement is highly variable for children in RTF. Some have intact, supportive families and their parents participate regularly in RTF treatment. More often, chaotic family living situations and maladaptive or abusive parenting contributed to the children's need for RTF care. Family disruptions also occur during RTF stays, including termination of parental rights; parents relocating out of state; caregiver relationships ending, with the child losing a long-standing relationship with the parent's significant other; or foster parents terminating fostering during RTF treatment. Any of these events may escalate children's behavioral problems in the milieu. Since direct milieu staff members' task is to manage children's problems in the RTF milieu, these workers must understand how trauma impacts children in RTF settings, how to minimize trauma reenactment in the milieu, and how to optimally support TF-CBT implementation. In this chapter, we focus specifically on direct milieu staff, but similar considerations apply to other RTF staff members (e.g., teachers) who have regular interactions with children in the RTF milieu.

Trauma Reenactment

Trauma reenactment frequently occurs in RTF settings. Trauma-informed care and TF-CBT aim to prevent trauma reenactment. Trauma reminders or triggers (cues that remind a child of one or more past traumatic experiences and then re-create negative aspects of the child's emotional, behavioral, or physical responses to the original trauma) are numerous in the RTF setting. For example, other children fighting or crying, a parent calling or failing to call, or a staff member redirecting a child in a loud voice may serve as trauma reminders. Because many children in the RTF milieu have trauma histories, multiple children may be "triggered" simultaneously and lead to one or more traumatized child losing behavioral and/or emotional control. When staff members acknowledge and validate how upset the child is and encourage him or her to use TF-CBT coping skills, the child is more likely to gain affective and behavioral regulation. However, when staff members intervene in a manner that the child perceives as a further trauma reminder (e.g., use a loud tone of voice or an intrusive or forceful physical manner), this will likely escalate rather than deescalate the child's trauma-related behavior. This response from staff members may trigger other children in the milieu, potentially leading to poor affective and/or behavioral regulation among several residents or an out-of-control situation in the milieu. The following clinical example illustrates a scenario in which direct milieu staff members failed to recognize trauma reenactment, with negative consequences for the milieu. Information sheets for direct milieu staff about how to support implementation of TF-CBT skills in the RTF milieu are included as appendices at the end of this chapter.

CASE EXAMPLE

Jared's mother didn't call when she promised him she would. Jared got increasingly angry as it became clear that she would not call. He kicked over a chair, yelling, "I hate my f---ing mother." A staff member yelled, "Jared! No swearing here! Now pick up that chair!" Two residents said, "Hey, he can be pissed off" and "You don't know what it's like," respectively. The staff member who had yelled and one other approached the boys, and the staff member who had yelled at Jared said in a loud, threatening manner, "You all just lost your levels." Jared picked up the chair and threw it at the staff member. The two staff members then put Jared into a therapeutic hold. Two other residents who were watching the scene became angry and tried to pull the staff members off of Jared, leading to them also being placed in holds. Three additional residents then tried to defend those who were being held down. Five residents and Jared were restrained during this incident. The staff members present recalled this incident as "bad kids acting badly" while all of the residents said that the staff members "disrespected us" and "didn't care how we felt." Jared later told his therapist that when the incident started he was thinking about all the times his mother had abused him and let him down. Not calling was "just one more time she screwed with me." Recognizing trauma impact and how to implement TF-CBT coping skills may have prevented this scenario from getting out of control.

Direct care staff members are often young, have had little or no professional education about child psychopathology, and have little prior experience working with troubled children. These individuals receive annual mandated training in techniques for conflict resolution and management of problem behaviors, but because they are often spat on, called names, and kicked and/or punched by residents, they may take this personally, viewing themselves as victims of abuse by the children in the RTF rather than seeing these children as reenacting trauma that they themselves have experienced. In the absence of a trauma-informed understanding of trauma triggers, traumatic reenactment, and specific behavioral training and early-intervention practice, direct milieu staff members often experience negative emotions toward residents. To their credit, RTF programs are increasingly seeking trauma-informed care training for staff. One example is the Sanctuary model (*www.sanctuaryweb.com*), an organizational approach to providing care for traumatized individuals. Using a trauma-informed care model such as Sanctuary in conjunction with TF-CBT likely provides an ideal approach for traumatized children in RTF settings.

UNIQUE TF–CBT ASSESSMENT STRATEGIES IN RTF

Many RTF programs now include questions about trauma exposure and trauma symptoms as part of their formal initial evaluation. However, this is not universally the case. RTF programs are required to conduct and document intake assessments in order to receive reimbursement and to meet a variety of regulations (e.g., state, county, child welfare, juvenile justice). In some cases, the assessment may be conducted by a psychiatrist or psychologist instead of the therapist, and for a variety of reasons the RTF assessment protocol may not include a formal assessment of trauma exposure or symptoms. In this case, the first challenge may be how to incorporate information about trauma exposure and symptoms into the assessment and treatment plan. In our experience, most RTF programs want to consider this information but do not have a mechanism to include it in the formal assessment protocol as a result of lack of resources. In these situations, the therapist can clinically interview the child and, if feasible, the parent or caregiver and administer the UCLA PTSD Reaction Index (RI), a freely available instrument, to assess the child's history of trauma exposure and trauma symptoms and determine whether the child has experienced trauma and whether this is a relevant focus of treatment. This information can then be incorporated with the initial evaluation at subsequent team meetings in order to update the diagnosis and treatment plan. A therapist who can conduct a trauma-informed assessment and provide TF-CBT integrated with other appropriate treatment as agreed upon by the treatment team will be a valuable addition to any RTF program.

Case Example

Merle was a 13-year-old admitted to RTF for participating in gang-related violence. She denied drug or alcohol use and urine toxicology screens were negative. Soon after admission, Merle was seen by staff apparently responding to auditory hallucinations. She initially refused to divulge the content of these voices, but eventually stated that they were coming from around the unit and the TV, and the voices kept saying that she was bad and should kill herself. She was isolative on the milieu and talked to herself. Merle slept less than 2 hours each night, and when peers approached her she became violent. Her initial diagnosis was schizophrenia, R/O atypical bipolar disorder, and Merle was started on antipsychotic medication. When conducting a thorough trauma assessment, her therapist found that Merle had a long history of domestic and community violence, had been sexually abused by her stepfather from 3 to 10 years of age, and had more recently experienced a series of gang-related rapes. As the therapist spoke more with Merle about these experiences, it became clear that Merle was intimidated by the older males on the unit, who reminded her of the perpetrators of the recent gang rapes. Merle said that she couldn't sleep because she had recurrent fears of being raped in the RTF. The therapist asked whether the voices started before or after these rapes. Merle said, "The voices are they all who did this to me telling me I'm no good. It's me saying I deserved what they all did to me (i.e., to be raped) so I should just kill myself and leave this life." After more questioning, the therapist clarified that the "voices" were dissociative and reexperiencing phenomena rather than psychotic symptoms. The therapist explained these symptoms to Merle and changed the diagnosis to PTSD and major depression. The antipsychotic medication was discontinued and TF-CBT was started, initially focusing on enhancing Merle's feeling of safety in the RTF setting.

The most significant challenge in assessing trauma impact in RTF settings is often determining whether or not children's severe behavior problems are related to past traumatic experiences. Often, children in RTF have long histories of multiple traumas and losses—such as placements in and out of multiple foster homes; chronic experiences of physical, sexual, or emotional abuse; and/or domestic violence—and when a thorough trauma assessment is performed, these children and/or their caregivers endorse multiple trauma symptoms. The therapist is often able to discern connections between the children's behavioral problems and the past traumas they experienced (e.g., sexual offending in a youth who experienced sexual abuse; physical assaultive behavior in a youth who experienced physical abuse or witnessed domestic violence), or that the behaviors are sometimes prompted by traumatic reminders (e.g., the youth started a fight when called the same name that his abusive father used to call him). These connections can be formulated as trauma reenactment (American Psychiatric Association, 2000, p. 468), and justify the use of TF-CBT for the youth's severe behavioral problems.

Case Example

Carl was a 14-year-old admitted to RTF for gang activity. His gang behavior included violence in school and toward multiple foster parents, bullying at school, and property destruction. Carl had a long history of witnessing extreme domestic violence, including the murder of his mother by his father, and having been bullied by his father and older brothers and at school. His father regularly and severely beat his mother and was rumored to have killed a man. Carl's older brothers were extremely emotionally and possibly physically abusive to Carl; the father encouraged this behavior, calling Carl a "sissy" and a "mamma's boy." When Carl was 9 years old, his mother and he ran away. The father came after them and shot the mother dead in front of Carl. The father was jailed, and Carl's oldest brother, because he was an adult, was given custody of Carl, and the abuse continued. At 11 years of age, Carl joined a gang "to protect me from my brothers." He ran away again at age 12 and was placed in a series of foster homes but was forced to visit with his brother. During the trauma assessment, Carl scored 14 (low) on the RI, but the therapist observed that Carl was extremely avoidant about talking about trauma experiences or symptoms during the clinical interview and she believed that Carl was minimizing these symptoms. The therapist began TF–CBT and after three sessions repeated the RI. At that time his score on the RI was 45 and he acknowledged severe physical abuse by his brothers.

While recognition of the central role of trauma reenactment in severely traumatized youth is crucial, it is also important that therapists not automatically attribute all behavior problems to trauma. Some youth only experienced trauma in the distant past and do not have any apparent trauma symptoms other than severe behavior problems, and there is no apparent connection between the current behavior problems and the past trauma. Unless more information becomes available to suggest trauma etiology, therapists should not assume that current behavior problems are related to or will be resolved by engaging in trauma narrative and processing work.

CASE EXAMPLE

Tom, a 16-year-old living with his single mother and two younger brothers, was admitted to RTF specializing in sexual offending after he raped his neighbor. He had also raped several other girls (acquaintances), but because of his gang activity, they had been afraid to report this. Tom was also displaying threatening behavior toward his mother. He had a history of trauma—being in a car accident as a young child and having witnessed community violence. His score on the RI was 13, but his primary trauma symptoms were irritability, gang-related hypervigilance, and angry outbursts. The therapist did not believe TF–CBT was appropriate.

UNIQUE TF–CBT ENGAGEMENT
STRATEGIES IN RTF

Engaging the family in TF–CBT while the child is in RTF may require unique strategies for several reasons. The child's severe behavioral problems may have exhausted the parents, leading them to feel both relieved and guilty about agreeing to residential placement for the child. The family may not understand why trauma should be a treatment focus for severe behaviors; if the family is chaotic or a parent experienced and/or perpetrated multigenerational trauma, the parent may feel blamed or defensive about the idea of trauma-focused treatment (e.g., "I went through this when I was a kid and I never acted up like this"). The RTF may be far from the child's home, making it difficult for the family to participate in therapy in person. Engagement strategies for these situations are described shortly.

Experiencing a child's severe behavior problems or having to place a child in a residential setting brings parents heartache and feelings of failure as parents. Therapists must first communicate that they do not negatively judge the parents based on the child's negative behaviors or the family's history. Providing TF-CBT is based on the premise that past traumatic experiences provide at least a partial explanation for the child's problematic behaviors. This "no shame and no blame" approach can be helpful for parents who feel that they have been ineffective or "bad" parents in not being able to control the child's problematic behaviors.

It is important to validate and acknowledge that the child's behavior has caused the parents significant distress. By relieving the parents' immediate burden of managing these behaviors, RTF admission may contribute to parental engagement over time. Psychoeducation about trauma impact may diminish child blame. Using the analogy of service members with violent outbursts after returning from the war in Iraq may be helpful to explain the behavioral impact of PTSD to parents who have never heard of this trauma manifestation. Pointing out that PTSD is both a response to trauma and a brain disorder (i.e., trauma causes biological changes that maintain behavioral and emotional changes) may help parents to better understand their child's behaviors. For the parent with a personal trauma history who says "I didn't act up this way," it may be helpful to first validate his or her resilience, drawing the parallel to the fact that most service members do not develop PTSD. The therapist can then point out ways in which children respond differently to benign experiences such as starting kindergarten (i.e., some do well, others have problems).

TF-CBT has been provided via phone to parents that live too far away to attend sessions regularly. In addition, newer technology is making it easier for RTF programs to engage parents long-distance. For example, Skype and similar free downloadable programs allow any family with a home computer to access the RTF therapist at the appointed therapy hour. Therapists can now schedule sessions remotely via computer with parents and conduct TF-CBT parent sessions in which the therapists can "see" the parent and during conjoint sessions the parent and child can "see" each other. Although not exactly the same experience as face-to-face therapy, for families who wish to participate in their children's TF-CBT treatment, this is a feasible alternative, and many families are happy to have choices through which to learn parenting and other skills during the therapy hour.

UNIQUE TF-CBT APPLICATIONS IN RTF

Unique considerations for applying TF-CBT in RTF settings include when to begin TF-CBT; how to combine TF-CBT with other RTF treatment modalities; how to include RTF direct care staff in TF-CBT; and how to optimally apply TF-CBT for children and youth in RTF settings.

When to Start TF-CBT

TF-CBT is typically started in RTF only after (1) the child has been integrated into and adjusted to the RTF setting (e.g., the child understands the milieu's level system and other basic rules); (2) the therapist or another clinician has completed the assessment and ascertained that trauma is relevant to treatment; and (3) stabilization of acute psychosis, suicidality, self-injury, or other acute conditions has occurred. In a very short-term RTF program (e.g., 4 months), there is often insufficient time to completely stabilize the child before starting TF-CBT. In this situation, the pacing of integration, assessment, and stabilization occurs much faster than in longer term RTF settings. Such programs can be extremely successful at providing TF-CBT if trauma treatment is well integrated into the structure of the program and a concerted effort is made to involve family members in treatment. For example, a 4-month RTF program for severely multiply traumatized Latino teens with comorbid substance abuse disorders in Laredo, Texas, has successfully implemented TF-CBT with more than 50 youth, who demonstrated significant improvement in trauma and substance abuse problems.

Integrating TF-CBT with Other RTF Treatment Modalities

Multiple mental health interventions are provided in RTF. Optimal methods and timing for integrating TF-CBT with existing RTF interventions are now being examined and developed. For example, one method for integrating TF-CBT into the RTF milieu or level program (developed and pilot tested in collaboration with RTF milieu staff and therapists) is through the use of TF-CBT coping cards (Figure 3.1). Staff members receive education about TF-CBT skills and how to support their implementation prior to using these cards. The therapist completes the coping card with children as they learn and practice new TF-CBT skills in treatment, and instructs children to carry the card with them wherever they are in the RTF. When a child shows signs

Name: _____

Relaxation skills (date learned):

Feeling management skills (date learned):

Behavior management skills (date learned):

Thought management skills (date learned):

FIGURE 3.1. TF-CBT coping card.

of regulation problems, any staff member asks the child for his or her coping card, identifies a TF-CBT coping skill the child is currently using, and encourages the child to use one or more skill. The child then earns points in the level system for successfully implementing any skill on the card to regain regulation. (The child loses points for not having the card with him or her.) This is also a good method by which to emphasize in an ongoing manner to residents, staff, parents, and other stakeholders the connection between implementing TF-CBT and improving children's behavioral problems.

Many RTF programs that are implementing TF-CBT already use a group trauma format. A typical approach is to delay starting TF-CBT until youth complete the trauma group. This decision is based on the premise that providing both individual and group trauma-focused treatment concurrently is likely to be redundant and also on concerns that youth may become overwhelmed by talking so much about trauma issues. These RTF programs do not provide evidence-based group trauma treatments but rather a variety of different untested approaches, and in our experience youth often continue to have high levels of trauma symptoms after the end of trauma groups, suggesting that starting with individual TF-CBT may be a more effective approach. However, to date RTF programs have not been amenable to starting with individual TF-CBT except for individual residents who missed the starting date for group or were deemed inappropriate to join the group.

In contrast, many other RTF interventions are effectively provided concurrently with TF-CBT. For example, many programs provide targeted treatment for juvenile sexual offenders who also have significant trauma symptoms, and some are implementing TF-CBT concurrently with treatment for offending behaviors. Therapists in these programs report that providing TF-CBT in conjunction with treatment that addresses the sexual offending behavior is optimal for these youth because it helps them to understand and feel understood regarding the connection between their personal traumatic experiences and their subsequent offending.

CASE EXAMPLE

John was a 14-year-old adjudicated to RTF as a result of sexual assault of a 13-year-old cousin during a weekend visit with his aunt and uncle. This was his first sexual offense. During the initial assessment, John acknowledged domestic violence and "other" traumas but would not disclose what these were. His RI score was 58, in the very severe range. He eventually disclosed severe chronic sexual abuse by his father and older brothers. His mother witnessed this on many occasions but never intervened. John received TF-CBT in conjunction with treatment for sexual offending. During the trauma narrative, he said, "The worst part of all was that my mother let my dad and brothers do that to me and she never lifted a finger to help me. That made me into nothing. I don't know why no one ever loved me in that house." Through this concurrent treatment, John was able to understand his own abuse, feel compassion from his therapist and other staff for these painful experiences, and also understand the process through which he abused his cousin and take responsibility for this abuse. This allowed him to make the connection between his own pain as a victim and what his cousin must have felt. He wrote a letter to his aunt, uncle, and cousin telling them about his previous abuse and asking them if they could ever understand and if there was a way he could somehow make amends.

Including Direct Care Staff in TF–CBT When Parents Are Not Involved

Although TF-CBT significantly improves symptoms when provided only to the children (Deblinger, Lippmann, & Steer, 1996; Weiner, Schneider, & Lyons, 2009), additional benefits are derived when a caring adult participates in TF-CBT with them. For example, including parents in TF-CBT significantly improves children's depression and behavior problems (Deblinger et al., 1996), and increased parental support is a strong predictor of children's trauma-related symptoms (Cohen & Mannarino, 1996, 2000). Despite efforts to engage parents, about half of the children in RTF do not have ongoing parental involvement in treatment. For these children, including direct care staff in TF-CBT treatment may be beneficial if both parties are agreeable. In situations where there is no parent participating in treatment, the therapist can ask the child whether he or she would like to ask a specific milieu staff member to participate. Usually, but not always, in RTF programs in which each child is assigned a primary milieu staff member, the child will select this individual to participate in treatment. The therapist should explain the guidelines for participation to the staff member and the child. Specifically, the child and staff member must agree that the worker will not break confidences shared during therapy and will still enforce the rules in the RTF fairly and impartially. During treatment sessions with the direct care staff member, the therapist works in a somewhat parallel manner as with a parent (i.e., identify the child's trauma triggers and plan how the staff worker might implement TF-CBT skills in the RTF). Direct care staff may need extra preparation and support for hearing children's trauma narratives before participating in conjoint sessions because they may not have previously heard these in such detail. However, many direct care staff report a new level of understanding and compassion for RTF patients after participating in TF-CBT treatment.

CASE EXAMPLE

Eleven-year-old Michael was admitted for violent acts (bullying, property damage, theft) at school. His foster parents gave notice that they were terminating foster care shortly after he came to RTF. He had experienced early exposure to domestic violence, severe neglect, physical abuse, and parental substance abuse prior to going to live with his great-grandmother at age 6. She became his legal guardian and adopted him the following year but 2 years later became too ill to care for him. Michael entered a series of foster homes, where he experienced violence and school bullying. His great-grandmother died 2 months ago, prompting serious behavior problems. During the trauma assessment, he identified this death as his worst trauma. He scored in the moderate range (37) on the RI but his therapist believed he was minimizing some symptoms. Since no caregivers were available to participate and loss was a significant issue for Michael, the therapist asked him if he would like one of the direct care staff members to participate in treatment with him. Michael chose his primary direct care staff member, Joanne, a woman who, like him, was African American. Joanne was a little nervous but very pleased that Michael wanted her to do this. During the first session with the therapist, she expressed the concern that Michael had asked her to participate so that he could "play" her in the RTF. As Joanne gained increasing insight about Michael's trauma history and triggers and how to use the TF-CBT skills to help him manage these, she looked back on that comment ruefully, saying, "I can't believe how little I understood him." Over time Joanne came up with her own ideas about how to help Michael in the RTF. For example, she became particularly adept at recognizing early signs that he was being triggered by other kids or situations and developing inventive techniques to distract him before he lost control. For example, she would sing his favorite rap songs to get his attention and then change the words (e.g., to "use your skills, baby, start to breathe"). This usually made Michael laugh. Joanne was shocked at hearing Michael's early experiences when the therapist read the trauma narrative to her. At first she didn't think she could do a conjoint session because she was "too angry at his parents to even be civil." She also told the therapist that it triggered her own issues of loss (her aunt had cancer and was dying). However, she insisted that "if that little boy lived through all this, I can listen to it." Joanne also talked to other staff members about how to recognize when Michael was having trauma reminders and how to help him settle himself down. This, in turn, helped Michael feel more supported and safe on the milieu. At the end of therapy, Michael thanked Joanne for being there for him, telling her she reminded him of his grandma (great-grandmother) because he knew "you're always here for me." Joanne said that doing TF-CBT with Michael "helped me understand what these kids have been through, and how to help them better."

TF-CBT for Youth with Extreme Family Trauma

Many children in RTF have experienced long histories of extreme family trauma, which contributes to serious impairments in establishing trust, safety, and/or attachments. RTF staff members frequently express the belief that because of their long experience with betrayal from adults such children will not be ready to directly address traumatic experiences until they have spent considerable time establishing trust with the RTF staff. However, there is no evidence to suggest that talking about traumatic experiences impedes the development of trust. To the contrary, Sanctuary's research (*www.sanctuaryweb.com*) documents that a trauma-informed RTF environment where discussion about trauma is actively encouraged *enhances* the development of trust and a sense of safety among children and staff. It stands to reason that children whose traumas have included extreme invalidation would benefit from direct acknowledgment that their experiences occurred and that their thoughts and feelings have a reality basis. This suggests that introducing TF-CBT early in RTF treatment for such children may be helpful. Because these children are also extremely reactive to trauma reminders, and even talking about what these reminders are may trigger extreme responses, therapists may find it very helpful to decrease these children's hyperarousal by changing the order in which they introduce TF-CBT components. For example, introducing and helping children master relaxation (without gradual exposure at first) before introducing psychoeducation may be very helpful for some children. Once children have mastered relaxation and possibly affective regulation skills without gradual exposure and are able to "turn down the volume" of their anxiety, they may be better able to tolerate discussion of trauma topics. Therapists can then revisit these skills components with the addition of gradual exposure.

Case Example

Jane spent the first 5 years of her life locked in an attic closet by her mother. When Jane's mother was out of the house, her boyfriend would come to the closet with a knife and sexually abuse Jane, telling her that if she made a sound he would kill her. When she cried, her mother would burn Jane with a hot iron. When she was discovered, at 5 years of age, Jane weighed 20 pounds and was covered in feces. She was placed in foster care, where she had severe aggression but was relatively stable for 2 years until her foster mother died of a heart attack. In her next foster placement, Jane was extremely aggressive and was physically abused by the foster mother in an attempt to get her to listen. Jane was then placed in a series of foster homes where sexual and physical abuse occurred. At 11 years of age, her behavior was out of control, leading to RTF placement. On admission, Jane endorsed physical abuse and said the worst thing that happened was her foster mother dying. She scored 71 on the RI (in the very severe range). The therapist and many staff members doubted that TF-CBT was appropriate since "her whole life has been trauma." Jane was aggressive and isolative on the milieu. After a month of nondirective therapy, the therapist found that Jane liked coming to therapy and decided to try some relaxation to address Jane's agitation and aggression. Jane was able to use relaxation during the therapy sessions, but she would not look at the therapist for more than several seconds before lowering her gaze. The therapist worked with Jane's primary milieu staff, Carlos, who also tried hard to engage Jane in milieu activities and encouraged her to use relaxation strategies on the milieu. Carlos was a muscular man whom all the residents looked up to. He dedicated himself to engaging Jane. Despite her aggression and persistent isolation, Carlos believed Jane was trying to use the relaxation strategies. The therapist noticed after two to three sessions of using relaxation that Jane seemed to be a bit more engaged in therapy. She decided to start TF-CBT at that point but to do so slowly. The therapist asked Jane whether she would like to include one of the direct milieu staff in therapy, and Jane chose Carlos. The therapist, Jane, and Carlos agreed that Carlos would participate in Jane's therapy in this way: Jane would decide what she wanted to share with Carlos, and the therapist and Jane would then meet with Carlos. If Jane gave permission, the therapist could also meet alone with Carlos to talk about what Jane was doing in therapy. The therapist started psychoeducation by introducing the What Do You Know? game, using only some of the safety cards and providing Jane with a piece of candy whenever she answered a question. Jane and the therapist talked about safety, and Jane said that she did not feel safe before coming to RTF. The therapist said, "It's hard to feel safe when the grownups who are supposed to take care of you don't keep you safe or even hurt you. But you are safe here." Jane became very anxious at this point but with the therapist's guidance was able to soothe herself using her relaxation skills. Jane then picked up one of the safety cards about "not OK" touches. Jane said, "I know all about that." When asked by the therapist what she meant, Jane said, "First Leroy (the mother's boyfriend) hurt me, then my mom burned me. They took turns." Jane briefly described the sexual abuse by her mother's boyfriend and her mother's physical abuse. The therapist told Jane how brave she was to talk about this and reassured her that she was safe in the RTF. The therapist was ready to end the session when Jane asked, "Aren't we going to tell Carlos?" The therapist followed up, asking Jane what she wanted to tell Carlos. Jane said that she wanted to tell Carlos about the abuse she had just disclosed to the therapist. After listening to Jane's disclosure, Carlos told her how brave she was and that he was really proud of her for sharing this. He also told her that he and the other staff would keep her safe in the RTF. Jane continued to make slow but steady progress in TF-CBT, including eventually creating a detailed trauma narrative of her early trauma experiences and sharing this with Carlos. However, Jane was not able to tolerate placement in a foster home (presumably because of her early extreme traumatic experiences in nuclear family settings) and was eventually placed in a long-term group home setting, where she did very well.

Unpredictable Discharges

In RTF discharges may occur unpredictably based on child protection, family, and/or insurance decisions, leading to poor or no discharge planning. Specific to TF-CBT, the therapist may have no opportunity to end treatment in an optimal fashion or to arrange for treatment transfer. If the child is in the middle of the trauma narrative, this would be the least optimal circumstance for ending treatment, and in such cases the therapist should try to have one to two final sessions in order to bring TF-CBT treatment to some sort of closure before the child leaves the RTF program. If this is not feasible, the therapist might be able to arrange for these meetings via phone or Skype after discharge.

CLINICAL CASE DESCRIPTION

Luisa, a 15-year-old Hispanic, was referred to a residential substance abuse treatment facility by her probation officer after having spent 2 weeks in a juvenile detention center. This latest stay in juvenile detention followed a long string of arrests. Adolescents referred by the legal system are typically accompanied to the facility by their probation officer rather than a parent; however, in this case, Luisa's mother and father were both present for the admission process. During this meeting, her parents informed the therapist of Luisa's legal problems, including running away, truancy, and other status offenses that began at the age of 11 and reportedly became an increasing source of concern because of the growing level of risk. They reported separate incidents of self-injury that on several occasions resulted in Luisa being admitted to psychiatric behavioral centers for evaluation. Now, at the age of 15, Luisa's other high-risk behaviors included inappropriate sexual relationships and drug use. Prior to the age of 11, Luisa experienced several traumatic events, including exposure to domestic violence throughout her childhood, community violence, and the loss of a close family member. After receiving this information, the therapist held an individual session with Luisa to introduce integrated substance abuse and trauma treatment. Luis identified her index trauma as losing someone who was like a second mother to her.

Psychoeducation

The average length of stay at the facility is 4 months, during which time the residents participate in individual, group, and family sessions. The first month of treatment focused on providing Luisa with psychoeducation on substance abuse and trauma, with each topic addressed in relation to the other. The therapist conducted group sessions that fostered a general understanding of trauma and substance abuse among Luisa and her peers. Group sessions also enabled the residents to share how they used drugs to manage distressing emotional states. Luisa adapted well to these sessions, talking openly about feelings of anger and sharing her understanding of how traumatic experiences might be influencing her current difficulties. In a later session, Luisa reported to the group that the discussions made her "feel understood and not crazy."

Individual sessions began with providing psychoeducation about Luisa's grief symptoms and trauma reminders. Luisa described that she had coped with grief by using Rohypnol to erase feelings of sadness and by becoming aggressive with family when she didn't have the drug. When arguments arose, feelings related to the loss of her family member intensified, and she would seek an escape through drug use. The therapist helped Luisa understand these behaviors as responses to trauma reminders. Withdrawal symptoms from Rohypnol and other drugs were identified, and relaxation skills were taught and incorporated as alternative ways of coping with trauma reminders. Reemergence of trauma symptoms and how to cope with these more positively was also discussed as a part of her recovery. This not only permitted Luisa to understand emotional dysregulation as a consequence of drug abuse but also opened up the need to address underlying trauma issues.

Parenting Skills

Parent sessions were conducted over the phone when the caregivers were unable to travel to the facility from their home out of town. During the initial calls, the therapist collected a great deal of information in the form of behavior analyses closely reviewing the severe parent–child conflicts experienced prior to Luisa's admittance to the RTF. Educating Luisa's parents about posttraumatic reactions was a new consideration for them because, until then, problematic behaviors had been attributed to Luisa's coexisting attention-deficit/hyperactivity disorder diagnosis and her seemingly chronic negative attitude. Familiarizing the parents with common trauma reactions was critical to enhancing their understanding of factors that may have contributed to Luisa's drug use and problematic behaviors. For example, her mother reported frequently reaching levels of frustration that led to screaming as a form of discipline. With a new appreciation for how screaming not only triggered trauma memories but also inadvertently reinforced the very behavior her mother was scolding, both parents were educated about how important their attention could be in influencing Luisa's behavior. The potential for parent–child conflicts was limited to weekend visits at the facility. Still, the parents were encouraged to plan their time with Luisa carefully to create structure and rituals that would be comforting, while also using praise and differential attention to focus on reinforcing Luisa's strengths and progress in the program. In collaboration with Luisa and therapist, specific rules of "no fighting" and "no foul language" were presented as a way of keeping order in the facility, and the facility consequences for breaking those rules even during parent–child visits were agreed upon. The therapist worked with all family members, encouraging them to practice keeping their voices down and addressing each other in a respectful manner. "I" statements were extremely effective in breaking communication barriers and creating an understanding of each other's concerns for safety. The parents also worked diligently to identify emotional cues in Luisa in an attempt to be more sensitive to her stress level and to trauma reminders. This consisted of allowing her "chill-outs" to collect herself, speaking in a calm tone, making encouraging statements in the form of praise for adaptive behaviors, and recognizing their own yelling as a trauma trigger for Luisa. The therapist highlighted Luisa's behavioral progress for the parents during all phone and in-person contacts. Luisa's improvements were attributed to consistent rule implementation throughout weekly interactions with staff and peers and to her hard work in facing and processing the traumatic loss of a family member as well as other trauma exposures she experienced at home and in the community. Luisa's parents were consistently encouraged to support Luisa's behavioral and emotional recovery by acknowledging her progress and hard work in participating in the RTF and therapy activities.

Relaxation and Stress Management

Relaxation techniques were successfully mastered in individual and group sessions. Morning yoga workouts, progressive muscle relaxation sessions, and art classes were weekly occurrences. A milieu staff member provided art lessons as a way to promote personal expression through a healthy medium. Luisa was able to ease her anxiety through physical activity while expressing her feelings through artwork. She reported feeling good about having something she could practice with others that wouldn't cause problems.

Breathing techniques were encouraged during individual sessions to calm her through a surge of negative emotion. This was an essential component for the management of unhealthy behaviors that could impede her treatment progress.

Affective Expression and Modulation Skills

During initial sessions an emotional struggle became apparent when Luisa continually shifted from crying to verbal aggressiveness. The therapist focused on keeping her in session despite the volatile nature of her words by acknowledging basic underlying feelings of grief. She would state that "all life had to offer was a puke-filled world." Such comments were considered as indicators of distress more than mere gross opposition. The therapist responded supportively to her tears, helping her to accept that crying could be healthy and a sign not of weakness but of strength, in terms acknowledging and facing painful experiences. Over time Luisa was encouraged to verbally share her distress in words, poetry, and artwork, and the therapist praised her for expressing herself without resorting to harmful behaviors.

Luisa continued to share her thoughts through disturbing imagery for several sessions. At times she would express to the counselor an emotional state through the description of what she would do to the person she was talking about. For example, if the client was talking about how her mother angered her by not taking her to visit her loved one's grave, she would describe how much physical pain her mother would feel as a consequence. Her mother would reportedly have Luisa's "blood on her hands," then realizing how she'd wronged Luisa. The therapist introduced affect expression cards to assist Luisa in identifying her dominant feeling by selecting the appropriate card. Gradually, she explored feelings elicited by general stressors as well as trauma reminders, including those that reminded of her deceased family member. The identification of positive and negative feelings associated with the lost loved one was an important part of therapy. Luisa was then able to remember positive characteristics of that person and the influence on her personality, thus providing her with a sense of connectedness. Often, the therapist encouraged Luisa to end such sessions with a self-soothing activity associated with remembering her loved one.

Cognitive Coping Skills

Luisa displayed unhealthy and volatile communication with her mother and father in the early stages of TF-CBT that indicated a need for significant work in developing cognitive coping skills. When her parents were unable to visit, Luisa expressed maladaptive beliefs that her parents were abandoning her. Through cognitive coping exercises, Luisa began to understand how her thoughts about her parents were influencing her feelings and behaviors toward them. Fortunately, Luisa and her parents began to practice communication skills during the substance abuse family groups that were held every Saturday. Adherence to the rules of the facility also helped with timely completion of treatment. Luisa initially had trouble complying with rules as a result of disobedience at home. By monitoring her daily interactions, the therapist was able to have Luisa process behaviors in relation to her feelings and later her underlying thoughts. This was facilitated by trauma-informed milieu staff who provided the consistency necessary for Luisa to develop healthy cognitive coping skills. The therapist helped Luisa identify several unhelpful coping styles, including (1) generalization, (2) jumping to conclusions, and (3) all-or-nothing thinking. The therapist explored the accusation of abandonment with her parents in terms of "all-or-nothing" thinking, for example, "If my parents don't do exactly what I expect, they don't love me at all and are abandoning me." Luisa was able to come to a more nuanced position regarding her parents' decision to place her in RTF, and in fact agreed that they may have done this for her benefit (because they love her). Although frustrated by her reactions toward them, the parents were able to be more patient by realizing that Luisa was no longer engaging in any self-injurious behavior.

Over time, family visits improved through the application of relaxation, affective modulation, and cognitive coping techniques. Reviewing past experiences with stressors was the start of managing unhealthy thought processes and behaviors. Similarly, daily interactions with peers and staff became an opportunity for practicing cognitive coping. Luisa at first described it as "seeing the future and keeping upsetting things from taking over." This task proved difficult at first because of her aggressive forms of expression; however, the implementation of relaxation and coping skills provided reinforcement to continue not to jump to conclusions about what her peers thought of her, but rather to explore the possibility that they were responding to her own behaviors to them. As Luisa used cognitive coping more, she noticed improved interactions with peers in the RTF and her aggressive behaviors decreased. Luisa noticed positive results through improved interaction with her parents and peers, problems that she once considered significant stressors. Client and parent sessions took place during the time that Luisa began to focus on her trauma narrative. A goal for each meeting was set to preserve a healthy understanding of her trauma-related issues.

Trauma Narrative

Luisa took a creative approach to developing her trauma narrative. Written in a mix of English and Spanish, she chose to write about her deceased loved ones in prose with accompanying drawings. The imagery she used aptly described her emotional states and associated thoughts about her multiple losses. Bound together like a book, the prose reflected her life changes through several specific traumatic experiences, including thoughts, feelings, body experiences, and how her behaviors and interactions with family and peers were affected as a result of each of these traumas.

The therapist spoke with Luisa's parents throughout the development of the trauma narrative. Concerns over her choice of words were normalized as a part of trauma and grieving. Accepting Luisa's appropriate expression of negative emotions ("feeling bad") was imperative for her parents to be able to support for full therapeutic benefits to occur. Her parents struggled with this as they still feared that these feelings would lead to self-injury; however, Luisa was able to reassure her parents that talking about these feelings openly was the best way to prevent such behaviors. The final chapter was more optimistic about her outlook on coping with the loss of her family members and other traumatic experiences. This demonstrated Luisa's capacity to cope with intense feelings of trauma and grief within the context of a supportive relationship and with the growing support she felt from her parents.

Luisa's progress in treatment resulted in her being allowed three separate visits home. The therapist would follow up after each visit in an attempt to assess potential risk factors. The parents reported some struggles with implementing house rules, yet noted significant improvement in Luisa's impulse control and their overall interactions with her. Luisa agreed, stating that she "is trying to make better decisions but it won't happen overnight." Luisa was also able to begin to acknowledge her parents' ongoing efforts to help her despite their own struggles and learned to express her appreciation to them as well through words of praise. Drug-related triggers were reportedly manageable for Luisa since she had decided to comply with probation for her well-being.

Enhancing Safety

Throughout treatment, residents keep a daily journal. Two weeks prior to graduation, the therapist and Luisa processed her efforts using the journal along with her trauma narrative. She was able to identify the development of safer modes of coping within her own writing. She remembered what she was feeling during each entry, speaking of it as a past form of expression. The therapist informed her that upon returning home these feelings had the potential to arise with the same intensity. Safety planning then became the primary focus of finalizing therapy. Luisa's safety plan included how to safely cope with future social stressors, accessibility to drugs, and emotional triggers. Luisa's parents were involved in her safety plan to help her implement coping skills. Upon her discharge from treatment, outpatient services were arranged for continued support her in substance abuse recovery. Luisa's safety plan included family and community support resources.

Treatment Progress

Luisa spent a total of 3 months at the facility. During this time, she experienced increased self-awareness in terms of personal safety by identifying emotional triggers related to her trauma. This helped transformed her communication style from verbal aggression to one of healthy expression. Her parents also displayed progress by becoming more sensitive to Luisa's trauma triggers and using improved parenting and communication skills learned throughout treatment. Her parents were also far more inclined than previously to be an active part of Luisa's substance abuse recovery process. Overall, the integration of substance abuse treatment and TF-CBT enabled Luisa to successfully address the two major issues of distress in her life in a trauma-informed manner and with a highly positive outcome.

CONCLUSION

While youth in RTF settings have very high rates of trauma exposure, only recently have treatment providers in these settings recognized the potential influence of trauma on the development and escalation of behavioral, emotional, and substance difficulties among RTF clients. Surprisingly, many youngsters who have had numerous outpatient and inpatient experiences report TF-CBT as the first therapy experience during which childhood traumas were acknowledged and directly and openly discussed. Despite their seeming fragility, many youth in RTF respond positively to addressing traumatic childhood experiences with the objective of helping them understand the relationship of these experiences to current difficulties, processing distressing trauma-related thoughts and feelings, and developing coping skills to manage everyday stressors as well as trauma reminders. Ideally, TF-CBT not only should be offered in the RTF setting but should continue at least briefly in aftercare, particularly if caregivers were not able to actively participate with the youth during their RTF stay. The case examples presented here highlight both the challenges and the extraordinary benefits of offering TF-CBT in RTF settings.

REFERENCES

American Psychiatric Association. (2000). *Diagnostic and statistical manual of mental disorders* (4th ed., text revision). Washington, DC: Author.

Cohen, J. A., & Mannarino, A. P. (1996). Factors that mediate treatment outcome for sexually abused preschool children. *Journal of the American Academy of Child and Adolescent Pschiatry, 35*, 1402–1410.

Cohen, J. A., & Mannarino, A. P. (2000). Predictors of treatment outcome in sexually abused children. *Child Abuse and Neglect, 24,* 983–994.

Cohen, J. A., Berliner, L., & Mannarino, A. P. (2010). Trauma-focused CBT for children with co-occurring trauma and behavior problems. *Child Abuse and Neglect, 34,* 215–224.

Copeland, W. E., Keeler, G., Angold, A., & Costello, E. J. (2007). Traumatic events and posttraumatic stress in childhood. *Archives of General Psychiatry, 64,* 577–584.

Debellis, M. D., Baum, A. S., Birmaher, B., Keshavan, M. S., Eccard, C. H., Boring, A. M., et al. (1999). Developmental traumatology: Part I. Biological stress systems. *Biological Psychiatry, 45,* 1259–1270.

DeBellis, M. D., Keshevan, M. S., Clark, D. B., Casey, B. J., Giedd, J. N., Frustaci, K., et al. (1999). Developmental traumatology: Part II. Brain development. *Biological Psychiatry, 45,* 1271–1284.

Deblinger, E., Lippmann, J., & Steer, R. (1996). Sexually abused children suffering posttraumatic stress symptoms: Initial treatment outcome findings. *Child Maltreatment, 1,* 310–321.

Steiner, H, Garcia, I. G., & Matthews, Z. (1997). PTSD in incarcerated juvenile delinquents. *Journal of the American Academy of Child and Adolescent Psychiatry, 36,* 357–365.

Weiner, D. A., Schneider, A., & Lyons, J. S. (2009). Evidence-based treatments for trauma among culturally diverse foster care youth: Treatment retention and outcomes. *Children and Youth Services Review, 31,* 1199–1205.

APPENDIX 3.1. TF-CBT TRAUMA PSYCHOEDUCATION FOR RTF MILIEU STAFF

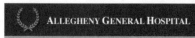 **ALLEGHENY GENERAL HOSPITAL**   Residential Treatment
                                                       Facility Series

TF-CBT Trauma Psychoeducation for RTF Milieu Staff

TF-CBT Psychoeducation helps children understand the impact that past traumatic experiences have on them in the present. You can support TF-CBT psychoeducation by recognizing when trauma reminders occur, understanding connections between trauma reminders and behavior problems, and preventing trauma reenactment.

Ramon was physically and emotionally abused by his father, witnessed domestic violence, and has a severe learning disability. He is in RTF due to physical aggression. Ramon gets into fights every day before school, which he refuses to attend. One of the other kids will call him "stupid," prompting Ramon to become aggressive, requiring you to physically intervene. This enrages Ramon, and he screams, "I'll kill you, get away from me!" One time you get so frustrated that you yell, "Cut the crap, Ramon!"

When children like Ramon have experienced severe early traumas, they often reenact those traumas in new situations and relationships. These episodes are frequently spawned by children coming into contact with a **Trauma Reminder**. Trauma reminders are things, places, situations, people, words, sounds, smells or other cues that remind children of their past traumatic experiences.

Trauma reminders can be internal to the child. For example:

- the child's thoughts
- the child's memories
- the child's feelings
- the child's behaviors
- the child's own body or body parts
- physical sensations or anything else internal to the child

Trauma reminders can also be external to the child. For example:

- another person
- a place
- a situation
- a smell
- a certain type of food
- a song
- a word
- a color
- a time of day
- a physical characteristic, mannerism, or behavior of another person
- anything else external to the child that reminds the child of the traumas experienced

Trauma reminders provide an important link between past trauma and current behavior problems. Understanding the impact of trauma reminders and preventing trauma reenactment will allow you to help children learn new ways to cope and to move forward.

Children work with their TF-CBT therapist to identify their personal trauma reminders. Therapists may write a child's trauma reminders on a PRACTICE Coping Card, which the child will carry on the unit. However, in the moment the children may not understand or forget that they are dealing with a trauma reminder. You can help children by being familiar with their trauma reminders, helping them appropriately manage them when they are encountered and, therefore, reduce trauma reenactments in the milieu.

When Ramon was living at home he was afraid to go to school because every day after school his father would call him a "retard". When his mother intervened, his father beat her, then would sit on Ramon and punch him and make Ramon say, "I'm a piece of crap".

Working with his therapist, Ramon identified the following as trauma reminders:

- being called names
- being held down
- being hit
- going to school

Now it is easier for you to understand Ramon's behavior as trauma reenactment. You thought he was being non-compliant in refusing to go to school, but the thought of going to school is really scary to Ramon. The other kids taunting him served as a second trauma reminder of his father's past emotional abuse, and triggered his past fear of being beaten up. He began to **reenact his past trauma by acting in the way most likely to prompt the abusive adult behavior he has come to expect.** You and other staff members unknowingly fulfilled these expectations by holding him down and yelling at him. You feel awful about this, but how could you know that this was trauma reenactment rather than bad behavior?

You can't always know every trauma reminder for every child. However, you can be calm, fair, and firm, to ensure that all children are treated with respect, and to implement the rules consistently. **If you are aware of each child's trauma reminders, you will be in a good position to recognize and prevent trauma reenactment.**

Here are some clues that trauma reenactment is occurring:

- Child's emotional response is extreme for the situation, e.g., a minor situation triggers extreme rage.
- Child's behavioral response is extreme for the situation, e.g., a minor disagreement prompts an immediate violent reaction.
- Child seems "out of it," unresponsive, or dissociative.
- Child seems to be responding to someone other than the person present, e.g., yelling "I'll kill you" did not seem directed at you in the above example.
- Child is engaging in "strange" behavior, things that don't seem to make sense under "normal" circumstances.

Once you understand trauma reminders and can connect these to behavior problems, you are in a better position to intervene and prevent trauma reenactment.

For example, now that you and Ramon's therapist have identified his trauma reminders, how can you help him prevent trauma reenactment every morning before school?

Idea #1 -- Change the routine.
Together, his therapist, you, Ramon and the teacher need to replace his current negative routine (get ready for school, refuse to go, get teased, get into a fight, get restrained) with a positive one. The routine can include elements such as some 1:1 time with staff he likes, acknowledgement and labeling by him of his feelings, use of his PRACTICE Coping Card strategies, and a special activity with the teacher when he arrives at school. These activities will make going to school more enjoyable or at least less upsetting, less of a trauma reminder. Changing his morning routine will

(continued)

likely take some time to accomplish, and will require a team effort until it becomes established, so be persistent.

Idea #2 – Change peer interaction.
Be on the lookout for peers who tease Ramon at breakfast or anytime before school. This behavior should not be acceptable at any time, but knowing that this is a trauma reminder, it should be followed immediately by consequences so that Ramon does not feel threatened or left to deal with it alone.

Idea #3 – Reinforce positive coping strategies.
Help Ramon recognize when he copes positively with trauma reminders. For example, if he is able to restrain himself from fighting when you give consequences to a peer who teases him, use this episode as an opportunity not only to praise his control, but also to educate him that trauma reminders are likely to occur in unexpected places, and he gets to be in charge of how he responds to trauma reminders, rather than trauma reminders controlling him.

Information about additional TF-CBT PRACTICE skills will also be helpful in supporting children to master trauma reminders and avoid traumatic reenactment.

APPENDIX 3.2. TF–CBT RELAXATION SKILLS FOR RTF MILIEU STAFF

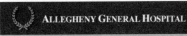 **ALLEGHENY GENERAL HOSPITAL**   Residential Treatment
                                                         Facility Series

TF-CBT Relaxation Skills for RTF Milieu Staff

TF-CBT Relaxation Skills help children "turn down the volume" of physical hyperarousal due to trauma. Common relaxation skills are listed below, but often TF-CBT therapists and children create individualized relaxation strategies for specific settings. You can support children in using these strategies in RTF settings by encouraging children to use relaxation skills before hyperarousal gets out of control.

Tracy was physically and sexually abused and neglected during early childhood. Tracy's mother was a drug addict and often absent. At 6 years old Tracy came to school with bruises and was placed in a series of foster homes where she experienced sexual abuse by older foster siblings. Tracy is in the RTF due to aggressive and self-injurious behavior. She is extremely jumpy, irritable, can't sleep and has angry outbursts towards males.

Chronically traumatized children like Tracy are like war veterans. Visible wounds include physical injuries and emotional or behavioral problems. **Trauma also causes less visible wounds to children's brains and bodies.** These may include:

- Elevated heart rate and blood pressure
- Smaller brain volumes
- Impaired immune functioning and increased physical illness
- Trouble sleeping
- Increased startle response
- Increased irritability and anger
- Impaired ability to distinguish between danger and safety
- Inability of brain to extinguish learned fear responses
- Dysregulated biological response to stress and trauma

Even when they are safe, traumatized children like Tracy function as if they are still in danger. Their bodies and brains remain "on alert".

"Every night when I got ready to go to bed, I never knew whether this was a safe night or a bad one. If it was a bad night, my father would be coming in to hurt me. If I cried he'd put his hand over my mouth and nose until I couldn't breathe. The worst feeling was not being able to breathe when he's tearing me up inside down there. I thought I was going to die. I couldn't get any breath. I still feel that way. Every night when I go to sleep it comes back on me. I thought foster care would be better but I was never safe."

Tracy's body reacts pretty much the same whether she is scared or angry—she becomes short of breath, her heart is pounding, her gut shuts down, and her muscles tense. She is ready to fight. To you she looks aggressive, but inside she is a scared kid. How can you help her calm the storm inside her body?

(continued)

Supporting TF-CBT Relaxation Skills
Some common TF-CBT relaxation skills that therapists will work with you to support children in using include the following:

- Focused (yoga) breathing
- Progressive muscle relaxation
- Visualization ("perfect day", ocean, sky, cloud, butterfly, etc.)
- Music
- Dance
- Going to room to relax or calm down
- Talking to you or another staff person
- Drawing, journaling, reading
- Going outside for a walk
- Nature
- Sports
- Blowing bubbles (younger children)

TF-CBT relaxation skills are individualized to meet the needs of each child. Therapists work with each child to identify what relaxation strategies work best in different situations. The child's therapist will communicate with you to keep you up to date about this as strategies change during therapy. This may be through writing the child's relaxation strategies on the child's PRACTICE Coping Card; through regular unit meetings; or other systematic ways of communicating with you.

Ask the child, *"What relaxation skills are you using to cope with stress?"* If the child says he or she is not using any or the child doesn't know what you are talking about, ask to see the child's PRACTICE Coping Card. If no relaxation skills are on the card, you might suggest that the child use one of the strategies in the list above in the moment. Check in with the child's therapist to let him or her know how this strategy worked and whether other relaxation skills should be added to the child's PRACTICE Coping Card.

If specific relaxation strategies are marked on the child's PRACTICE card, encourage the child to use these skills. If you aren't familiar with the particular skill on the card, ask the child to show the skill to you. This approach is a great way for the child to show you that they have special "expertise" in something, to potentially share this skill with you, and for you to praise them for remembering, demonstrating, and using it. Providing positive feedback (e.g., *"Wow, I never saw that before. That's a great idea. I'm going to try that myself when I'm stressed out"*) is a great way to show appreciation for the child's special knowledge and skill and reinforce the use of effective strategies in daily life.

You also can model appropriate relaxation skills by staying calm and "keeping your cool" in the milieu setting, even when things get stressful. When you model "walking the walk", children may ask you how you manage to stay so relaxed and easy-going under pressure. Then you can share some of your personal favorite stress reduction strategies with them.

APPENDIX 3.3. TF–CBT AFFECT REGULATION SKILLS FOR RTF MILIEU STAFF

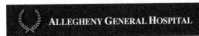

ALLEGHENY GENERAL HOSPITAL

Residential Treatment
Facility Series

TF-CBT Affect Regulation Skills for RTF Milieu Staff

TF-CBT Affect (feeling) Regulation Skills help children recognize and talk about their upsetting feelings rather than showing these feelings through problematic behaviors. Often therapists and children create individualized affect regulation skills during TF-CBT treatment. In the moment, it may be especially helpful to validate, acknowledge and inquire about the child's feelings as described below.

At 5 years old Anthony witnessed his father's death from community violence. Two older brothers died in gang-related shootings. Last year his sister was raped. Anthony was sent to the RTF after stabbing one of the brothers of his sister's rapist.

Many children in RTF settings have experienced repeated traumas like Anthony. These children often have severe difficulty with emotional and behavioral regulation. That is, they cannot appropriately manage their feelings and related behaviors. When something reminds traumatized children of their past traumatic experiences — a **trauma reminder** — they often decompensate. The process that typically occurs is that a trauma reminder causes significant negative feelings, which lead to acutely agitated, dissociative, self-injurious, disorganized, aggressive and/or destructive behaviors. However, this process may occur very quickly with seemingly little warning between the reminder and the behavior. This diagram illustrates the process:

Trauma reminder ➡ **Negative feeling** ➡ **Negative behavior**

Anthony overheard two boys talking while watching TV, shouting to the TV character, "Kill him!" Anthony became enraged, and with narrowed eyes and clenched fists, stomped over and started punching the boys.

Your goal is to prevent children's negative feelings from progressing to negative behaviors, that is, to interrupt this progression **as early as possible in the process**. It is helpful to:

- Recognize and intervene when trauma reminders occur in the milieu (e.g., when Anthony's peers said *"Kill him!"*)
- Recognize early signals of emotional distress or dysregulation (e.g., Anthony's narrowed eyes and clenched fists)
- Help children recognize their distressing feelings (e.g., Anthony's anger, grief)
- Help children use affect regulation skills to "turn down the volume" of distress before it leads to out-of-control behavior (use TF-CBT skills described below)

Recognizing early warning signals of distress

The higher a child's emotional response, the more out of control their behavior usually is and the less able they are to listen, reason, think clearly, or use coping skills. When rating behavior problems on a scale of 1-10, with 1 = perfect behavior control and 10 = behavior totally out of control, interventions are more effective when children's emotional and behavior responses are at 4-5, not at 8-9. Using the analogy of traffic signals, green (1-3) is "safe"; yellow (4-7) is "warning—slow down" and red (8-10) is "danger—STOP!". You need to put on the brakes when problems are in the yellow zone. By the time they are in the "red" zone it is too late.

(continued)

Green	Yellow								Red
1	2	3	4	5	6	7	8	9	10
Good control				Losing control				Lost control	

Some things to look for in trying to detect **early warning signs** are:

- Trauma reminders that may set off the above process

- Changes in facial expression or body language suggesting increased distress

- Changes in verbal expression suggesting distress: increased volume, change in tone, increased irritability, escalation of arguing, etc.

- Changes in physical agitation level, e.g., increased shaking of extremities, fidgeting, pacing, tapping feet or fingers, etc.

- Angry face, clenched lips or fists, muttering, narrowed or rolling eyes

- Requests or demands for staff attention, stomping away when requests are not granted

- Increase in silent, withdrawn, moody behavior, seeming more "out of it", talking to self, seeming more confused, dissociative or psychotic than previously

You may be thinking, *"This describes every child in RTF. What am I supposed to do, pay attention to every early warning sign in every child?"* You can't be perfect at recognizing early warning signs of emotional or behavioral regulation problems. However waiting to intervene until *severe* problems occur is "the squeaky wheel gets the grease" model. That is, the children with the most severe problems get the most staff attention. Since staff attention, even negative attention, is often reinforcing for children, this approach will result in children developing more, not less, severe behavior problems. The RTF will become crisis-driven rather than focused on developing children's coping skills.

The goal is to interrupt the process early, in the green or early yellow periods, when interventions will be most effective. When you instead focus on identifying problems at a lower level of intensity, children learn to use coping skills earlier in the process. The milieu will become skills-focused, not crisis-driven. Over time, children will have less severe behavior problems. Everyone in the RTF milieu benefits from this approach—children, families, administration, and you, the front line milieu staff.

Interrupting escalation using TF-CBT feeling identification skills

Imagine you see the early warning signs of Anthony's distress in the above example (i.e., his clenched fists and angry face) before he stomped over to the boys watching TV and started punching them. How could you interrupt this process? Here are some ideas:

- **Acknowledge and inquire.** Ask the child about the feelings you are observing. *"Anthony, you look really mad. What's going on?"* Anthony will hopefully respond to your acknowledgement with a response that shows just how angry he is. This response is exactly what you hope for, a verbal response instead of angry behavior. He may say something like, *"F—king right, I'm mad. My brothers are dead. They f—ked with my family. How the f—k do you think I feel?"*

- **Validate the feeling.** Tell the child you understand why he is feeling the way he is and what he believes is going on: *"Of course you're angry. You're thinking about your brothers and how they died. You're right, I'd be mad too if that had happened to my family."*
- **If the child denies the feeling, ask what he *is* feeling.** If instead of describing their feelings, the child denies a feeling such as, *"I'm not mad, leave me alone"*, reflect what you see, as if you were holding up a mirror: *"I only asked that because your fists are clenched and your face looked angry. I guess I'm way off base. What are you feeling?"*

Using TF-CBT affective modulation skills to "turn down the volume"

Once children have acknowledged feelings you have already started to defuse the situation. However, it is still not a "done deal" that the child won't escalate to out of control behavior. At this point it is crucial to help children use affective modulation skills to "turn down the volume" to prevent further escalation. At this point you can:

- **Model affective modulation skills.** Continue to keep your voice calm. Speak slowly and softly even if the child is yelling. Raising your voice to match his volume will not help the child to calm down. Raising your voice will only make him angrier and escalate the situation. Do not reprimand him for swearing. This is the time to model affective regulation, not to establish your authority.
- **Offer options for affective modulation.** Offer the child options for affective modulation, for example, offer distraction options such as asking if he would like to play a game with you, go to a quiet place and talk with you, take a walk, or whether there is another affective modulation skill on his PRACTICE Coping Card he would like to use. Your knowledge of the particular child, his interests and mood, and your intuitive judgment of what will work best to defuse a given situation is critical to success in the moment.
- **Offer praise for not escalating.** Once the child is able to respond to you calmly, praise him for successfully avoiding further escalation: *"Anthony, you've done a great job of keeping your cool even though you're really angry. That's hard to do and I hope you're really proud of this."*

APPENDIX 3.4. TF–CBT COGNITIVE COPING SKILLS FOR RTF MILIEU STAFF

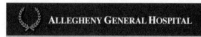
ALLEGHENY GENERAL HOSPITAL

Residential Treatment
Facility Series

TF-CBT Cognitive Coping Skills for RTF Milieu Staff

TF-CBT Cognitive Coping Skills help children understand connections between maladaptive thoughts and negative feelings and behaviors. By helping children to examine and change unhelpful or inaccurate thinking patterns, children learn to modify their negative feelings and behaviors.

Maladaptive thoughts may be factually inaccurate. For example, Anthony from the Affect Regulation Skills handout may think, *"I should have been able to save my father's life."* Maladaptive thoughts may also be somewhat accurate, but unhelpful. For example, Anthony may think, *"You can never tell who belongs to the gang that raped my sister."* Either one of these thoughts may contribute to negative emotions, increased physiological arousal, and to Anthony quickly going from zero to ten in behavior problems when triggered by a reminder of gang behavior.

TF-CBT therapists work with children to examine such thoughts and replace them with more accurate and helpful thoughts, and how this might affect their feelings and behaviors. The idea is that less upsetting thoughts lead to less upsetting feelings, which prevent negative behaviors. The connections between thoughts, feelings, and behaviors are usually shown as a triangle, but they can just as accurately be shown this way:

More accurate/helpful thoughts ➡ Less negative feelings ➡ Less negative behaviors

- A more accurate thought for Anthony might be, *"Even the EMT and the doctors couldn't save my father's life. I wish I could have done something to save him, but I was only 5 years old. It was really painful to see him die."*

- A more helpful thought might be, *"Most guys do not rape girls."*

Therapists will work closely with you to keep you informed of each child's cognitions and how they are addressing them in therapy. This information will help you to reinforce more adaptive cognitive coping by the child in daily life situations.

Often kids in a RTF have negative thoughts about non-trauma-related things as well. For example, they may assume that other kids are laughing at them, that their peers don't like them, or that staff is angry at them. Instead of doing a "fact check" (e.g., asking the kids why they are laughing, asking the peer if there is a problem, or asking the staff member if they have done something wrong), kids will typically get angry, isolate, explode, or withdraw without bothering to see whether their assumptions are accurate. You can help children in the milieu examine these negative cognitions by checking with children when you see this sort of situation happen and helping them to check out the facts and examine the evidence rather than jumping to conclusions.

When kids learn to have more accurate and helpful thoughts about non-trauma-related issues, this practice will help them to "turn down the volume" of their negative feelings, which in turn will decrease their negative feelings.

PART II

TF-CBT
DEVELOPMENTAL
APPLICATIONS

4

Play Applications
and Skills Components

ATHENA A. DREWES
ANGELA M. CAVETT

OVERVIEW OF TF–CBT PLAY
APPLICATIONS AND SKILLS COMPONENTS

Play is as natural to children as breathing. It is intrinsically motivating, an end in itself, transcending differences in ethnicity, language and culture, and it is associated with positive emotions (Drewes, 2005, 2006, 2009; Lidz, 2006; Tharinger, Christopher, & Matson, 2011). Play is perhaps the most developmentally appropriate and powerful medium for young children to build adult–child relationships, develop cause–effect thinking critical to impulse control, process stressful experiences, and learn social skills (Association for Play Therapy, 2011; Chaloner, 2001).

Play not only is essential for promoting normal child development but has many therapeutic powers as well (Russ & Niec, 2011; Schaefer & Drewes, 2009). Empirical literature (Reddy et al., 2005; Russ, 2004; Russ & Niec, 2011) has found that play relates to or facilitates problem solving, which requires insight ability, flexibility, and divergent thinking ability; the ability to think of alternative coping strategies in coping with daily problems, to experience positive emotion, to think about affect themes (positive and negative), and to understand the emotions of others and take the perspective of another; and aspects of general adjustment.

Description of Population

Utilizing play-based techniques within structured cognitive-behavioral therapy (CBT) can be a very useful modality for children 3 years of age and older depending on their emotional and developmental maturity. Children and teens who are challenging to engage in treatment may respond well when the therapeutic environment is playful and when play-based techniques are utilized by a playful therapist, all of which can offer relief from intensely emotionally charged work in dealing with feelings and trauma experiences.

Blending play and play techniques into CBT (Drewes, 2009) allows effective delivery of CBT while not affecting its theoretical underpinnings. Knell (1993; Knell & Dasari, 2009) demonstrated that CBT could be modified for use with young children utilizing puppets, stuffed animals, bibliotherapy, and other toys with which cognitive strategies could be modeled. Over the past 10 years, there has been increased attention toward adaptation of CBT for use with preschoolers (Knell & Dasari, 2011). Consequently, the use of a CBT play approach with children between 2½ and 6 years has developed incorporating cognitive, behavioral, and traditional play therapies (Knell & Beck, 2000; Knell & Dasari, 2011). Thus, play-based activities developed by creative play therapists may be integrated into CBT components to support engagement and enhance participation when working with children and teens (Knell, 1993; Knell & Dasari, 2011; Meichenbaum, 2009).

Play Applications with Young Children

Although the change mechanisms of play and play therapy are not fully researched, Singer and Singer (1990) see play as reinforcing when it allows expression of positive affect and appropriate control of negative affect. Golomb and Galasso (1995) found this to be the case in their research with preschoolers. Research has shown that developing a coherent narrative is central to the structured techniques that Gaensbauer and Siegal (1995) used with toddlers who had experienced traumatic events. These researchers believed that the change mechanisms of play among younger children were similar to those among older children with PTSD.

In the 20-plus years since trauma-focused cognitive-behavioral therapy (TF-CBT) was developed (Cohen & Mannarino, 1996; Deblinger, McLeer, & Henry, 1990), it has become "clear that children respond very differently to therapy than adults, and the element of play became a crucial ingredient in engaging children in the therapy process as did the important involvement of parents" (Briggs, Runyon, & Deblinger, 2011, p. 169). Difficult and emotion-laden trauma material can be more easily digested, with play and play-based techniques becoming a sort of "enzyme" (Goodyear-Brown, 2010) that dissolves the painful connection to traumatic memories, thereby easing the discomfort and increasing control and confidence within the child. A new pairing can then occur whose basis becomes associated "with laughter, playful competition, pride and feelings of courage and confidence" (Briggs et al., 2011, p. 174; Deblinger & Heflin, 1996).

Traditionally, TF-CBT has utilized structured and educational play over nondirective, child-led, or pretend play. Play is used to help engage children and parents in treatment; create a playful, safe, and therapeutic environment; help facilitate communication between the therapist and child; and teach specific skills (Briggs et al., 2011). It is important to note that nondirective or child-led free play is only included in TF-CBT for a few minutes at the end of sessions, as a reward or for relaxation and self-soothing transition from intense feelings that may have been aroused during the session.

A core value of TF-CBT is flexibility, which allows the clinician to utilize a playful approach in order to reach children and develop a therapeutic relationship. Indeed, "the success of the evidence-based model (TF-CBT) is founded on the creativity, adaptability, and playfulness of the clinician. The use of diverse structured play approaches highlights the flexible and adaptable nature of TF-CBT" (Briggs et al., 2011, p. 174). Therefore, the application of play and play-based techniques are consistent with and have increasingly been incorporated into TF-CBT for use with young children to assist in engagement along with the educational and skill-building components that make up TF-CBT.

Special Considerations

Challenges may exist in implementing TF-CBT with young children who are verbally and/or cognitively limited and perhaps have more difficulty using TF-CBT components. Using developmentally appropriate play to implement TF-CBT components allows children and parents to feel more relaxed and engaged. Because play is the language of children (Landreth, 2002), it can be utilized to help gain their interest and maintain attention as well as process and comprehend each of the components through a multimodal approach that developmentally and culturally taps into the natural learning style and life experiences of children. Without a playful aspect to the components, young children may view treatment activities as though they were formal, academic tasks and may become disinterested or refuse to participate. Play also allows children to learn concepts that may be difficult when described verbally but better understood when visually and experientially processed. Furthermore, because trauma is not always processed on a verbal level, play allows children to use a multisensory approach to access their trauma memories and create their trauma narrative (e.g., by playing out the trauma through the use of a dollhouse rather than trying to articulate horrific images and memories verbally). Thus, playful interventions structured to achieve the goals of the TF–CBT components are engaging and invite children to more readily and easily communicate their experiences with their therapist and overcome common difficulties encountered during treatment. However, it is important for the TF–CBT therapist to be comfortable directly addressing trauma while simultaneously being playful in order to be authentic and believable.

APPLYING PLAY-BASED TECHNIQUES TO ASSESSMENT AND ENGAGEMENT

All of the techniques that follow may include the parent as needed or indicated during the treatment process. Having the child practice the various techniques in many different settings, incorporating repetitions within the therapy sessions and over time, and having the child teach the techniques to the parent helps to ensure generalization and the likelihood of mastering and using them.

Assessment Strategies

TF–CBT identifies biopsychosocial problems common among children who access treatment and who have been traumatized by the CRAFTS spectrum: Cognitive problems, Relationship problems, Affective problems, Family problems, Traumatic behavior problems, and Somatic problems.

Several play interventions that may be used to assist in assessment include Stepping Up to Success and the Caterpillar to Butterfly Treatment Plan (Cavett, 2010). In Stepping Up to Success, the child and parent think of the three to eight main presenting problems and treatment goals on which they want to focus. They are then encouraged to make stairsteps from construction paper or foam representing the problems to be addressed, and on each step the child writes the problem identified. Treatment goals for each of the presenting problems are then written on footprints, which are attached to the step.

Caterpillar to Butterfly Treatment Plan utilizes a simple story played out with a butterfly puppet. The story tells of a big, fuzzy caterpillar that creates a cocoon in the trees after eating a full meal of leaves. It dreams of having beautiful wings and being with other butterflies, but wonders how it could change. The caterpillar realizes that it has, within itself, the ability to become all that it wanted to be, but getting out of the cocoon would require working very hard in order to become free. The child is told that therapy is like the caterpillar making a cocoon and changing into a butterfly. The child is helped to identify what behaviors need to be changed (represented by the caterpillar), what needs to be learned (the cocoon), and what the positive behaviors would be (the butterfly). The child then creates a butterfly from construction paper and decorates it, along with making a caterpillar out of pipe cleaners and a cocoon from construction paper.

Activities during the assessment phase can also include directed play using, for example, painting, dollhouses, storytelling, clay, and puppets. These allow exploration of the child's strengths, talents, worries, and problem areas as well as an informal assessment of his or her emotional, cognitive, and developmental levels and the ability to use imagination and pretend play.

Unique Engagement Strategies

The *"Talking Ball" Game* (Leben, 2008) involves the therapist having members taking turns rolling a ball from one (the sender) to another (the receiver) across a table. The sender asks the receiver a question—for example, "What is your favorite food?" or "What is your biggest worry?"—to explore likes, dislikes, interests, hobbies, ways of coping with worries, and so on. The game continues for 5 to 10 minutes or until every player has a chance to ask three questions.

Feeling Balloons (Drewes, 2011; Horn, 1997; Short, 1997) can be utilized to help explain the therapy process. The therapist has the child blow up a balloon (or does it for the child if he or she is too young or is allergic to latex), and as the balloon is blown up all the negative feelings (e.g., anger, sad, mad, hurt) are put into the balloon. Once it is blown up, the therapist, using a marker, writes on the balloon the various feelings the child indicates that are "inside," along with names of people whom the child may have negative feelings about. The therapist explains that the balloon is much like a person's head, with many feelings that fill it up. The therapist explores with the child what would happen if the balloon kept getting bigger, and that indeed it would pop. In real life, though, heads don't pop; instead, all the angry and strong feelings that build up might make the child "pop" inside, making him or her become aggressive or physical toward others. These strong feelings get in the way of learning and feeling happy. The therapist explains that in each session the child will get to let out his or her feelings and experiences a little at a time, not all at once, in a way that the child can handle. The child is encouraged to let out some air from the balloon and note its progress in getting smaller, until finally all the air is released.

The *Scavenger Hunt List* (Cavett, 2010) requires the children to search their home for various items that will ultimately be used in the therapy process. They are asked to find a special stuffed animal to bring to sessions as well as something that helps them relax—maybe a picture of someone important to them, a picture of their room, something they do when they are bored, or a favorite book. The stuffed animal can be utilized during future sessions to help ease the children's anxieties or discomfort encountered in the session and for practicing various techniques.

TF–CBT Components

Psychoeducation and Parenting

Using playful interventions allows the parents to communicate with their child in a developmentally appropriate manner as well as help in engagement and gaining of skills. Difficult and anxiety-provoking topics such as sexual and physical abuse, domestic violence, and healthy sexuality can be processed in a playful way, lessening discomfort and making the psychoeducation component fun. When the parents and child learn playful interventions that are consistent with the TF-CBT model, the parents are more apt to use them with the child and the child more likely to be receptive and willing to practice and utilize the skill.

To better understand the relationship between children and their nonabusive parent, the play intervention *Me and My Mom* (Crisci, Lay, & Lowenstein, 1998) is effective. With this technique, young children make a collage of magazine pictures of women or men and children who remind them of their relationship with the nonoffending parent before the trauma and at the beginning of treatment. At the end of treatment, this intervention is utilized again to help provide insight into the children's perception of what has changed in the parent–child dyad.

Special question-and-answer games that playfully explore the child's trauma while correcting subsequent cognitive distortions, misperceptions, and gaps in information are a fun way to help the child and parent become comfortable in talking and asking questions about uneasy topics while learning important information. For example, the What If Game (Budd, 2008) has the therapist make up cards with different questions that tap into various misconceptions and probe for the child's strengths. Examples of these explorative questions include "What if you could ask anyone a question? What might you want to know?"; "What if you could go back in time? What would you want to change?"; or "What if your pet could share something about you? What would it say?" The questions can be adapted to fit the child's trauma situation. The child can play the game with the therapist and, once comfortable talking about the trauma, can then play the game with the parent, sharing his or her knowledge and reinforcing skills. The parent is encouraged to praise and reward the child's efforts in playing the game and answering the questions. The What Do You Know? card game (Deblinger, Neubauer, Runyon, & Baker, 2006) facilitates dialogue on difficult topics such as sexual and physical abuse, domestic violence, and personal safety. Questions such as "Why don't children tell about sexual abuse?" or "What can a child do if he or she has been sexually abused?" allow the therapist to help clarify misinformation and dysfunctional beliefs and thoughts. The card game can then be set up as a friendly competition between child and parent (after the parent has had an opportunity to prepare for the joint session), with teams competing for stickers and using a bell to ring and earn points. Adding to the fun component, on the back of each card there are small pictures of animals, along with a picture of one-quarter of an animal, so that when four cards are put together, like a puzzle, it makes the whole animal. A talk or game show format can also be utilized (Kaduson, 2001) whereby the child is empowered and becomes the "expert" who shares the newly learned information with imaginary callers who ask, via "questions" relayed by the therapist, about similar situations and concerns that the child has. Use of these games offers the child gradual exposure to the trauma material along with practice opportunities for learning new information. The child is praised and reinforced for participation.

Bibliotherapy can be helpful especially with young children. General books related to the specific trauma are powerful as are books related to the concept of a "bad thing that happened," such as *Brave Bart* (Sheppard, 1998); *No-No and the Secret Touch* (Scott, Feldman, & Patterson, 1993); *The Adventures of Lady: The Big Storm* (Pearson & Merrill, 2006); and *A Very Touching Book* (Hindman, 1983). Books can help in opening discussion related to the concept of trauma, psychological symptomatology, and healing. They can be read to a child along with use of puppets for storytelling and enactment, which can help deepen the child's understanding. The parent and child can also use the books at home to help gradually expose the child to the trauma material and help in desensitization.

Relaxation

Utilizing animal postures, such as that of a lion, cat, snake, bird, or fish, can be appealing to younger children and can help in both relaxing them and reinforcing positive traits (Drewes, 2011; James, 1989). The children are directed to see themselves as a lion (or other favorite animal), feeling the lion energy moving up from the earth, through their feet, and up throughout their bodies, letting it rise up into a powerful roar. They practice roaring loudly and then slowly lowering it to a whisper. They are then encouraged to silently move into a stretching posture, creating within themselves the quiet strength of the lion as it relaxes. The children then practice the stretching and slow breathing of the calm lion. The therapist can process with the children their inner strengths and power and, using the lion metaphor, explain how the lion does not always roar and use up its energy and that there are times to "roar" and times to save energy and stretch and relax.

Using the guided relaxation Safe Place (Drewes, 2011; James, 1989) is an effective way to teach deep breathing while offering the children a relaxation tool to use at any time. While sitting with eyes closed, they imagine being a movie director and visualize themselves making a movie. They are directed to breathe in and out slowly and to think of a time and place when they felt safe—maybe lying in the sun at the beach, hiding under their bedcovers, or snuggling with a favorite pet. They zoom in with their camera and film the location, taking in all that is there. They then freeze the camera shot. Continuing their slow breathing in and out, they look around in their imagination and notice what they see, smell, hear, feel, and whether or not there are any people or animals there. As they continue deep breathing, they are instructed to feel how safe they are and how relaxed they feel in their body while in their safe space. Next, they give their special safe place a name, preferably one word. It is the key that will get them back to their safe place anytime they wish to go. All they have to do is remember the name. The children continue to breathe in and out slowly, focusing on how relaxed and safe they feel. After a few minutes, they are directed to slowly move their camera back, and in another minute they will be back in the room with the therapist with their eyes open. The goal is to link the deep breathing with the experience of feeling safe and with the word chosen. At times when they feel upset or anxious, they can remember the word and help their body begin to relax.

The *Tighten and Relax Dance* (Cavett, 2010) incorporates movement to facilitate relaxation. The therapist models a tight dance, dancing stiffly in a circle with tight muscles. The child is invited to participate in the dance and follow along. The dance next shifts into a tight march, with stiff muscles. The therapist switches into a floppy dance/march, with a floppy, relaxed manner, ultimately flopping into a beanbag or a chair. This series is repeated several times at a comfortable rate for the child. Relaxation can also be done while playing Simon Says, with "Simon" asking the person to tighten and relax different muscle groups. The parent, child, and therapist take turns tightening and relaxing.

Personalized Pinwheels (Goodyear-Brown, 2005) or bubbles are useful in practicing deep breathing. The children are instructed to take a deep breath in and slowly blow it out, making the pinwheel turn or making as big a bubble as possible. While thinking of a favorite color, the children inhale and imagine this color going to all the areas in their body where they are feeling tense, angry, or worried and replacing the feelings with calm and relaxation. Then they can blow out and see how many bubbles they can make or how long they can make their pinwheel turn. A simple mantra that can be taught young children to assist with deep breathing is "Smell the flowers and blow out the candles" (Henriquez, personal communication, March 17, 2011). Bubbles are also a great way to teach boundaries

(Drewes, 2011). The children imagine they have an invisible bubble around them, which extends out one arm length. They hold their arm straight out to measure the distance. They are asked what happens when bubbles meet, and they blow bubbles to see what happens. When the bubbles pop, the therapist reinforces that when their invisible bubble gets too close to another child's, even an adult's, personal bubble space, it may make the child angry and want to strike out. By remembering the arm's length of their invisible bubble, they can keep themselves safe and allow for personal space. Also, using bubbles as a ritual, at the end of each session, helps in relaxing the children and allows for an easy transition from therapy.

Affective Expression and Modulation

This component allows for the skill development of expression and modulation of feelings, helping both the child and the parent become able to recognize, identify, express, and effectively modulate emotions. There are numerous play-based techniques useful in helping young children with a limited affective vocabulary to identify and quantify emotions as well as modulate them.

The Gingerbread Person Feelings Map (Drewes, 2001) is a variation of the Color Your Life technique (O'Connor, 1983) but uses the drawing of a gingerbread person with arms outstretched and with eyes, nose, and smile. It is used to assess (1) the overall vocabulary range of feelings the child or adolescent has and can identify; (2) how aware the child is about where he or she physiologically feels the emotions; and (3) how well integrated these emotions are. Because it takes just a few minutes, the Gingerbread Person Feelings Map allows for a quick gathering of information in a nonthreatening and play-based way.

Next to the shape of a gingerbread person, the words *happy*, *sad*, *afraid*, *angry*, *love*, and *worried* are listed, one under the other. The child is asked to include a few additional feeling words (one is often surprised at what they include, e.g., *petrified*, *stupid*, *anxious*, "wishing I was somebody else"), which are written underneath the other standard emotions. This helps the child to expand his or her "emotional vocabulary." It also helps to give the child some control over the task and feel like an active participant in the process. The child then chooses a color for each feeling and puts a little color line next to each feeling (like creating a legend for a map). It does not matter what color the child uses for each feeling. The child is asked to color inside the gingerbread person the parts where he or she may physically experience each feeling listed. The child can shade it in, scribble, draw hearts—whatever he or she chooses. The therapist goes through each feeling and has the child imagine where he or she feels each one (so none are omitted).

Once completed (usually less than 5 minutes), the therapist and child process the drawing, paying particular attention to where in the body anger is expressed and how that might play out in the child's world in responding to situations. The therapist looks for how many feelings are integrated, how much color is used, and where, and also for discrepancies, such as where the child may have colored in happy feelings on the face but anger in the hands or feet or body, or having placed a spot of color representing anger outside of the figure. The therapist and child process how the child may present to others as calm but inwardly is seething or perhaps manifesting anger through hitting or restlessness in the legs. Together, they identify where the child puts love (often drawn as a heart) and how it may be walled off by layers of scared, hurt, or angry feelings. The therapist explains how we all can have more than one feeling at a time within us, sometimes feeling ambivalent—feeling angry and loving at the same time toward someone. Sometimes one feeling is so strong that it can hide other feelings, which makes people feel confused and unsure about their feelings. This technique can also be used with the parent and the child together, each working independently of the other. At the end parent and child can share their finished product and compare similarities and differences in the ways anger is felt. Younger children (preschool age) are directed to use one color/feeling at a time rather than integrating all of them into one figure at the same time.

An adaptation of this technique uses two gingerbread figures (Gil, 2006). Children color in each figure based on the various feelings experienced in the presence of each parent. Children who may be uncomfortable thinking about their body and using a person-like shape (especially if they were sexually abused) might prefer using a heart shape. Heartfelt Feelings Coloring Card Strategies (Crenshaw, 2008) uses preprinted cards with a drawn heart and feeling words to add colors to in order to help children identify, label, and express their feelings about heartfelt issues and relationships with the important people in their lives. Similar to the Gingerbread Person Feelings Map and Color Your Life, children pick colors to match various feelings listed and fill in the amount of feelings they have, thereby quantifying how they are feeling at the moment or at a particular other point in time. They can also write on the card a response to a time when they had this feeling. *Color Your Heart* (Goodyear-Brown, 2002) is another variation utilizing a heart shape, which is colored in proportion to the amount of each feeling in the children's heart.

For younger or preschool children, *Basket of Feelings* (Drewes, 2011; James, 1989) allows for quantifying feelings using plastic game chips, crayons, or markers. Two or three sheets of plain paper are cut or ripped into fours, creating 8 to 12 squares. The therapist and child alternate in naming a feeling, which the therapist (or child) writes down on each square. The therapist then demonstrates by relaying a scenario in which many feelings occurred. An example would be recounting coming out of a store and seeing a big dent in the car. The therapist puts a handful of chips on mad (explaining how angry the therapist was), then a few on sad (that the car got damaged), a few more on worried (about how to get it fixed), and maybe a few on happy (that perhaps the therapist would have an even nicer looking car after it was fixed). The therapist then "decides" to add even more plastic chips to the angry feeling so that it has a larger amount. The child is then encouraged to think of a situation that was upsetting or the time when the trauma occurred and to put corresponding amounts of chips to show the intensity of and contradictory feelings experienced. The therapist explains how people can have more than one feeling at a time about a person or situation.

With Feelings Memory (Cavett, 2010), the therapist introduces two sets of index cards. In one set, each card has one feeling written on it, such as *annoyed, excited/surprised, sad, angry, happy, scared, worried*, or *calm*. Each card in the second set contains a scenario and physiological responses for the heartbeat, mouth, eyes, and muscle tone. The child can contribute the scenario, and the therapist writes down the various physical responses that are felt or can prewrite various scenarios and corresponding physical responses. The cards are then placed face down. The goal is for the feeling word to be matched to the corresponding physiological response. The players (therapist and child) put back the cards that don't match and try to remember their location. They keep selecting cards until they successfully remember the matching pairs, at which time they put the correct match in their pile until all the cards are matched.

Feeling Charades (Drewes, 2011) allows the child and parent to practice expressing feelings. A variety of positive and negative feelings are written on index cards. Each person takes a turn picking a card, and using pantomime only—no words or sounds—tries to get the other to guess the feeling. Another version involves taping a feeling card on the back of one person. The other "player" reads the feeling card and acts it out, with actions and facial expressions, for the other person to guess what the feeling is. Feelings Photo Shoot (Cavett, 2010) helps in feelings identification in self and others. The child makes a scrapbook of magazine pictures of people and animals expressing different feelings. They can be commercial pictures or cartoonish characters and can represent a variety of ethnic backgrounds, ages, and genders. These feeling pictures can open up discussion of common behaviors associated with the feelings and potential coping skills. The child lists several feelings and a book of five or more feelings is created. The therapist processes how the child looks when the feeling is expressed; how the parent looks; how a friend might show the feelings; where in his or her body it is felt; and some of the things the child typically does when he or she has the feeling.

Play-based techniques that integrate physical activity are helpful in engaging the young child and allow for physiological release and encoding, which may enhance learning. Mad Maracas (Goodyear-Brown, 2005) allows the child to experience sound volume related to the intensity of feeling. Weighing Things Out (Kenney-Noziska, 2008) lets the child visualize the intensity of the emotion and how it relates to coping skills. The Feelings Abacus (Cavett, 2010) provides an easy means for communicating about the intensity of feelings. The clinician can easily track the child's distress, based on the Subjective Units of Distress Scale, using this intervention. While used early in TF-CBT when implementing affective modulation, the same intervention may be understood and utilized during the processing of the trauma narrative.

Practicing feelings identification and expression through a variety of playful ways encourages the child to continue practicing them at home with family members, thereby increasing generalization and skill mastery.

Cognitive Coping

Puppet play, in general, can be used to enact scenarios common for the child, such as peer conflict, fears related to the bedroom, and being able to say "no" and be assertive as well as those addressing defiance and other behavioral issues. Role modeling in play is often met with less resistance than simple discussions. The clinician's playfulness allows for the message to be heard while adding details and alternative solutions. The child can feel empowered while rehearsing and enacting scenarios and practicing assertiveness skills.

Learning what a thought is and its connection to feelings and behaviors is often too complex for a young child to understand. Use of a three-headed dragon puppet (Drewes, 2011) visually shows the child that what we think, feel, and do are all interconnected. The goal is to help the "thought" dragon slow down or go to sleep so that the "feelings" and "acting" dragons can be heard or calm down. Alternatively, the Magnetic Cognitive Triangle (Cavett, 2010) uses a large magnetic board and colored magnet shapes for the same purpose. A large triangle is drawn on the board, with the corners labeled "feeling," "thinking," and "doing/actions," with a different shape used for each (e.g., heart for feeling, brain for thinking, and body for doing). Yellow octagon-shaped magnets are for feelings, red trapezoid magnets for behaviors, blue triangles for feelings, and orange diamonds for triggers or antecedents. A particular scenario can be used, with the child or therapist writing on the various magnets the corresponding thought, feeling, and behavior that ensued. Particular triggers or antecedents can be added, and all the magnets are arranged in a hierarchy of events along with solutions.

Creating a coping box (Drewes, 2011) also allows the child tools to use when thoughts or feelings become overwhelming. The therapist and child brainstorm about his or her favorite activities that make the child feel better and write each down on separate index cards. To each card the child adds a corresponding magazine picture or personal drawing. Ideas can include petting the family dog, listening to music, jumping rope, and asking for a hug, for example. The child then decorates a small box or an envelope where the coping strategies can be kept and referred to as needed. Creating personal affirmations (Drewes, 2011) can also be created in a similar way using magazine pictures and drawings. The child then has a set of index cards created with positive, helpful thoughts—such as "I am one of a kind," "My smile can make others smile back," "I am special," "I am brave"—that can counter his or her negative self-image and be empowering.

CLINICAL CASE DESCRIPTION

Jason: A 5-Year-Old Who Experienced a Natural Disaster/Flood

Jason is a 5-year-old white boy who presented with symptoms of anxiety following the flooding and destruction of his home. He exhibited crying and whining, and verbalized that he was afraid. He avoided stimuli that reminded him of the flood, and exhibited clinging behaviors when he sensed any indication of a storm. His sleep was especially disturbed because he had not been able to sleep in his own bed since the flood. His family was initially referred to the American Red Cross, where they were provided with resources to meet their basic needs, which were not addressed by the time of treatment onset despite the flood having occurred 3 months prior. The family was also encouraged to seek respite from family and friends to assist with Jason's care when his parents were involved with addressing insurance and clean-up needs.

Psychoeducation included a coloring book from the American Red Cross that included descriptions and information about several natural disasters as well as information about how to cope with stressors. In addition, *The Adventures of Lady: The Big Storm* (Pearson & Merrill, 2006) was utilized for bibliotherapy to show common responses and recovery/healing following a natural disaster. The therapist introduced bubble breathing, during which Jason inhaled slowly for 4 seconds, held his breath, exhaled slowly for 4 seconds, and then did nothing for 4 seconds. During his exhalation he blew bubbles. He also did "bear breathing," with a long, flat stuffed bear on his chest to watch going up and down. He utilized Cool and Calm Feather Breathing Dragon (Gobeil, 2010) to learn breathing techniques as well. This playful intervention was more engaging to him, and he was reminded in future sessions, sometimes with the dragon puppet, that he could change his breathing to decrease anxiety or anger. The therapist had Jason show these skills to his mother, who helped Jason practice them at home.

Jason utilized games including Feelings Ring-Toss (Cavett, 2012) and Feelings Hide-and-Seek (Kenney-Noziska, 2008). Feelings Ring-Toss is a five-spoke ring-toss game with colored rings. Each spoke had a different feeling depicted on a magnetic card. When the rings landed on the spokes, Jason and his mother showed the feeling on their own faces and talked about times when they had felt that way. Physiological responses to different feelings as well as both positive and negative behavioral reactions to feelings were processed.

The Magnetic Cognitive Triangle—Picture Version (Cavett, 2012) was utilized with Jason to explain the cognitive triangle and relationships among feelings, thoughts, and behaviors. Pictures of behaviors common to Jason were taken. Several incidents, both positive and negative, were reviewed using the Magnetic Cognitive Triangle to allow Jason practice with the concepts of the connection among his feelings, thoughts, behaviors, and triggers. The therapist also worked with the mother during individual parent sessions to help her learn about cognitive coping and to support Jason in using positive cognitive coping related to everyday situations.

Natisha: A 7-Year-Old Biracial Girl who Experienced Sexual Abuse

Natisha is a 7-year-old Native American girl who was referred by child protective services for TF-CBT following sexual abuse. She disclosed sexual abuse, including fondling and digital penetration by her mother's boyfriend. Natisha's half-sister was referred to a fellow TF-CBT clinician, allowing for collaboration on the case. Natisha's mother initially seemed overwhelmed by the therapy process and was resistant to commit to the TF-CBT sessions. She felt that Natisha was doing well since the boyfriend left the home, and the severe symptoms and sexual behavior problems had decreased. She also did not feel that Natisha would respond well to "talking about it" and acknowledged that in the past talk therapy had not been helpful for Natisha. Natisha exhibited anxiety related to the sexual abuse. Initially, she demonstrated some sexualized behaviors with other children, such as touching a peer's private parts in the school bathroom. She continued to have nightmares and times during the day when she seemed to "zone out," after which she indicated that she was thinking about the abuse. She had somatic complaints, including stomachaches and refusal to urinate, which may have been related to a history of pain with urination caused by a urinary tract infection while the abuse was occurring.

As Natisha and her mother discussed the areas of concern and the treatment goals, they worked on a playful treatment planning activity. First, they cut six colorful steps from construction paper, with Natisha writing the problem on each step. They cut out six feet from the construction paper, and for each one Natisha, along with her mother and therapist, identified skills that could help them meet the respective goal.

Natisha enjoyed books, and the vehicle for psychoeducation was often bibliotherapy. *A Very Touching Book* (Hindman, 1983) was utilized after getting permission from her mother. Natisha and her therapist played Paper Airplanes, a game developed to help children think about what is sexual abuse (Crisci, Lay, & Lowenstein, 1998). When introducing relaxation, *A Boy and a Bear* (Lite, 1996) was utilized to show Natisha an example of progressive muscle relaxation. Afterward, Natisha, her mother, and the therapist acted out the steps. Each of them also had a stuffed bear beside them as they tightened and relaxed their muscles.

Relaxation exercises included Natisha singing a song with her mother at night. It was a traditional song that was soothing and connected Natisha to the culture. While Natisha and her mother sang, they would take turns drumming a wooden and leather drum. Natisha's mother expressed appreciation for the culturally sensitive aspects of TF-CBT after feeling that social services had not always provided such sensitivity.

When learning about feelings and as a positive nurturing experience, Natisha and her therapist utilized the *Mood Manicure* (Goodyear-Brown, 2002), which consists of choosing colors of fingernail polish that Natisha matched with feelings and discussing the feelings while having the therapist paint her nails. She also utilized the Feelings Abacus (Cavett, 2010), which allowed Natisha to learn about labels for feelings and measuring the intensity.

The *Magnetic Cognitive Triangle* was utilized to teach about cognitive behavioral concepts and introduce how feelings, thoughts, and behaviors are related. Natisha spent time talking about different feelings that were on the board and added a couple that were not on the board. She was introduced to the behaviors on the board and discussed several positive and negative behaviors. She was also introduced to common feelings that children have after experiencing sexual abuse. Being able to manipulate the magnets to show the flow of feelings, thoughts, and behaviors was helpful for Natisha. The concept of changing one's thoughts and having feelings change as a result was introduced with the Magnetic Cognitive Triangle. During individual sessions with the mother, the therapist also introduced the cognitive triangle and started to address some of the mother's personal maladaptive cognitions related to Natisha's sexual abuse (e.g., "I should have known my boyfriend was sexually abusing Natisha").

CONCLUSION

Integrating play with TF-CBT skills components can be highly beneficial, particularly for young children. Moreover, encouraging children to choose from alternative play interventions supports their feelings of control, joy, and mastery while simultaneously achieving the specific TF-CBT component goals. Therapists, however, must maintain the structural integrity of the TF-CBT model—that is, use play to implement specific TF-CBT components in a systematic and planned manner consistent with the TF-CBT model rather than allowing child-directed or nonstructured play to replace this structure. Otherwise, the fidelity of the TF-CBT model will be compromised.

REFERENCES

Association for Play Therapy. (2011). *Play therapy makes a difference!* Retrieved June 2, 2011, from *www.a4pt.org/ps.index.cfm?ID=1653*.

Bratton, S., Roy, D., Rhine, T., & Jones, L. (2005). The efficacy of play therapy with children: A meta-analytic review of the outcome research. *Professional Psychology: Research, and Practice, 36,* 376–390.

Briggs, K.M., Runyon, M. K., & Deblinger, E. (2011). The use of play in trauma-focused cognitive-behavioral therapy. In S.W. Russ & L.N. Niec (Eds.), *Play in clinical practice: Evidence-based approaches* (pp. 169–200). New York: Guilford Press.

Budd, D. (2008). What if game. In L. Lowenstein (Ed.), *Assessment and treatment activities for children, adolescents, and families*: Practitioners share their most effective techniques (pp. 34–36). Toronto: Champion Press.

Cavett, A. M. (2010). *Structured play-based interventions for engaging children and adolescents in therapy.* West Conshohocken, PA: Infinity.

Cavett, A. (2012). *Enhancing cognitive behavioral therapy with children with the magnetic cognitive triangle.* West Conshohocken, PA: Infinity.

Cavett, A. (2012). *Play-based cognitive behavioral techniques for children.* West Conshohocken, PA: Infinity Press.

Chaloner, W. B. (2001). Counselors coaching teachers to use play therapy in classrooms: The play and language to succeed (PALS) early, school-based intervention for behaviorally at-risk children. In A. A. Drewes, L. Carey, & C. E. Schaefer (Eds.), *School-based play therapy* (pp. 368–390). New York: Wiley.

Cohen, J. A., & Mannarino, A. P. (1996). A treatment outcome study for sexually abused preschool children: Initial findings. *Journal of the American Academy of Child and Adolescent Psychiatry, 35,* 42–50.

Crenshaw, D. A. (2008). Heartfelt feelings coloring cards strategies. In L. Lowenstein (Ed.), *Assessment and treatment activities for children, adolescents, and families: Practitioners share their most effective tchniques* (pp. 80–81). Toronto: Champion Press.

Crisci, G., Lay, M., & Lowenstein, L. (1998). *Paper dolls and paper airplanes: Ther-*

apeutic exercises for sexually traumatized children. Indianapolis, IN: Kids-rights.

Deblinger, E., Neubauer, F., Runyon, M. K., & Baker, D. (2006). *What do you know?: A therapeutic card game about child sexual, physical abuse, and domestic violence.* Stratford, NJ: CARES Institute.

Deblinger, E., & Heflin, A. H. (1996). *Treating sexually abused children and their nonoffending parents.* Thousand Oaks, CA: Sage.

Deblinger, E., McLeer, S. V., & Henry, D. E. (1990). Cognitive behavioral treatment for sexually abused children suffering post-traumatic stress: Preliminary findings. *Journal of the American Academy of Child and Adolescent Psychiatry, 29,* 747–752.

Drewes, A. A. (2001). Gingerbread person feelings map. In H. G. Kaduson & C. E. Schaefer (Eds.), *101 more favorite play therapy techniques* (pp. 92–97). Northvale, NJ: Jason Aronson.

Drewes, A. A. (2005). Play in selected cultures: Diversity and universality. In E. Gil & A. A. Drewes (Eds.), *Cultural issues in play therapy* (pp. 26–71). New York: Guilford Press.

Drewes, A. A. (2006). Play-based interventions. *Journal of Early Childhood and Infant Psychology, 2,* 139–156.

Drewes, A. A. (2009). *Blending play therapy with cognitive behavioral therapy: Evidence-based and other effective treatments and techniques.* New York: Wiley.

Drewes, A. A. (2011, April). *A skill-building workshop: Effectively blending play-based techniques with cognitive behavioral therapy for affect regulation in sexually abused and traumatized children.* Paper presented at the annual conference of the Canadian Association for Child and Play Therapy, Guelph, ON, Canada.

Drewes, A. A., Bratton, S. C., & Schaefer, C. E. (2011). *Integrative play therapy.* New York: Wiley.

Gaensbauer, T., & Siegal, C. (1995). Therapeutic approaches to posttraumatic stress disorder in infants and toddlers. *Infant Mental Health Journal, 16,* 292–305.

Gil, E. (1991). *The healing power of play:* Working with abused children. New York: Guilford Press.

Gil, E. (2006). *Helping abused and traumatized children: Integrating directive and nondirective approaches.* New York: Guilford Press.

Gobeil, J. (2010). Cool and calm feather breathing dragon. In L. Lowenstein (Ed.), Assessment and treatment activities for children, adolescents, and families: *Practitioners share their most effective techniques* (Vol. 2, pp. 82–83). Toronto: Champion Press.

Golomb, C., & Galasso, L. (1995). Make believe and reality: Explorations of the imaginary realm. *Developmental Psychology, 31,* 800–810.

Goodyear-Brown, P. (2002). *Digging for buried treasure: 52 prop-based play therapy interventions for treating the problems of childhood.* Nashville, TN: Author.

Goodyear-Brown, P. (2005). *Digging for buried treasure 2: Another 52 prop-based play therapy interventions for treating the problems of childhood.* Nashville, TN: Author.

Goodyear-Brown, P. (2010). *Play therapy with traumatized children: A prescriptive approach.* New York: Wiley.

Haworth, M. R. (1964). *Child psychotherapy: Practice and theory.* Northvale, NJ: Jason Aronson.

Hindman, J. (1983). *A very touching book for little people and for big people.* Ontario, OR: Alexandria Associates.

Horn, T. (1997). Balloons of anger. In H. Kaduson & C. Schaefer (Eds.), *101 favorite play therapy techniques* (pp. 250–253). Northvale, NJ: Jason Aronson.

James, B. (1989). *Treating traumatized children: New insights and creative interventions.* New York: Free Press.

Kaduson, H. G. (2001). Broadcast news. In H. G. Kaduson & C. E. Schaefer (Eds.), *101 more favorite play therapy techniques* (pp. 397–400). Northvale, NJ: Jason Aronson.

Kenney-Noziska, S. (2008). *Techniques—techniques—techniques: Play-based activities for children, adolescents, and families.* West Conshohocken, PA: Infinity.

Knell, S. M. (1993). *Cognitive-behavioral play therapy.* Northvale, NJ: Jason Aronson.

Knell, S. M., & Beck, K. W. (2000). Puppet sentence completion task. In C.E. Schaefer (Ed.), *Foundations of play therapy* (pp. 175–191). New York: Wiley.

Knell, S. M., & Dasari, M. (2009). CBPT: Implementing and integrating CBPT into clinical practice. In A. Drewes (Ed.), *Blending play therapy with cognitive behavioral therapy. Evidence-based and other effective treatments and techniques* (pp. 321–352). New York: Wiley.

Knell, S. M., & Dasari, M. (2011). Cognitive-behavioral play therapy. In S. W. Russ & L. N. Niec (Eds.), *Play in clinical practice: Evidence-based approaches* (pp. 236–262). New York: Guilford Press.

Landreth, G. (2002). *Play therapy: The art of the relationship* (2nd ed.). New York: Routledge.

Leben, N. (2008). The "Talking Ball" game. In L. Lowenstein (Ed.), *Assessment and treatment activities for children, adolescents and families: Practitioners share their most effective techniques* (pp. 2–3). Toronto: Champion Press.

Lidz, C.S. (2006). *Early childhood assessment.* New York: Wiley.

Lite, L. (1996). *A boy and a bear.* Plantation, FL: Specialty Press.

Meichenbaum, D. (2009). Foreword. In A. A. Drewes (Ed.), *Blending play therapy with cognitive behavioral therapy: Evidence-based and other effective treatments and techniques* (pp. xxi–xxiii). New York: Wiley.

O'Connor, K. K. (1983). The color your life technique. In C. E. Schaefer & K. J. O'Connor (Eds.), *Handbook of play therapy.* New York: Wiley.

Pearson, I., & Merrill, M. (2006). *The adventures of Lady: The big storm.* Orlando, FL: The Adventures of Lady, LLC.

Reddy, L. A., Files-Hall, T. M., & Schaefer, C. E. (2005). *Empirically based play interventions for children.* Washington, DC: American Psychological Association.

Russ, S. W. (2004). *Play in child development and psychotherapy: Toward empirically supported practice.* Mahwah, NJ: Erlbaum.

Russ, S. W. (2007). Pretend play: A resource for children who are coping with stress and managing anxiety. *NYS Psychologist, XIX,* 13–17.

Russ, S. W., Fiorelli, J., & Spannagel, S. C. (2011). Cognitive and affective processes in play. In S. W. Russ & L. N. Niec (Eds.), *Play in clinical practice: Evidence-based approaches* (pp. 3–22). New York: Guilford Press.

Russ, S. W. & Niec, L. N. (Eds.). (2011). *Play in clinical practice. Evidence-based approaches.* New York: Guilford Press.

Schaefer, C. E. (1993). The therapeutic powers of play. Northvale, NJ: Aronson.

Schaefer, C. E., & Drewes, A. A. (2009). The therapeutic powers of play and play therapy. In A. A. Drewes (Ed.), *Blending play therapy with cognitive behavioral therapy: Evidence-based and other effective treatments and techniques* (pp. 1–15). New York: Wiley.

Scott, D., Feldman, J., & Patterson, S. (1993). *No-no and the secret touch: The gentle story of a little seal who learns to stay safe, say "no" and tell!* San Rafael, CA: National Self-Esteem Resources & Development Center.

Sheppard, C. H. (1998). *Brave bart: A story for traumatic and grieving children.* Grosse Pointe Woods, MI: Institute for trauma and loss in children.

Short, G. F. (1997). Feelings balloons. In H. Kaduson & C. Schaefer (Eds.), *101 favorite play therapy techniques* (pp. 59–60). Northvale, NJ: Jason Aronson.

Singer, D. G., & Singer, J. L. (1990). *The house of make-believe: Children's play and the developing imagination.* Cambridge, MA: Harvard University Press.

Tharinger, D. J., Christopher, G. B., & Matson, M. (2011). Play, playfulness, and creativity in therapeutic assessment with children. In S. W. Russ & L. N. Niec (Eds.), *Play in clinical practice: Evidence-based approaches* (pp. 109–145). New York: Guilford Press.

ADDITIONAL RESOURCES

Huebner, D. (2008). *What to do when your temper flares: A kid's guide to overcoming problems with anger.* Washington, DC: Magination Press.

Kaduson, H. G., & Schaefer, C. E. (Eds.). (1997). *101 favorite play therapy techniques,* Northvale, NJ: Jason Aronson.

Kaduson, H. G., & Schaefer, C. E. (Eds.). (2001). *101 more favorite play therapy techniques.* Northvale, NJ: Jason Aronson.

Kaduson, H. G., & Schaefer, C. E. (Eds.). (2003). *101 favorite play therapy techniques: Volume III.* Northvale, NJ: Jason Aronson.

Sunderland, M. (2003). *Helping children locked in rage or hate.* Oxon, UK: Speechmark.

Whitehouse, E., & Pudney, W. (1996). *A volcano in my tummy: Helping children to handle anger.* Gabriola Island, BC, Canada: New Society.

5

Play Applications and Trauma–Specific Components

ANGELA M. CAVETT
ATHENA A. DREWES

OVERVIEW OF TF-CBT PLAY APPLICATIONS
AND TRAUMA-SPECIFIC COMPONENTS

In the initial work with trauma-focused cognitive-behavioral therapy
(TF-CBT), clinicians utilized a playful approach, and incorporated many
art activities, games, and songs that were engaging and developmentally
responsive. Yet clinicians sometimes find implementing TF-CBT with their
youngest clients challenging. The directive play therapy literature describes
additional play interventions that can be effectively incorporated into the
treatment process to support and individualize the implementation of each
of the TF-CBT components (Cavett, 2009a, 2009b). Directive play therapists have described in detail structured, play-based interventions that fit
in the TF-CBT framework (Goodyear-Brown, 2002, 2005; Cavett, 2010,
2012a, 2012b; Kenney-Noziska, 2008; Lowenstein, 2002, 2006a, 2006b,
2008, 2010a, 2010b, 2011). In the previous chapter, Drewes and Cavett
outlined the use of play in TF-CBT for the skills-based components. This
chapter addresses the use of play for the more intensive trauma-related components, including developing and processing the trauma narrative.

The skills learned from the skills-based components, discussed by
Drewes and Cavett (Chapter 4, this volume), are foundational in implementing TF-CBT. The more intensive trauma-related components included in this

124

chapter focus on assisting the child in developing the trauma narrative and processing it as well as safety planning and *in vivo* exposure. As with the skills components, the more intensive trauma-related components can be enhanced with the use of play. The use of play allows the child a developmentally appropriate method of communicating and processing the trauma narrative. Using play is consistent with the core values of TF-CBT because it is flexible and allows for the development of the therapeutic relationship. Indeed, from the development of the model, the originators of TF-CBT have encouraged the use of art, games, role plays, music, and playfulness in its implementation.

Challenges may exist for clinicians treating young children with TF-CBT related to the more intensive trauma-related components. Using play to tell and process the narrative is engaging. Play is the language of children (Landreth, 1991), and allowing them to process and learn about each of the TF-CBT components through play is developmentally appropriate. Although children may not have words to express themselves, often in play narratives they communicate more thoroughly. Play is also helpful for children using TF-CBT because it allows for the concrete representation of abstract concepts. A concrete object may be manipulated, which facilitates learning. Play may help children to learn concepts that may be difficult when only described verbally. However, when understanding the concept through visual and experiential processing, learning may occur at a deeper level of understanding. Play is adaptive to the individual child's developmental level, cultural identity, and individual interests. Young children do not experience trauma primarily as a verbal experience, which is especially important during the telling and processing of the narrative. Play allows children expression that is multisensory. Their expression is also limited when it is restricted to verbal responses. Case in point: Processing a trauma narrative in the dollhouse allows the child to act out aspects of the trauma that may not have been articulated in a verbal narrative.

INTRODUCING NARRATIVES

Older children utilizing TF-CBT are often introduced to the trauma narrative with the "cut metaphor." The therapist discusses how the trauma is like a cut, which needs to be taken care of to keep it from getting infected. The cut is cleaned out with soap and any rocks or dirt in it are removed so that the cut does not get infected. The parent also helps with the cut's healing by being loving and nurturing during this process, gently cleaning the cut, wiping away tears, and giving hugs. With young children, the verbal telling of the cut metaphor may be enhanced with toys. Reparative toys are valuable resources to use while verbalizing the concept of cleaning, medicating, and covering a wound in order to assist in the healing process. Children who have been traumatized often gravitate toward toys that represent healing, such as medical kits. Children use the toys as receptive and expressive language tools. Using the "fixing" toys example, children process what it means to help someone heal and show how they feel a need for fixing or healing. Children at times verbalize their experience of the trauma as a time when they felt hurt. The therapist hears the spoken language and responds empathically. Likewise, the therapist may also appreciate the unspoken themes communicated by children through play, such as using bandages and a medical kit to express that they have been hurt. The clinician then empathically encourages further verbalization of the once unspoken experience.

Baseline Narrative

With the older child or the child who verbalizes the trauma narrative without play, the clinician initially has the child tell a less emotionally intense, baseline narrative. Likewise, it is important for clinicians to observe the young child creating and processing a different story with his or her play. Play of nontraumatic events facilitates the child's telling of the trauma at a later point in therapy. Playing out nontraumatic events also places the trauma into the context of the child's life as a part of the total experience but not the one defining moment. After the skills-based components are adequately covered in sessions, the therapist observes play by asking the child to show an incident that has occurred in his or her life. The therapist and child can discuss recent events and choose a positive experience for the child to reenact with the toys (i.e., dollhouse). This reenactment, as with the verbal baseline narrative, provides the clinician valuable information about how the child typically communicates and plays. This baseline allows the therapist to note any significant changes in the child's style of communication or play when traumatic memories are evoked during the trauma narrative process.

Enhancing the Trauma Narrative with Bibliotherapy

Psychoeducation through bibliotherapy may be utilized throughout the treatment and often during the development and processing of the narrative. Children often benefit from hearing stories that provide information about characters who have undergone similar traumas or that depict an unnamed trauma that could be generalized across traumas. It allows children and parents to understand the trauma and common responses. Books related to the specific trauma, such as *The Adventures of Lady: The Big Storm* (Pearson & Merrill, 2006) or *No-No and the Secret Touch* (Scott, Feldman, & Patterson, 1986), are beneficial for opening discussion related to the concept of trauma, psychological symptomatology, and healing. However, more general books related to the concept of "something bad happening," such as that described in *Brave Bart* (Sheppard, 1998), are also helpful. Playing out the concepts in the book with puppets or toys either during or after the reading of the book deepens children's understanding and allows them to integrate the concepts.

Pacing the Narrative

Pacing the development and processing of the trauma narrative is crucial in enhancing the child's positive experience. The child who has been traumatized may either want to tell what happened soon after initiating therapy, even in the first session, or more typically indicate that he or she does not want to talk about it ever. Pacing of the trauma narrative begins by setting the telling/playing out of the trauma narrative within a therapeutic context that provides the structure to make the narrative a healing experience. This pacing allows the therapist to communicate that certain skills need to be learned and used before the telling of the narrative. Using a playful intervention such as the Nested Boxes: Building Coping Skills Prior to Processing Trauma intervention (Cavett, 2010) allows the therapist, child, and parent to understand the sequential process of TF-CBT. The Nested Boxes intervention provides the opportunity for each of the steps, representing the TF-CBT components, to be discussed in terms of building on earlier skills throughout therapy. By using such a visual representation, the child and parent understand that there are steps that will be taken in therapy prior to telling the trauma narrative. The steps are important for emotional safety and processing of the trauma. However, it is important to avoid placing too much emphasis on any single component, particularly with respect to the trauma narrative. Exposure to traumatic memories occurs throughout the treatment process, making the transition to the trauma narrative component very gradual and natural, like taking just one more "step" in the journey.

Later, pacing of the narrative is essential in facilitating the gradual exposure work as a beneficial experience. Therapeutic discretion should be utilized to decide whether the skills-based components have been acquired to the degree necessary to be helpful during the narrative. The therapist must also observe the children and the play for cues as to how they are feeling. Setting a specific amount of time, as is done with verbal narratives (Cohen, Mannarino, & Deblinger, 2006), can be helpful with play narratives as well. An increase in distress is natural during this process, and most children can endure some distress and "play" through it, allowing them to ultimately learn that it is okay to cry and express upset feelings. In addition, through this process, children learn that the distress is not enduring but naturally subsides on its own. Monitoring their responses and levels of distress is important because it often helps children recognize that each replaying of the traumatic experience becomes less distressing over time. Using a nonverbal tool such as the Feelings Abacus (Cavett, 2010) before, during, and after the trauma narrative provides the opportunity for children to communicate how anxious, scared, or upset they feel without interrupting the play, and helps the therapist pace the telling/playing of the trauma narrative. For some children, however, it may help to encourage the use of coping skills such as relaxation when necessary during the telling of the narrative. Beforehand, the therapist and child can agree that if the child shows anxiety elevated to a certain degree, the narrative will be stopped briefly so the child can practice calming using relaxation techniques such as drawing a picture of a calm, peaceful place. Balancing Out Your Feelings technique (Kenney-Noziska, 2008) is a play-based intervention helpful in matching coping skills with level of anxiety. In the intervention, a scale is used to show intensity of affect while the other side represents coping skills used. Play used in this way to help children face traumatic memories and associated fears builds feelings of mastery.

Creating the Trauma Narrative with Young Children

Some young children may resist a verbal narrative or talking about the trauma but may be willing, even eager, to tell the story through play. Typically, older children tell their trauma narratives or may use other forms of expression, including drawings or songwriting. Younger children may be asked to play out the narrative or use another means of expression that the therapist feels is consistent with their interests and abilities. Often initial trauma narratives are simple and short, and this is especially true for very young children. The narrative includes words that the children have heard from others through the process of investigation by social services or the court system or by parents who have spoken about the trauma. Even for adults and older children, putting a traumatic event into words may be extremely difficult. For young children it is often even more challenging.

The narrative is most effective if the process is adapted to allow children their personal most comfortable form of expression. The recording of the events of the narrative should also reflect their communication strengths. Some older children feel empowered by writing all or parts of the narrative. Typically, young children benefit from having the therapist act as the "secretary" as they dictate the narrative. Even for children who are capable of writing, having the therapist act as the secretary results in more details of the trauma being shared. The method of telling the narrative is adapted for each child based on their personality and interests. To illustrate, some children enjoy using a microphone and clap board, whereas others will resist the suggestion and may become more anxious. Clinical discretion should determine what tools may be helpful based on individual needs. As children play out their narrative, the therapist writes their stories from beginning to end, with as many details as possible. The therapist can use statements from children's verbal narrative, told earlier, to prompt the play. Reflecting their play verbally and then writing it into the narrative allows children to clarify any mistakes and misinterpretations. To illustrate, a child may show a male figure in the dollhouse using a toy frying pan to hit the female character. If the child has already identified the male and female figures as his or her own parents, the therapist may refer to them as such in the reflection. The therapist also reflects using a nonspecific term to describe what the child played out, such as "Your dad did that to your mom with that." The child will usually fill in the specifics, and if not, a hesitant pause while verbalizing the statement allows the child an opportunity to state what happened. The child may say "My dad hit my mom with the shovel over and over." As the trauma narrative is told repeatedly, the child is encouraged to tell what he or she was feeling and thinking at different points.

While the child is preparing to tell the narrative, the therapist is attentive to his or her verbal, emotional, and behavioral responses. This allows the therapist to determine what options may be helpful in allowing expression of the trauma narrative for each child. The process typically begins with a verbal narrative or description of the trauma. The therapist dances between verbal and play interventions to deepen the narrative. Several play interventions are provided as options to the child. These include the sand tray, play buildings (dollhouse, police station, court house, and fire station), puppets, and songs. Alternatively, if a therapist feels confident that a child uses a certain means of expression naturally, this may be offered as a way to tell about the narrative. If during the free play time during earlier sessions the child often gravitated to the dollhouse to play out scenarios, the therapist may say that the child can use the dollhouse to show what happened during the trauma. Examples in Angela Cavett's practice are children who were impacted by the trauma of flooding. Often during the free play at the end of the sessions focusing on the skills components of TF-CBT, the children play in the sand. This may provide a minimal level of exposure to a sensory trigger related to their traumatic experiences, which included sandbagging. When one's community has millions of sandbags around, children and adults often feel sand and this later reminds them of the time when their homes flooded or were close to flooding. As the children play in the sand, it is evident that this may allow for a deeper processing, which includes sensory memories.

Puppets may be made for and by the child and may represent the child, perpetrator, and/or other important figures in the narrative. Puppets may also represent figures related to the fantasies (i.e., rescue or retaliation) of the child related to the trauma. Homemade puppets created from lunch bags, muslin, or tongue depressor craft sticks (Cavett, 2010; Drewes, 2011) can be used to depict each person, from the child's perspective, who was involved in the trauma or the events following it. Often a greater depth of emotion and other aspects of the person are revealed through the puppets the child creates than through the words the child expresses. Case in point: In Angela Cavett's practice, a child created puppets of both of his parents, himself, and his siblings for his trauma narrative. Although he did not indicate verbally that his mother was sad, he drew her puppet character with tears. As the trauma narrative was developed and resolution discussed, which occurred several sessions later, the child asked for another puppet to decorate and made a new mother puppet that was smiling. When initially discussing his sharing of the narrative with his mother, he indicated that he did not want his mother to see the crying puppet. As he processed his feelings and she was able to communicate that she was sad during the traumatic events, they both found more resolution to an unspoken concept: "My mom could not handle this and I must protect her from it." As he used the puppets, he was able to allow her to see the crying mother puppet, and she processed with him how scary her response of hopelessness and depression had been. They also processed how she has learned to share her feelings and thoughts and now feels hope for the future while accepting the traumatic event as a part of their shared history.

Some children use music as a form of expression that is natural for them and may incorporate music into the trauma narrative. Taking another example from Cavett's practice, to tell her trauma narrative, one child adapted a country singer's song about losing a loved one in war and added verses to describe her own father's death in Afghanistan.

Some children, Native American and non-Native American, have gravitated toward expressing their narratives through journey sticks (BigFoot & Schmidt, 2010). With this intervention, children use a stick to represent their lifeline and decorate it to symbolize different times in their lives. For children with multiple traumas, this can allow a visual and experiential processing of life and how the traumatic events have fit into their lives overall.

Richard Gardner's The Story Telling Game is helpful for children telling their narratives. The game provides paper doll characters across developmental levels and racial identities. Background scenes—for example, homes, bedrooms, schools, playgrounds—are provided. The game can be offered as an alternative for children telling their trauma narrative.

Children may create a scrapbook as part of their trauma narrative and processing to help understand the trauma. It is helpful for them to include photos or drawings of different tasks representing each of the trauma and nontrauma components that were taught and utilized in the session. This may be done in a similar sequence as the order of the components presented in sessions. Including copies of pictures the children drew in therapy can be helpful if clinically indicated. Pictures may include scenes from the play narrative if it seems this would be helpful. Given the depth of psychological information contained in a scrapbook or other narrative, the therapist should use discretion about the content of a written or pictorial narrative given to the children to keep at the end of treatment.

Deepening the Narrative through Play

Cohen and colleagues (2006) suggest that children retell their narratives after each segment to provide additional exposure. The narratives are told over the course of sessions in order to have the experience communicated more fully and to assess feelings and thoughts related to the experience. One of the most important challenges for young children derives from their lack of verbal skills to communicate details and address feelings, thoughts, behaviors, and sensory experiences related to the trauma narrative. It seems likely that the more detailed the trauma narrative is, the more reparative it may be for the children.

The verbal narrative of young children may include words that they have heard from others. Often when the trauma was experienced, the initial description was sensory in nature, not verbal. Children may not know the descriptive words related to their traumas until after it has occurred. However, as parents, police, social workers, and others become involved, they begin to hear words that are associated with the trauma. Often children's first narrative is vague, such as "I was sexually abused" or "My dad touched my private parts." These may be the words or phrases that adults have used to describe the traumatic experience.

The therapist may incorporate the same words the child used as a description in the narrative to prompt the child's playful narrative. The child may be told, "When you were telling me your story of what happened, you said 'I was sexually abused,' but I am wondering if you could use the dollhouse to show me what happened when you were sexually abused." The child's verbal ability may be enhanced by the stimuli provided by play materials. One of the most important benefits of using play is that experiences that cannot be verbalized can be reenacted. Toys, such as a dollhouse, allow a child to show the context in which the trauma happened. In the dollhouse the child may show details that were not offered verbally, such as "Mom was standing behind the corner when dad was walking down the hall." The words may be beyond the verbal ability of the child, but by using the dollhouse and with the therapist's reflection the narrative is told through the child's play and the therapist's recording. The therapist may comment on the play that "Mom was standing behind the corner and dad was walking down the hall." Young children interact with the therapist and provide corrections. The child may say, "She was in the closet because she was hiding from him." The child often asks for props that resemble those he or she remembers from the trauma and comments on the differences between the toys available for reenacting the trauma and how he or she recalls it. At times, videotaping of the narrative is helpful. The child and therapist may watch the play narrative and process feelings and thoughts related to it.

Including Sensory Memories in the Narrative

Trauma may be experienced through the child's senses. Therefore, sharing sensory memories is essential. The child's telling of the trauma and the clinician's witnessing and verbalizing it through descriptive comments about the child's play allow the child to begin to process a nonverbal, sensory-based traumatic experience in a verbal manner. Increasing sensory-based verbalizations allows the therapist to understand how the child lived through and processed the trauma. The child feels heard by the therapist as the therapist better understands what it was like to be in the child's shoes. Play, therefore, seems to enhance the child's efforts to share traumatic memories in words.

Given a young child's limitations of verbal communication, using play to assist in the expression of the trauma and how it was experienced sensually is often beneficial. Therefore, a play intervention such as Putting the Pieces Together (Goodyear-Brown, 2005) or Re-Building Mr. or Mrs. Potato Head: Processing Traumatic Sensory Memories and Providing Healing Sensory Memories (Cavett, 2012b) may be helpful as details are added to the initial trauma narrative. Using either of these interventions allows for dialogue about what the child sensed (i.e., heard or tasted) during the trauma. The child plays with a toy, such as Mr. Potato Head, while the trauma narrative is read, and as he or she puts in each piece of the puzzle or each part on Mr. Potato Head, the child adds details to the trauma narrative about what was heard, felt (hands), seen (glasses or eyes), or tasted (tongue or lips). Placing the hat on the Mr. Potato Head opens up an opportunity for the child to discuss thoughts during the narrative.

TRAUMA PROCESSING

The processing of the trauma blends together with the telling of the narrative. As the children express their memories of the trauma, feelings and thoughts related to it will be expressed. The categorization of feelings and thoughts may be confusing to young children. Using a tool like the Magnetic Cognitive Triangle is helpful in differentiating feelings from thoughts. As with the other TF–CBT components, understanding the Magnetic Cognitive Triangle prior to beginning the narrative is beneficial.

Considering Themes of Play as Insight into Unspoken Feelings and Thoughts

Children likely benefit most when more emotionally intense aspects of the trauma are processed. Therefore, with verbal narratives for older children, one may ask them to make sure they share the most difficult aspects of the traumatic event. With young children, there may be times during the play narrative when they seem "stuck," and this must be assessed and processed. At times, children may play out the initial aspects of the narrative, and then nonrealistic things appear that may indicate overwhelming affective and cognitive responses, likely both at the time of the trauma and during the processing. By reflecting the children's behaviors in the play narrative, both the children and the therapist can explore how the play reflects thoughts and feelings. To illustrate, when a child figure begins falling off the house or floating, this may indicate a feeling/cognitive state, the therapist can explore to better understand the child's experience. Feelings may include a sense of numbness or being in a dissociative state, or the cognition may be "I wish I could escape/float away." It is especially important to introduce and acknowledge the sense of numbness when teaching feelings during the skills phase because this is common among children who have experienced trauma. However, it is infrequently included in standard feeling posters or commercially processed feeling cards. The play narrative allows children to tell what the trauma was like from their perspective more accurately and completely. Four important themes of play are common with children who have experienced trauma: symbolism, rescue/revenge fantasies, blame/responsibility, and fixing.

Symbolism

Cohen and colleagues (2006) suggest that if a child expresses inaccurate (verbalized) thoughts about the trauma, these should be included in the narrative and later explored and processed. In the play narrative, this is especially true as the child may express his or her trauma with play that reflects his or her perceptions of the experience. When asked to use play to develop the narrative, a child may begin to show what happened but then add details that seem unrealistic. The perceptions this play suggests can provide powerful insight into the child's difficulties and can facilitate healing as they are processed. At times the child may use toys to express the experience in a nonverbal manner that is not factual. Toys may be used to represent the experience or the people involved (e.g., an abusive stepfather may be represented in the play narrative by a monster figure when the abuse is being played out but by an adult male figure when nonabusive). An adult may say, "My stepdad was a monster when he abused me," while a child may "say" this through his or her play. Play gives insight into the unspoken thoughts that are too complex for a child to express verbally. The clinician observes play to gather information about thoughts too confusing or complex to verbalize initially. After witnessing play behaviors, the therapist encourages and supports the child in sharing the details of the traumatic events through play and further communicating feelings and thoughts with words.

Rescue/Revenge Fantasies

In verbal narratives, children may express fantasies of rescue or revenge. Such fantasies are also noted when children develop play narratives. A trauma narrative may include other figures (i.e., superhero, police, fantasy parent) that depict rescuers, or children may show in their play a desire to have been able to rescue themselves or others. Children may also depict revenge (the perpetrator being put into a jail or a box) in their play. When narratives depict events that did not occur, the therapist can note verbally what he or she is observing in the play and encourage the children to further communicate their perceptions. To illustrate, a child may depict a perpetrator as having gone to jail by placing the figure in the play jail. The therapist then notes the play behavior and encourages the child to expound on it, typically with reflective statements. Doing so enables the child to express thoughts such as "He did something that hurt me" or "My mom thinks he should be in jail." As with verbal narratives, play narratives that include such fantasy play should be considered part of children's perception of self, others, and the experience. The details of such play inform the processing of the trauma experience by allowing children expression of complex thoughts and feelings that without play might be beyond developmentally normative language.

To illustrate, a child who was sexually abused by her father feels that her mother, if present at the time of the abuse, would have been able to rescue her. Since her mother was not there, the child may feel that she did not deserve protection and cannot expect to be protected in the future. The rescue fantasy can allow the therapist to articulate that the child did deserve to be protected and that efforts will be made to reduce the chances of something similar happening in the future (i.e., enhancing safety component).

Blame/Responsibility

When included in the processing of the narrative, play can be helpful in assessing self-blame and reprocessing it. Children often feel responsible for traumas that are not within their control. At times, there may be instances when a trauma occurred and the children, although not responsible, may have exhibited a behavior that impacted the situation. When discussing behaviors that are important for safety, it is imperative that the children are not blamed. However, as part of safety planning, some behaviors may be suggested in the future to reduce their risk of further trauma or victimization. To illustrate, a child who is bitten by a strange dog after running up to it and grabbing at its eyes while making noise is not to blame for the dog bite but should learn appropriate behaviors related to being around dogs and other animals. Using role play to act out scenarios is a playful activity that can reduce the risk of future harm through education and modeling.

Fixing

Cohen and colleagues (2006) discuss children's need to have a reparative activity related to traumatic grief (e.g., a child visualizing a deceased loved one, whose body was not found or was severely damaged at the time of death, as being repaired in a hospital). This reparative theme in the play is evident both in nonfatal traumas and fatalities. Children's need for fixing and repairing themselves or loved ones who suffered in the trauma is healing. To help children process the trauma, and incorporating the reparative theme, at different points during the narrative it is helpful to consider with them what actually helped or might have helped them feel safe.

ASSESSING PLAY AS INSIGHT INTO THE CHILD'S THOUGHTS AND FEELINGS

Young children's difficulties with separating feelings and thoughts are especially pronounced when working on the narrative. Therefore, understanding the cognitive triangle is essential prior to processing the narrative. Young children sometimes have difficulty saying what they are thinking. However, their thoughts may be revealed in their play. Their trauma-specific play provides a view of their perspective of the trauma, which can be processed using play-based interventions.

Often when children, and especially younger ones, first tell the trauma narrative, they do not verbalize cognitive distortions. Instead, they often tell cognitions that are adaptive. Upon further exploration, the therapist may discover that they are parroting a "correct answer" that well-meaning adults have given them. However, without allowing young children time and developmentally appropriate means to express their thoughts, providing a parroted but not felt response is not helpful. Often children tell a verbal narrative that includes the corrective verbal responses, but their play narratives provide deeper access to their true thoughts and beliefs. To illustrate, a child may verbally indicate that the sexual abuse was not his fault, but while processing the narrative at a deeper level with play he may label himself as "naughty" or "sexy," which may reflect his true but nonadaptive thoughts.

With verbal narratives, the therapist processes the child's thoughts throughout the narrative as it is reread. This may include asking the child if the thoughts expressed were helpful or accurate. A similar intervention may be done as the child acts out the narrative.

The Magnetic Cognitive Triangle (MCT; Cavett, 2010, 2012a) is a play-based intervention that can help explain the cognitive triangle. In this intervention, children learn about feelings, thoughts, and behaviors as well as the connection between them. The MCT initially allows children to begin to explore feelings and to increase the breadth of descriptors for their internal experience of feelings. The MCT may be implemented in a joint session so that both child and parent understand their individual expressions of different feelings. Thoughts that are common for children who have been abused are also processed using the MCT. Spending a portion of a session discussing common thoughts (cognitive distortions, inaccurate cognitions, unhelpful thoughts) provides the children permission and understanding about their own experience. The MCT should include both positive and negative behaviors common for survivors of trauma. When the children process the trauma in their play, it may be helpful to utilize the MCT to explore feelings, thoughts, and behaviors.

Using the MCT, the child may be able to sort out feelings, thoughts, and behaviors more easily than if they were processed only verbally. As the narrative is read, the therapist and child identify feelings and thoughts and depict on a board how the thoughts impacted the feelings. A child who was sexually abused, for example, may have the thought, "I was a bad girl because I let him touch my privates," which may lead to her feeling guilty and sad. However, when the thought is changed to "I was just little and he tricked me into letting him touch me," the child might still continue to feel sad but less so. She also may not feel guilty and will assign blame to the perpetrator. When the thoughts and feelings are changed, her behaviors may also change (e.g., from isolating to seeking out support). Thus, the MCT allows for a visual representation of an internal process as well as more organized processing. Often children, even adolescents, say they cannot remember or do not want to tell more details when actually they need some assistance in communicating their thoughts, feelings, and behaviors, which is facilitated by the MCT.

DIRECTIVE PLAY THERAPY INTERVENTIONS

The processing of the narrative is a challenging stage of therapy, and engaging children in playful interventions that allow for deeper processing while maintaining their commitment to the process is essential. Children may benefit from matching play interventions to trauma-related cognitions, feelings, and behaviors. Play techniques have been developed to assist in identifying and changing cognitive distortions, developing coping skills, and conducting exposure to innocuous stimuli.

Several play interventions assist in the process of exploring thoughts and their impact on affect. Thinking Caps (Goodyear-Brown, 2005) and My View of the World (Cavett, 2010) facilitate the processing of thoughts that lead to positive and negative affect. With My View of the World, children use paper eyeglasses to look at how they see the world (cognitions) and explore more helpful cognitions that may result in improved mood. With Right Address/Wrong Address: Message from Self and Others (Cavett, 2010), children explore thoughts and consider what makes the message either helpful or not helpful. For example, if the thoughts a child writes in a letter to him- or herself are extreme, such as "I never make good choices," that message is rejected as a thought that has the wrong address. The clinician and child may playfully explore how such an extreme message should be sent to the North Pole, not to the child. By using play in talking about the messages sent to someone by him- or herself or others, the child is able to start looking at common cognitive distortions. The play intervention Erase the Place (Goodyear-Brown, 2005) can be utilized to address negative thoughts and replace them with positive ones.

Positive Thinking Checkers (Anderson, 2011) provides the opportunity for children to assess their thinking and learn to make positive self-statements. The game is based on checkers, with pieces determining whether or not the child makes a positive statement about him- or herself or draws a card with a negative self-statement, which the child then counters. Positively Painted Desert (Engberg & Schumann, 2011) is another cognitive reprocessing technique. Children discuss filling up their container with large rocks, which represent negative thoughts. Positive thoughts are represented by sand. Children learn that, by filling the container with positive thoughts about the self, there is no room for the negative thoughts. Both these activities allow children to consider and create positive thoughts about self and practice them. When children have negative or unhelpful thoughts in their trauma narratives, those are added to the games to practice making alternative thoughts.

Children who have been traumatized often did things during the event that they feel responsible for but that are not their fault. Children who have been sexually abused experience these events as "their" behaviors. Moral development precludes their understanding and processing that the behavior may have been a result of the trauma. For instance, sexually abused children who behaved in a specific way may not understand that the abuser "made," coerced, or forced them to perform the behavior. *Puppet on a String* (Goodyear-Brown, 2005) is a playful intervention that allows young victims to understand that the actions they performed during a trauma were not their fault and not "their" behavior.

Children who have been sexually abused and responded physiologically with pleasurable feelings often feel they are to blame. The clinician may observe evidence of this while the children are telling the narrative. Often children feel embarrassed and do not share this information in therapy. The clinician may ask open-ended questions about physiological responses and provide psychoeducation related to the normal responses to sexual touching. Cavett's (2010) *Pfffft—That's Just What Bodies Do* intervention provides humor and playfulness in processing pleasurable physiological reactions to sexual abuse. *The Bag of Tricks* (Crisci, Lay, & Lowenstein, 1998) provides "magic trick" opportunities to discuss the tricks that perpetrators use during different phases of sexual abuse. Young children especially are drawn to these interventions.

The decision as to when a narrative has been sufficiently processed is often challenging for clinicians. They may err by not encouraging deep enough narratives or by not providing exposure for a sufficient length of time. When a child continues to be symptomatic, or emotionally reactive or has indications of cognitive distortions, the narrative has not been adequately processed.

IN VIVO MASTERY: USING PLAY WITH HIERARCHIES AND EXPOSURE

The more intensive trauma-related components of TF-CBT are utilized to provide gradual exposure for the children related to their traumatic event. *In vivo* exposure allows the children to decrease their reactions to innocuous stimuli associated with the traumatic experiences in their actual environment. The engaging quality of play with *in vivo* exposure may encourage children to participate more willingly in a difficult therapeutic task. *In vivo* exposure is helpful when a hierarchy of related stimuli is created and the children are progressively able to face the innocuous stimuli successfully and reduce the anxiety response. For some young children, it is best to create a hierarchy only with the parent because focusing on the ultimate goal of the hierarchy or the more anxiety-provoking steps may lead to noncompliance. Most children, however, may enjoy participating in the development of a hierarchy with the therapist and parent.

Developing a hierarchy in play can be done using orange road construction cones (available in the automotive section of department stores). Each cone represents a subjective unit of distress. Clinicians choose to use different ranges of scores (i.e., 5, 7, or 10 cones), and the number may vary depending on age. Younger children may do better with five cones representing a range of anxiety level, from 1 to 5, while older children may do better with 10 so that more variance in the level of anxiety is represented. Faces can be drawn and attached to the cones to help the child visualize each level of anxiety. The therapist and parent may write down different scenarios related to the anxiety-provoking stimuli, or the child may draw a picture of each level. The child then takes each statement or picture and places it beside the cone that represents the level of anxiety it evokes. The child and parent talk with the therapist about the level of anxiety that could be tolerated with the use of coping skills. The child may use play to act out each level of the hierarchy, such as showing it in the dollhouse or acting it out with the parent in the office. The inclusion of the child in the playful development of the hierarchy may improve compliance with the *in vivo* exposure. The playful approach simply allows the child to feel more engaged in the process, which is followed by the actual *in vivo* exposure.

Play is also helpful when exposing the child to innocuous stimuli that occurred at the time of trauma. As an example, a ringing phone may remind the child of the environment following his father's suicide and may lead him or her to avoid answering and/or talking on the phone. The child and therapist may initially play out this aspect of the trauma by acting out the phone ringing and what the child's mother said to people at that time. Role-playing the exposure or including it in a play reenactment may be helpful. For example, the child and therapist may act out the roles of child and parent in the week following the suicide. The therapist may act as the mother and answer the phone and pretend to answer questions. The responses to the pretend questions are beneficial, as is exposure to the sound of a ringing phone, an innocuous stimulus associated with the suicide. Through exposure provided by the play, the child is able to process and reduce his anxiety. This process may be sufficient to help a child overcome avoidance and can also prepare the child for *in vivo* exposure if needed. The *in vivo* hierarchy might include steps such as listening to the phone ring at home, practicing answering the phone, actually answering the phone when it rings, and talking on the phone for increasing amounts of time. The therapist would then recommend the parent set up *in vivo* exposures by encouraging her child to listen for the phone at at time when someone was going to call. Once the child responds more calmly to the ring, he would be ready to respond to a call, finally working toward answering and talking on the phone again at home. The *in vivo* process is designed to help this child face his feared associations so that he could see that not every call will lead to tragic news.

ENHANCING SAFETY
AND FUTURE DEVELOPMENT

Children who have been victims of trauma may fear being traumatized again. Discussing safety issues with them is important to their long-term mental health. Frequently, children are traumatized repeatedly, highlighting the need for safety education and planning related to revictimization. As with the other TF-CBT, future safety concerns can be addressed through play-based interventions. Safety instruction can be done with worksheets and discussions about possible situations. However, discussion of safety issues through play typically engages the children to better comprehend and integrate the message.

Fabulous Frogs (Brace, 2011) is a play-based intervention that allows children to consider what type of environment is safe by developing a safe environment for frogs. This intervention allows the therapist to process what makes children feel safe. Children also make up rules they think will help the frogs to be safe, and this allows processing of what boundaries and rules make their own lives safe.

Boundaries are a vital part of safety planning for all traumatized children. To process boundaries, one may utilize bibliotherapy in addition to playful interventions. Many play interventions relate to interpersonal boundaries. As children learn about boundaries, it is helpful to use concrete objects or other visuals. A body drawing on butcher paper can be helpful in showing public (i.e., hands) or private (i.e., breasts) parts as well as those parts children identify as acceptable for touching by close friends or family (e.g., the shoulders, back) in certain situations (i.e., a backrub, shoulder massage). *Respect My Space* (Kenney-Noziska, 2008) is an intervention that uses hula hoops to create boundary bubbles, which can be implemented while processing strategies related to communicating with others about one's boundaries. A similar intervention, *Hula Hoop Boundaries* (Janis-Towey, 2010), also uses hula hoops to process personal space and the variations according to the nature of the relationship or situation. Finding one's voice and being empowered to tell someone when feeling uncomfortable or when in an abusive or dangerous situation is important to discuss during the safety planning portion of therapy. With play, children can act out calling a loved one, the police, or social services for help. Using possible scenarios along with play phones makes the abstract plan more integrated into the children's repertoire of behaviors. Children can also utilize megaphones while practicing saying "No" or telling others about inappropriate situations. In Goodyear-Brown's (2005) adaptation of this megaphone intervention—*Megaphones to Make a Point*—children practice saying "No" and setting boundaries. Using Goodyear-Brown's *Door Hanger* intervention (2005), children create foam door hangers to help them process both allowing people into their space and setting limits. Alternatively, *Keep Your Hands Off Me* (Goodyear-Brown, 2005) provides a kinesthetic experience for processing setting limits around personal space.

The clinician's approach to safety planning must consider the child's possible interpretations of the plan. Most importantly, the child may feel blamed for previous abuse if told that he or she is responsible for saying "No" in the future. The clinician may want to discuss how behaviors that enhance future safety may not have been known when the child was initially abused.

Building a community for support is an important skill for traumatized children and their supportive caregiver. Toward this end, children and adolescents can engage in an art project in which they create and depict their support system. The children typically have communicated their interests throughout the therapy, and the clinician uses this information to suggest options for them to consider when depicting their support system. For example, an adolescent who plays basketball structures his support system as a team, and uses art supplies to draw the players, coaches, and supports (managers). Each person he feels is a part of his support system is identified and depicted based on the role of that person in his ongoing support. The adolescent's mother, for example, may be labeled as a coach or the point guard. The art project allows insight for both the children and the therapist into the people whom the children see as supportive. Children can visualize their support system using any structure that works best for them: a sports team, a band or orchestra, a classroom.

For the very young child, having puzzles of helpers (e.g., police, doctor) while discussing safety planning can be very beneficial. Scenarios that depict safety situations can be read to the child, with the child responding by indicating to whom he or she would go and what would be told in order to receive the help needed. Puppets of helpers are also useful for engaging the child in safety discussions. The My Helpers technique (Crisci et al., 1998) was developed to provide information about safety planning. In the activity, the child matches scenarios with pictures of different helpers, such as doctors or parents. This paper-and-pencil activity allows the child to process more at home. My Safe Neighborhood (Cavett, 2010) encourages the child to play out different scenarios with toys such as a fire engine or police car while processing future safety.

Safety across different settings may be addressed during this component. Peer concerns such as bullying can be included in the safety planning, if indicated. Several games related to bullying (e.g., The Bully Free Game, Girls Games) are helpful in teaching bully reduction skills.

THE CHILD AS VICTIM, THEN SURVIVOR

As with older children and adults, the young child may see the trauma as an important, or even the most important, aspect of his or her life for a period of time after the trauma. He or she may identify with the label of victim. As the narrative proceeds, the child's play often goes from the perspective of a victim to one of an empowered survivor. Eventually, as with older children, the child is able to integrate the trauma as a part of him- or herself but not the main thing that defines him or her. Looking toward the future and integrating the trauma into the child's life is essential in processing the narrative. With the verbal narrative, the therapist helps the child write details about what may be helpful for the child or what activities or thoughts may help the child move forward from the trauma. In the play, this is developed at an experiential level. Play-based interventions during termination may be utilized to help the child process what he or she learned in therapy and how the trauma fits into the rest of his or her life.

CLINICAL CASE DESCRIPTION

Jason: A 5-Year-Old Who Experienced a Natural Disaster/Flood

Verbal Narrative

Jason began his narrative with a brief description of himself. He then discussed his experience with the flood.

> A storm came. We were getting ready for the storm. There were so many people around our house and outside. I felt worried. Our house was flooded and we had to live in a hotel. When we got back there was a mess.

Play Narrative

Using the sand tray, Jason re-created his trauma narrative. It was during the play narrative that the details about the Black Hawk helicopter and the animals that died became part of the narrative. Other important details were also communicated for the first time. He also gave more details about the preparations for the flood, such as taking toys upstairs. Using toy vehicles in the sand tray, he was better able to communicate his experience of he and his mother going in one vehicle while other family members went in another. The details provided deeper information about his experience with the traumatic event and what he felt and thought about it. He also offered comments during the play, such as his thoughts about wishing that someone would have helped rescue the animals, thoughts that were not revealed in the verbal narrative. The following verbalization of his trauma narrative was made utilizing play.

> A storm came. We were getting ready for the storm. We took things upstairs to stay dry. My parents were busy all the time trying to get the house ready. They knew it may flood. Then a storm started. My mom

and dad felt worried and I felt worried. It was hard to be with my parents 'cause they were worried and crabby. Mom and Dad started to build dikes around our house. There were volunteers who helped build too. Lots of helpers came. The police were there in cars. They only let people in who lived by us. The Natural Guard [National Guard] was there too. They were in Humvees and flew Black Hawk helicopters. I was scared when the Black Hawks were there 'cause Mom said that they only fly where the dikes might break. I saw deer and turkeys that were trapped in areas where the flood was. After the flood many of them were dead and I saw them on the fields. It made me sad that they died. I wish someone could have saved the animals, but they were too busy saving people. I wanted to do something other than watch the sandbagging. I asked Mom if I could go do something. She said that I could get hurt if something happened. I felt annoyed and mad. I wanted to go on a play date with my friend Jeremy. Mom said I couldn't go. I was scared when Mom said I had to stay home. If the dikes broke I would not be able to go back home and they would not know where I was. I thought, "I am never going to be able to do anything!" I was mad and scared. We couldn't go on the bridge. It was covered up with water. I wanted to help sandbag but I was too little. At first I sat and watched through the window. Mom kept telling me to go to my room so that I would be safe. Finally, she let me help make sandwiches for the volunteers. Then I felt better. Everyone was helping. Mom said I could help too but only with some things. The dike broke at 2 in the morning. I was sleeping and Mom came in and got me. I was scared and sleepy. She took me in the car and Dad followed with Jared. We went to a hotel. The people talked to Mom and Dad on the phone and said that our house was under water up to the first floor. My room was in the basement and I didn't get my other toys. Some toys we took upstairs and they were wet too 'cause the water was high enough to get things on the floor. Mom said we could not keep them 'cause water from a flood is taminated [contaminated]. We got some of them that were higher when Mom and Dad went back to the house. They brought them to the hotel. We stayed in the hotel for 3 weeks and then we decided to go to Grandma's house until our house was fixed. When we got back our house was a mess. I could not have my old toys. I wish I had my DSi games and the Wii and all my Legos that were downstairs. I feel sad that we lost them. But I can get new toys again. I feel happy about that. Mom and Dad said we can fix the house and in about 9 months we can move back in. I get to pick out the new carpet and get a new bed set. I feel happy.

Cognitive Processing

Jason was able to use the MCT between his verbal and play trauma narratives. This allowed him to explore the connection among thinking, feeling, and doing. The triggers, including the flood, news/TV, and parental emotions, were discussed. The MCT allowed him to realize that when he changed his thoughts he could change his feelings. For instance, on the MCT he used a thought magnet to represent "I wanted to do something other than watch the sandbagging" and another to represent "I can help with some things." By focusing on what he could do, he felt more positive. He also realized that his safety was important and he and his parents had that as a priority. He used pictorial magnets to represent behaviors that were positive and negative. Examples of positive behaviors included the relaxation activities he learned earlier.

In Vivo *Exposure*

Jason continued to express fears related to flooding. He was triggered by inclement weather, including rain/storms. He also was highly anxious about the sound of helicopters as there had been Black Hawks in the area during the flooding to monitor dikes. Jason listed scenarios that related to the weather and created a hierarchy based on subjective units of distress ranging from 0 to 10. Distress scores were represented by orange cones, which were placed on the office floor, with a space between each. Jason and his mother discussed each step and agreed that they could begin working on his anxiety related to rainstorms beginning with imaginal storms, which he depicted as being at a moderate level of anxiety (5) and thought he could confront with coping skills. In therapy he and his mother made a rice shaker, using two paper plates glued together and grains of rice in between. Shaking the rice shaker resulted in an auditory stimulus similar to the sound of a rainstorm. By playing with the shaker, taking turns being the shaker and having the therapist shake it while pretending to be in a storm, Jason was able to gain mastery. His controlling the intensity of the initial "storm," by shaking it harder or softer, increased his feelings of mastery. Jason's grandmother was committed to helping him learn coping skills and tolerate the anxiety, and together they recorded storms over the next couple of weeks and watched a movie depicting a storm. During the course of treatment, several storms, including a significant thunderstorm, allowed for *in vivo* exposure. Jason used the coping skills he learned prior to the exposure to gain success over his fears. After reducing the distress scores of different scenarios to tolerable levels, he then addressed fears related to helicopters. His initial exposure included play in the sand tray, where he used and manipulated toy Black Hawks and the other stimuli that reminded him of the flood, and was essential in his reducing anxiety to innocuous stimuli. Recordings and an eventual visit to an air museum allowed for increased levels of exposure.

Safety Planning/Termination

Jason created a My Safe Contacts (Cavett, 2010) list during his final sessions. The list of contacts, which was written on his drawing of a cell phone, allowed him to visualize several people to whom he could turn when he needed support. He then drew pictures of four of the contacts with whom he felt closest. The pictures depicted him doing something with each person that makes him feel better/safe/loved.

Natisha: A 7-Year-Old Biracial Girl Who Experienced Sexual Abuse

Natisha's original trauma-related narrative was simply "I was sexually abused." She developed the nontrauma as well as the trauma-specific chapters more fully through her play-based narratives across sessions. She utilized the dollhouse to show the trauma, with details that included sensory memories. She was also able to verbalize feelings and thoughts through her play. She indicated that the perpetrator called her his "little angel" and at times told her that she was bad because she touched his genitals. He indicated that it was her fault because she did it. This was not a part of the verbal narrative, and the fact that Natisha continued to feel some responsibility for the sexual abuse was not evident until she exhibited it in the play. In the play, the character that she identified as the perpetrator said to the character that she identified as herself, "You are touching me, look what you did! You made it get bigger. If you tell your mom, she will be angry with you." Although verbally Natisha was able to state that she knew she was not responsible, it was not known until she acted it out in the play that she had been told she was responsible and had internalized it. During the play, she also indicated that the character identified as her perpetrator stated that he would hurt her mom if she told.

After Natisha acted out her trauma narrative, it became evident that the perpetrator had made statements that can be considered "tricks" to get her to not tell. Therefore, Natisha and her therapist played the Trick Hat game (Crisci et al., 1998). The tricks used by the perpetrator included telling Natisha that her mother would not believe her and that he would hurt her mother if she told. Natisha was able to process blame, responsibility, and power issues through the Trick Hat game. After playing with the therapist, Natisha's mother was asked to join in the game to process Natisha's feelings (guilt, fear) and thoughts ("It was my fault because I touched his privates"). Playing the game together allowed Natisha to process her fears of her mother not believing her. As scenarios were acted out and Natisha was able to role-play possible scenarios, she was validated by her mother, and her mother reinforced that she would believe and protect Natisha.

Natisha's family utilized the family bed and co-sleeping had occurred in the context of the extended family. The therapist initially felt that Natisha's sleeping with her mother or grandmother was related to the sexual abuse and fears resulting from abuse. However, as the therapist became educated in the traditions of the family, and Natisha's mother expressed her acceptance of the co-sleeping as a choice and not a symptom, the location of sleep was not maintained as a therapeutic concern.

Natisha utilized the Crowing Community (Goodyear-Brown, 2005) intervention during the final sessions of therapy. This intervention allowed her to consider those who are supportive of her and how she can access them.

CONCLUSION

Play and playful interventions are frequently utilized in the context of TF-CBT to motivate and enhance children's participation in the various TF-CBT components. When TF-CBT therapists encourage children to engage in play that realistically depicts their traumatic experiences, they are achieving the important goals of gradual exposure to traumatic memories that are might otherwise be avoided and/or suppressed. More specifically, in the context of the trauma narrative and processing component, play can help children more comfortably bring to mind the details of highly traumatic experiences, while also revealing sensations, feelings, and thoughts that can later be processed with the help of their therapist and parents. In sum, as demonstrated in the prior examples and case studies, play is often an integral aspect of effective TF-CBT with children.

REFERENCES

Anderson, S. N. (2011). Positive Thinking Checkers. In L. Lowenstein (Ed.), *Assessment and treatment activities for children, adolescents, and families: Practitioners share their most effective techniques* (Vol. 3, pp. 155–157). Toronto: Champion Press.

BigFoot, D. S., & Schmidt, S. (2010). Honoring children, mending the circle: A cultural adaptation of trauma-focused cognitive-behavioral therapy for American Indian and Alaska Native Children. *Journal of Clinical Psychology, 66,* 847–856.

Brace, A. (2011). Fabulous frogs. In L. Lowenstein (Ed.) *Assessment and treatment activities for children, adolescents, and families: Practitioners share their most effective tchniques* (Vol. 3, pp. 109–111). Toronto: Champion Press.

Cavett, A. M. (2009a). Playful trauma focused-cognitive behavioral therapy with maltreated children and adolescents. *Play Therapy, 4*(3), 20–22.

Cavett, A. M. (2009b). *Playful trauma focused-cognitive behavioral therapy with traumatized children.* Retrieved from *www.lianalowenstein.com/cavett.doc.*

Cavett, A. M. (2010). *Structured play-based interventions for engaging children and adolescents in therapy.* West Conshohocken, PA: Infinity.

Cavett, A. M. (2011b). *Play-based cognitive behavioral techniques for children.* West Conshohocken, PA: Infinity.

Cavett, A. M. (2011b). *Enhancing cognitive behavioral therapy with children with the Magnetic Cognitive Triangle.* West Conshohocken, PA: Infinity.

Cohen, J. A., Mannarino, A. P., & Deblinger, E. (2006).*Treating trauma and traumatic grief in children and adolescents.* New York: Guilford Press.

Crisci, G., Lay, M., & Lowenstein, L., (1998). *Paper dolls and paper airplanes: Therapeutic exercises for sexually traumatized children.* Indianapolis, IN: Kidsrights.

Deblinger, E. &, Heflin, A. H. (1996). *Treating sexually abused children and their nonoffending parents: A cognitive behavioral approach.* Thousand Oaks, CA: Sage.

Drewes, A. A. (2011, April). *A skill-building workshop: Effectively blending play-based techniques with cognitive behavioral therapy for affect regulation in sexually abused and traumatized children.* Paper presented at the annual conference of the Canadian Association for Child and Play Therapy, Guelph, ON, Canada.

Engberg, K., & Schumann, B. (2011). Positively painted desert. In L. Lowenstein (Ed.), *Assessment and treatment activities for children, adolescents, and families: Practitioners share their most effective techniques* (Vol. 3, pp. 158–159). Toronto: Champion Press.

Gil, E. (2006). *Helping abused and traumatized children: Integrating directive and nondirective approaches.* New York: Guilford Press.

Gobeil, J. (2010). Cool and calm feather breathing dragon. In L. Lowenstein (Ed.), *Assessment and treatment activities for children, adolescents, and families: Practitioners share their most effective techniques* (Vol. 2, pp. 82–83). Toronto: Champion Press.

Goodyear-Brown, P. (2002). *Digging for buried treasure: 52 prop-based play therapy interventions for treating the problems of childhood.* Nashville, TN: Author.

Goodyear-Brown, P. (2005). *Digging for buried treasure 2: Another 52 prop-based play therapy interventions for treating the problems of childhood.* Nashville, TN. Author.

Janis-Towey, A. P. (2010). Hula hoop boundaries. In L. Lowenstein (Ed.), *Assessment and treatment activities for children, adolescents, and families: Practitioners share their most effective techniques* (Vol. 2, pp. 61–62). Toronto: Champion Press.

Kenney-Noziska, S. (2008). *Techniques–techniques–techniques: Play based activities for children, adolescents, and families.* West Conshohocken, PA: Infinity.

Landreth, G. (1991). *Play therapy: The art of the relationship.* Muncie, IN: Accelerated Development.

Lowenstein, L. (1999). *Creative interventions for troubled children and adolescents.* Toronto: Champion Press.

Lowenstein, L. (2002). *More creative interventions for troubled children and adolescents.* Toronto: Champion Press.

Lowenstein, L. (2006a). *Creative interventions for bereaved children.* Toronto: Champion Press.

Lowenstein, L. (2006b). *Creative interventions for children of divorce.* Toronto: Champion Press.

Lowenstein. L. (Ed.). (2008). *Assessment and treatment activities for children, adolescents, and families: Practitioners share their most effective techniques.* Toronto: Champion Press.

Lowenstein, L. (Ed.). (2010a). *Assessment and treatment activities for children, adolescents, and families: Practitioners share their most effective techniques* (Vol. 2). Toronto: Champion Press.

Lowenstein, L. (Ed.). (2010b). *Creative family therapy techniques: Play, art, and expressive activities to engage children in family sessions.* Toronto: Champion Press.

Lowenstein, L. (Ed.). (2011). *Assessment and treatment activities for children, adolescents, and families: Practitioners share their most effective techniques* (Vol. 3). Toronto: Champion Press.

Pearson, & Merrill, M. I. (2006). *The adventures of Lady: The big storm.* Orlando, FL: Adventures of Lady, LLC.

Scott, D., Feldman, J., & Patterson, S. (1993). *No-no and the secret touch: The gentle story of a little seal who learns to stay safe, say "no" and tell!* New York: Random House.

Sheppard, C. H. (1998). *Brave Bart: A story for traumatized and grieving children.* Grosse Pointe Woods, MI: Institute for Trauma and Loss in Children.

6

Children with Developmental Disabilities

CHRISTINA A. GROSSO

OVERVIEW OF TF-CBT WITH CHILDREN WITH DEVELOPMENTAL DISABILITIES

As we look at the emerging demographics in society today, we cannot ignore the need for specialized treatment for traumatized children with developmental disabilities. Developmental delays impact one in six children in the United States (Boyle et al., 2011), and these children are up to 10 times more likely to be maltreated than those who are not disabled (Goldson, 2002; Sobsey & Doe, 1991). With the prevalence of trauma in developmentally disabled children and the lack of trained professionals who are able to provide treatment (Charlton, Kliethermes, Tallant, Taverne, & Tisherlman, 2004), we are looking at a crisis in our mental health system. We need to understand how to adapt existing best practice to address the specific needs of the developmentally disabled.

The applications presented in this chapter are a result of the work done over the last 6 years implementing trauma-focused cognitive-behavioral therapy (TF-CBT) in several residential treatment facilities in New York State with children and adolescents with complex trauma and psychopathology (Cohen, Mannarino, & Deblinger, 2006). Of these children, many also suffered from various developmental disabilities, including but not limited to mild mental retardation, learning disabilities, receptive and expressive language disorders, and autism spectrum disorders, namely pervasive developmental disorder. As TF-CBT was initiated, the challenges of this population emerged as did the need for adaptations that addressed their impairments in cognition, communication, and affect management.

DEVELOPMENTAL DELAYS

The Centers for Disease Control and Prevention (2011) define developmental disabilities as "a diverse group of severe chronic conditions that are due to mental and/or physical impairments. People with developmental disabilities have problems with major life activities such as language, mobility, learning, self-help, and independent living. Developmental disabilities begin anytime during development up to 22 years of age and usually last throughout a person's lifetime."

The prevalence of developmental disabilities in children has increased significantly in the last decade. According to a 2008 survey, over 15% of children ages 3–17 have diagnoses of such disabilities, including "attention deficit hyperactivity disorder; intellectual disability; cerebral palsy; autism; seizures; stuttering or stammering; moderate to profound hearing loss; blindness; learning disorders; and/or other developmental delays" compared with 12.84% a decade earlier (Boyle et al., 2011, p. 1034). The occurrence of developmental delays in boys was nearly twice that of girls, with Hispanic children showing significantly less prevalence than white non-Hispanic and black non-Hispanic children. Children with families below the poverty line and children with access to Medicaid or other public health insurance also showed higher rates of developmental disabilities compared with middle-class children with private insurance (Boyle et al., 2011).

Limitations and Challenges

Children with developmental disabilities often have difficulty in areas of cognition, communication, and affective regulation (see Table 6.1). It is important to understand these deficits in order to create adaptations in treatment.

Strengths

As with all children, those with developmental delays also have strengths, a fact that may often be overlooked by caregivers and clinicians as a result of the severity of the developmental challenges. It is imperative that we identify these strengths and use a strengths-based approach to treatment. Children with developmental delays will often have an ability to retain information related to events. They may think in pictures and recall this

TABLE 6.1. Areas of Impairment in Developmentally Disabled Children

Cognition	Communication	Affect dysregulation

• May have difficulty with:
  ▪ Abstract thinking
  ▪ Critical thinking
  ▪ Sequencing events
  ▪ Prioritizing
  ▪ Task breakdown
  ▪ Ambiguity
• Concrete thought process
• Fixations
• Black-and-white thinking
• Think in pictures
• Highly focused areas of interest and expertise
	• Delays in receptive and expressive language
	• Idiosyncratic speech
	• Echolalia
	• Poor social skills
	• Engage in one-sided conversation
	• Difficulty engaging with and responding to others
	• Lack of boundaries, intrusive behaviors
	• Trusting of others
		• Difficulty identifying emotions in self and others
		• Difficulty expressing emotion via facial gestures and/or verbal statements
		• Sensory sensitivity
		• Impulsive
		• Easily agitated
		• More prone to anxiety
		• More behavioral issues; may be quick to hit, punch, kick when agitated
		• Tendency for rote behavior when anxious
		• Difficulty and/or discomfort with change

Note. Based on Charlton, Kliethermes, Tallant, Taverne, and Tisherlman (2004)

information with great clarity and detail. They may also have domains of interest and expertise, with special talents and insights in specific areas such as math, art, and music as well as spatial and mechanical abilities (Grandin, 2010).

TRAUMA AND DEVELOPMENTAL DISABILITIES

Children with disabilities are at higher risk to experience abuse than those without disabilities (Ryan, 1994). According to Sullivan and Knutson (2000), they are 3.79 times as likely to be victims of physical abuse, 3.14 times more likely to be victims of sexual abuse, and 3.76 times more likely to be neglected than their nondisabled cohort. Overall, the literature points to rates of maltreatment among children with disabilities of 1 to 10 times greater than among children without disabilities (Goldson, 2002; Sobsey & Doe, 1991). Studies indicate that 22–70% of abused children have developmental disabilities (National Research Council, 2001). Rates of abuse and maltreatment are thought to be much higher than the statistics just presented as a result of underreporting in this population because of communication issues, reliability of victim reporting, and the judicial system seeing reports as being of questionable credibility (Charlton & Tallant, 2003). Children with developmental disabilities are also more likely to be in out-of-home placement (i.e., residential treatment, day programs, and assisted-living facilities where rates of sexual abuse are two to seven times higher than in the community) (Overcamp-Martini & Nutton, 2009).

Because of the limitations and challenges discussed earlier, disabled children are at risk for increased victimization. They may not understand what is happening to them and may not have the capacity to communicate effectively with someone who can help. Children with disabilities are often dependent on multiple caregivers for learning and supervision as well as assistance in activities of daily living, including eating, bathing, and toileting, thus increasing exposure to potential boundary violations. They are taught to trust caregivers, adults, and authority figures. As such, they can be easier to manipulate because of decreased capacity for critical thinking and the inability to differentiate safe from unsafe persons and situations. Thus, children with developmental disabilities are more likely to experience trauma, and trauma exposure also increases the likeliness of developmental delays. Severe trauma and neglect can impact children's developing brain and affect problem solving, affect regulation, and comprehension. Prolonged abuse can result in permanent damage to these brain functions. The impact of the trauma on the children may be further compounded by the lack of response and understanding from society (Charlton et al., 2004).

TREATMENT ISSUES AND RECOMMENDATIONS

With the prevalence of trauma in developmentally disabled children, it is probable that clinicians will be finding these children on their caseloads. However, as a result of underreporting, these children may not receive appropriate therapy or may be misdiagnosed (Boyle et al., 2011; Goldson, 2002). Children may exhibit behavioral disruptions that are in reaction to trauma exposure but not report the incident of abuse. This behavior may then be seen as a symptom of the developmental issue alone, and the trauma may go unrecognized and untreated. Compounding this issue further is a twofold problem: (1) a lack of trained professionals who are able to assess for trauma exposure and provide trauma treatment to developmentally disabled children and (2) society's belief that the developmentally disabled do not benefit from verbal psychotherapy (Charlton et al., 2004; Reaven, 2009).

Children with developmental delays present some unique challenges to traditional verbal and cognitive-behavioral therapy (CBT) (Moree & Davis, 2010; Reaven, 2009). Because of their impairments in cognition, language, and emotion, adaptations are needed to help them access the concepts and develop appropriate skills (Moree & Davis, 2010; Wood et al., 2009). Some general strategies include those listed in Table 6.2.

Based on some of these unique challenges that children with developmental disabilities present, CBT offers inherent structure and skill building

TABLE 6.2. Treatment Strategies for Children with Developmental Disabilities

Strategy	Purpose	Examples	Goals
Provide structure, create routines.	Children with developmental delays will often have difficulty and discomfort with change.	• Have a consistent meeting day/time. • Create a routine for sessions with opening and closing rituals. • Help family and caregivers create schedules/routines in the home and school (e.g., set times for meals, homework, bed)	• Creates consistency and expectation. • Enhances predictability and comfort. • Increases capacity for autonomy. • Increases opportunity for repetition.
Shorten sessions.	Children with developmental delays will often have shorter attention spans and can be easily agitated.	• Adjust session time according to attention span. • Adjust dosage and pacing of gradual exposure.	• Increases sense of competence and success. • Increases capacity for self-control and affect regulation.
Slow down.	Children with developmental delays have difficulty breaking down tasks and interpreting complex and compound messages.	• Slow speech down. • Give simple messages. • Present one topic at a time. • Be specific.	• Increases comprehension and competence.
Use art/ visuals.	Children with developmental disabilities are often visual thinkers and "think in pictures."	• Provide images to illustrate directions and tasks. • Utilize visual aids when teaching skills. • Encourage children to draw, paint, sculpt their thoughts and feelings.	• Increases comprehension. • Increases ability to communicate.
Use play.	Children with developmental disabilities are visual thinkers and require movement and activation to remain focused.	• Use puppets, figurines, sand play, and dollhouses to create stories and metaphor.	• Increases comprehension. • Increases ability to communicate.
Provide repetition.	Children with developmental disabilities have cognitive limitations, including poor comprehension and retention and decreased capacity for generalization.	• Repeat skills and concepts in session. • Assign homework to practice skills taught in session. • Use consistent praise and rewards as reinforcement of positive behavior.	• Creates consistency and expectation. • Enhances predictability and comfort. • Increases capacity for autonomy.

(continued)

TABLE 6.2. (*continued*)

Strategy	Purpose	Examples	Goals
Use interests and fixations.	Children with developmental disabilities often have fixations or special interests.	• Ask, discover children's special interests. • Use fixation on favorite character, person, place, thing to teach skill. • Use shared interests to increase socialization.	• Increases engagement in treatment. • Increases communication. • Increases retention of skill. • Increases socialization.

Note. Based on Charlton, Kliethermes, Tallant, Taverne, and Tisherlman (2004); Grandin (2010); and Reaven (2009).

to directly address these needs (Reaven, 2009). CBT has shown to be an effective intervention with children with a variety of functional difficulties because of its capacity to provide structure and self-management strategies. The need for an integrated treatment approach is also emphasized, specifically the use of art therapy and visuals to create concrete, tangible resources to accompany verbal interventions (Moree & Davis, 2010; Oathamshaw & Haddock, 2006; Reaven, 2009; Taylor, Lindsay, & Wilner, 2008; Wahlberg, 1998).

APPLICATIONS OF TF–CBT SKILLS AND TECHNIQUES

As we begin to address these issues in TF–CBT, we must recognize the need to enhance our clinical knowledge and skill in assessing for trauma and developmental delays as well as adapting treatment to fit the needs of our clients. TF–CBT is a highly flexible model and lends itself well to diverse adaptations (Cohen et al., 2006). However, as with any adaptation, it is important to be mindful of the goals of treatment and the purpose of each component so that any alteration is congruent with the philosophy and fidelity of treatment. An effective strategy in achieving this is to ask the question "Why?" Why do we provide psychoeducation to a child who has experienced sexual abuse? Why do we teach grounding and relaxation strategies to survivors of trauma? These questions will help us maintain the fidelity of treatment while creating and adapting our methods/interventions on how to achieve the goals of TF–CBT. Children with developmental disabilities may move through the model more slowly and require more time to understand concepts through repetition and application. Change occurs slowly but does happen. One must be mindful of setting treatment goals to reflect this incremental progress and provide praise for accomplishments in a specific and immediate manner.

The remainder of this chapter is dedicated to the direct application of skills and techniques for use with children with developmental disabilities. A foundational working knowledge of TF-CBT is assumed and is a prerequisite for fully understanding this discussion, which is built upon original fidelity of the PRACTICE components. Each component is broken down by goal, challenge(s), and skill(s). The goal of each component—the "why"—is delineated as well as the unique challenges of the population and the reason for implementation strategies that are developmentally appropriate. Last, the specific skills and activities utilized to teach each component are discussed. In essence, a "toolbox" of interventions will be accessible to the readers for immediate and direct use with their client population.

Similar to creating a toolbox for the clinician, we also want to create a toolbox of skills for clients. The skills and activities discussed will provide useful and practical tools for the children as they progress through treatment. Clinicians can concretize the toolbox by creating a folder, binder, or box for these materials and use it as a resource and refer back to it to as needed. This will also provide a transitional resource when treatment concludes, to be used by the children at home and school with caregivers.

Assessment

As we know, the role of assessment is extremely important in TF-CBT (see Table 6.3). We need to screen for trauma exposure and symptoms as well as other psychiatric disorders to develop case formulation and treatment goals. At the onset of treatment, we need to determine trauma type and begin to develop a hierarchy of experiences. In addition to psychosocial history, we also complete standardized measures, such as the UCLA PTSD Reaction Index (Steinberg, Brymer, Decker, & Pynoos, 2004) to determine trauma exposure and symptoms and the Child Behavior Checklist (Achenbach, 1991) to reveal behavioral, emotional, and thought problems. Standardized measures are important in rating change over time from pre- to post-treatment. In working with developmentally disabled children, we may also want to consider administering cognitive scales to determine the degree of cognitive impairment and developmental level (Oathamshaw & Haddock, 2006). By completing these various instruments, we can begin to formulate a symptom picture and a differential diagnosis. Some symptoms may overlap across trauma and developmental domains, such as the ability to focus, regulate affect, and control impulses. Are these symptoms a result of avoidance, hyperarousal, and/or hypervigilance resulting from exposure to trauma? Are the symptoms in reaction to an attention-deficit/hyperactivity disorder? Or are these symptoms due to a cognitive delay?

TABLE 6.3. Why Do We Assess Clients?

Goals
- To assess for trauma, psychiatric disorders, and developmental level in order to develop case formulation and goals for treatment
- To monitor progress over course of treatment

Challenges
Children with developmental disabilities have:
- Overlapping symptoms of trauma and developmental delays
- Difficulty understanding language of assessments
- Limited capacity for sequencing and difficulty understanding frequency
- Difficulty engaging and responding to others

Skills
- Shorten sessions—complete assessment over multiple sessions
- Use visuals to illustrate concepts and aid in communication

Note. Based on Charlton, Kliethermes, Tallant, Taverne, and Tisherlman (2004) and Cohen, Mannarino, and Deblinger (2006).

Standardized measures may present an obstacle to children with developmental issues. They may have difficulty understanding the questions, organizing their thoughts, and communicating their answers (Avrin, Charlton, & Tallant, 1998) and may require one-on-one verbal administration to ensure comprehension. As clinicians, we may need to reframe or explain questions while remaining conscientious in maintaining their integrity. Using behavioral definitions and visuals to illustrate concepts can be helpful. For instance, the clinician can present a drawing of a fire, tornado, flood, or hurricane when asking the child, "Have you ever been in another kind of disaster, like a fire, tornado, flood, or hurricane?" (Pynoos et al., 1998). Children with developmental disabilities may also have difficulty completing an assessment within a standard session. Administering the assessment in sections may help with pacing, maximizing attention and minimizing agitation. The children may also have trouble responding verbally. The clinician should have paper, crayons, colored pencils, or a dry-erase board in the office for children to write responses. This can be a fun, interactive activity that also promotes engagement. Illustrations of people or characters nodding their head and saying "Yes" in a talk bubble or shaking their head and saying "No" can be a useful tool as well.

Completing assessments with intensity ratings and Likert scales, such as the UCLA PTSD Index for DSM-IV (Pynoos et al., 1998), may require additional explanation. Because of issues with sequencing and understanding frequency, children with developmental disabilities may have difficulty with this concept and require visual aids and metaphor. The Rain Cloud Likert Scale, for example (Figure 6.1), uses rain clouds to illustrate this continuum, with a response range of 0, or "none," to 4, or "most" (Grosso, 2011). In developing a hierarchy of negative stimuli, an illustration of a mountain can be used, with the top of the mountain as the event that "bothers me the most" and the bottom of the mountain as the least distressing event. One should keep in mind that children with developmental disabilities will often have a lower threshold for negative stimuli, and this should be considered when formulating hierarchies (Reaven, 2009).

CASE EXAMPLE

Johnny, a 12-year-old boy with pervasive developmental disorder, mood disorder not otherwise specified, and posttraumatic stress disorder, presented with a history of physical and sexual abuse by his father from age 4 to 7, failed foster care placements, and multiple hospitalizations for highly aggressive behaviors. Johnny had an IQ of 68 and scored a 43 on the UCLA PTSD Index for DSM-IV (Pynoos et al., 1998). Johnny had no contact with his father, who was in prison for his abuse of Johnny, or his mother and siblings. The family moved away when Johnny was placed in foster care and abandoned him, stating that he was "too difficult to care for." In residential placement, he was often shunned by peers because of his poor social skills and high impulsivity. Johnny would also engage in fantastical game play and appear in "his own world" with little to no awareness of others.

During our first session of TF-CBT, Johnny presented with a fixation on the cartoon Dragon Ball Z (Funimation Entertainment, 1999–2003). He discussed this cartoon at length, with particular attention to the character Goku. Johnny described Goku as a boy who knew "karate" and had "superpowers." Upon further investigation, I also learned that Goku was an odd, monkey-tailed boy who did, in fact, have superhuman strength as he was born from a race of extraterrestrials called the Saiyans, said to be the strongest warriors in the universe. However, Goku was separated from this family as a result of death and ambiguous loss. It became apparent to me that there were many similarities between Johnny and Goku and that Goku

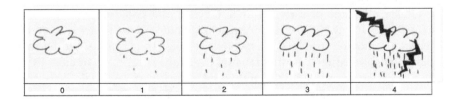

FIGURE 6.1. Rain Cloud Likert Scale (Grosso, 2011). Copyright 2011 by Christina A. Grosso. Reprinted by permission.

represented both an ego ideal and reflection of self for Johnny. His fixation on Goku was a coping strategy because it offered him a relatable figure with a means for self-protection. We began to use Goku in treatment from this moment forward.

Baseline Trauma Assessment

During the baseline trauma assessment, Goku's story served as a foundation for creating narrative. Johnny was able to recite with emotion and interest stories of Goku's adventures. However, Johnny had more difficulty reporting incidents and events from his own day-to-day life with the same intensity. When I asked him to tell me a story about the baseball game he attended a few days earlier, he recalled: "I went to the baseball game with my staff and some kids. The game was long. I ate a hot dog. We came home." When I asked him to tell me more about it and paced him through the story with encouragement to add thoughts and feelings, he added, "It was hot." When asked to tell me a story about his father and the abuse he suffered, he responded, "My dad is like Godzilla. I don't see my dad anymore." When prompted with similar questions, he slammed his fist on the table and stated, "I don't want to talk about it anymore."

After this clinical assessment and in combination with his standardized assessment scores, I realized that Johnny had limited language and cognition to describe what happened to him as well as difficulty identifying and expressing affect. His avoidance of thoughts, feelings, and details related to the trauma were substantiated by his score of a 43 on the UCLA PTSD Index for DSM-IV as well as his decreased detail in his baseline trauma narrative. The level of detail in his baseball story and his ability to tell Goku's story with emotion revealed his ability to complete a trauma narrative with a similar level of detail. However, he required a great deal of emotional and cognitive skill building in order to do so.

Many of the existing skills and activities outlined in TF-CBT for PRAC (Psychoeducation and Parenting, Relaxation, Affect expression and modulation, and Cognitive coping) can be used with children with developmental disabilities because of their highly interactive and visual nature (Cohen et al., 2006). During the PRAC components, children are developing competency and moving from a sense of powerlessness to control. Children with developmental issues are often reliant on caregivers for tasks of daily living and have a sense of diminished autonomy (Charlton et al., 2004). This, coupled with their traumatic experience, can leave children feeling even more dependent and helpless. Therefore, during PRAC it is essential for them to develop mastery and competence through skill-building activities that they can learn in session but then practice and use both in school and at home.

The repetition of these skills will also aid in retention and comfort with the material.

Psychoeducation and Parenting

During psychoeducation, our major goal is to normalize reactions to trauma (see Table 6.4). As with beginning treatment with any child, we want to begin by introducing the goals of therapy, review assessments, and learn more about the child. In working with a child with a developmental disability, we want to pay particular attention to his or her interests and the presence of any fixations because we can utilize this to support the child's learning. Existing strategies in TF-CBT for psychoeducation, such as bibliotherapy and games, are highly effective. Utilizing sources that contain illustrations to describe concepts are most successful, such as the book *A Terrible Thing Happened* (Holmes & Mudlaff, 2000). This book chronicles the behavior of Sherman the raccoon after he experiences "a terrible thing," and captures the raccoon's emotional, cognitive, and behavioral symptoms of trauma through both words and pictures. The "terrible thing" is depicted as a black cloud floating over Sherman's head in a thought bubble and can easily be substituted by the child's index trauma. This book offers a sufficient level of gradual exposure to the trauma through metaphor and provides a direct conduit to the subsequent TF-CBT components. This book can also

TABLE 6.4. Why Do We Provide Psychoeducation to Children Who Have Been Traumatized?

Goals
- To normalize responses to trauma
- To reinforce accurate cognitions

Challenges
Children with developmental disabilities have:
- Poor comprehension and retention
- Decreased capacity for generalization—are black-and-white thinkers
- Fixations or special interests
- Limited attention spans

Skills
- Use visuals to illustrate concepts and aid in communication
- Use favorite characters, cartoons, puppets, figurines, sand play, and dollhouses to create stories and metaphor
- Use active play and games to engage and maintain attention
  - What Do You Know? (Deblinger et al., 2006)
- Bibliotherapy
  - A Terrible Thing Happened (Holmes & Mudlaff, 2000)

Note. Based on Charlton, Kliethermes, Tallant, Taverne, and Tisherlman (2004) and Cohen, Mannarino, and Deblinger (2006).

be used to stimulate discussion by pausing at various intervals through-out the story and asking questions such as "What happened to you?" and "Have you ever felt like that?"

During psychoeducation with Johnny, we were able to use Goku as a vehicle for learning. As we discussed results from the assessment and began to review symptoms of trauma, I drew parallels to Goku and asked Johnny questions about some of the reactions Goku might have to scary events. This appeared to interest Johnny because he became engaged in this activity around trauma symptoms that both he and Goku experienced. Playing the What Do You Know? game (Deblinger, Neubauer, Runyon, & Baker, 2006), I asked Johnny, "How can you tell if a child has been sexually abused?" He responded, "You can just tell—you can see it." We were able to discuss further that unlike Goku, who had a monkey tail, we could not see Johnny's trauma. This direct discussion of trauma being invisible appeared to increase his understanding that he could feel and think about his trauma but others did not know or understand his thoughts, feelings, and experiences unless he shared them.

Providing support to parents of children with developmental disabilities is of utmost importance during TF-CBT (see Table 6.5). Research shows that these parents have increased stress because of the cognitive,

---

TABLE 6.5. Why Do We Provide Parenting Skills?

Goals
- To normalize responses to trauma
- To teach parents strategies for addressing problematic behaviors, including praise, selective attention, time-outs, and contingency reinforcement strategies

Challenges
Parents/caregivers of children with developmental disabilities have:
- Increased stress and feelings of overwhelm as a result of:
  - Increased supervisory demands
  - Lack of education and preparation to deal with disability
  - Lack of appropriate educational and treatment services for their children
  - Lack of response from child to traditional means of discipline and reinforcement

Skills
- Provide structure/ create routine
  - Help family and caregivers create schedules/routines in the home and school (e.g., set times for meals, homework, bed)
- Provide repetition and reinforcement
  - Repeat skills and concepts in session
  - Assign homework to practice skills taught in session
  - Use consistent praise and rewards as reinforcement of positive behavior
- Create supportive family groups

Note. Based on Cohen, Mannarino, and Deblinger (2006) and Hibbard and Desch (2007).

emotional, and behavioral issues presented by their children and a lack of support to effectively address them (Hibbard & Desch, 2007). These developmental issues coupled with the child's emotional, cognitive, and behavioral reactions to trauma creates a significantly stressed, overwhelmed family system. Parents will require creative adaptations to traditional parenting strategies and a flexible and patient clinician to help them after failed attempts. Some basic tenets to focus on with children with developmental disabilities are their need for structure, repetition, and reinforcement. Many children have multiple caregivers because of their increased need for supervision. Treatment may include not only the parents but aides, teachers, and other caregivers to establish safety and increase communication. In essence, the clinician will be working with a multidisciplinary team of individuals who need to understand the impact of the trauma on the children and have consistent skills and strategies to reinforce in their respective roles and environments. It is recommended that the clinician share the children's toolkit with all caregivers, with additional copies made to be kept at home and school.

Relaxation

As we look at the role of relaxation and grounding in trauma treatment (see Table 6.6), we recognize the need to regulate physiological responses, such as increased heart rate, shallow breathing, tension in the body, sweating, stomachaches, and headaches. This regulation is needed in order to manage trauma reminders and later tolerate increased exposure during the trauma narrative. Children with developmental disabilities may have a higher baseline of anxiety and agitation and encounter difficulties remembering and utilizing relaxation strategies (Wood et al., 2009). They may require more repetition of skill with little to no exposure as they learn and practice. Once the skill is acquired, it can be gradually paired with exposure to their negative stimulus hierarchy with support and prompts from both caregivers and therapist.

In order to determine where stress and tension exist in the body, a doll or a drawing of a human figure can be used to have children point to areas of the body that feel activated. The children should be encouraged to use this as a starting point and identify areas on their own body that become dysregulated and then asked, "How does your body feel when you think about scary things?" Relaxation strategies can then be introduced, such as deep breathing using bubbles. Blowing bubbles provides a concrete, focused task for children in that they need to blow the bubble in a slow, steady manner in order to form a full, round bubble that is able to float off the wand. If they blow too hard and fast the bubble will break; and if they blow too slowly the bubble will not form. The therapist can then extend the relax-

TABLE 6.6. Why Do We Teach Relaxation Strategies to Children Who Have Been Traumatized?

Goals
• To reduce physiological symptoms of stress and trauma

Challenges
  Children with developmental disabilities have:
  • Sensory sensitivity
  • Impulsivity
  • Agitation and greater proneness to anxiety
  • More behavioral issues; may be quick to hit, punch, kick when agitated

Skills
  • Relaxation
    ▪ Bubble breathing
    ▪ Goku Squeeze
  • Grounding
    ▪ Sensory toolkit
    Pocket Pal

Note. Based on Charlton, Kliethermes, Tallant, Taverne, and Tisherlman (2004) and Cohen, Mannarino, and Deblinger (2006).

ation exercise to include watching the bubbles float in the air and gently pop on surfaces they contact.

When I began the relaxation phase of treatment with Johnny, some of the exercises, such as squeezing lemons to make lemonade, lost his attention (also note that he appeared confused that lemonade was made from lemons and not from a container of powder). Johnny held a great deal of tension and emotion in his body and would explode with aggression when triggered. In an effort to gain his attention, I created the Goku Squeeze. Goku was able to reach his full superhuman strength when he entered super-Saiyan mode, which he achieved by squeezing his hands into fists and tensing his body. Johnny stated that Goku was strongest then and able to "do good." Johnny was able to visualize Goku and tense his muscles in his body, beginning with his fists, then moving to his arms, shoulders, face, torso, legs, and feet. He would practice this and hold for a count of 10. He then would release his muscles, and we would reflect on how his body was feeling. He expressed having a sense of calm and that he could "do good" like Goku rather than explode and get into fights.

Grounding

Children with developmental disabilities may also have issues with sensory integration and sensitivity. They may become overwhelmed with loud noises or be soothed by the feeling of cool water on their hands. When working with these children, it is beneficial to explore how they react to various sensory stimuli and to develop a toolkit with items they find soothing and can use for grounding. Items such as bubble wrap, sandpaper, cotton, felt, Model Magic, playdough, water, and sand can be explored.

People, places, and things can also be used as grounding strategies. Very often, Johnny would rely on his milieu counselor, Pat, to help himself regulate. This worked well when Pat was available but was not an effective strategy when Pat was in a meeting, was off grounds, or had a day off. When Johnny experienced a trigger that was overwhelming, he often relied on Pat to prompt and model the use of a relaxation and/or grounding strategy. As Johnny's autonomy and proficiency in relaxation increased, he still relied on Pat to be present, even though he could do these skills on his own. We soon discovered that Pat himself was a grounding strategy and became part of Johnny's routine when triggered. We wanted to increase Johnny's independence and create a new routine, which prompted us to create a pocket pal, named Pocket Pat. Pocket Pat was a pocket-sized, felt cutout of a gingerbread-shaped person. Johnny was able to create this during session and fill in the facial features and clothing to resemble those of Pat. On the reverse was his "safety plan": a list of his relaxation and grounding strategies. After completing Pocket Pat, he kept it in his pocket for retrieval whenever he felt triggered or upset to prompt him to use his relaxation strategies. As Johnny used Pocket Pat, his dependence on the real Pat decreased.

Affect Identification and Modulation

As stated earlier, there are many wonderful activities already embedded in TF-CBT that utilize visual and interactive learning that can be used with children with developmental disabilities (Cohen et al., 2006). Affective identification and modulation skills, such as Feeling Faces, Feelings in My Body, and emotional thermometers are highly effective tools to use with developmentally disabled children (see Table 6.7). Additional time may be needed to teach and practice skills to ensure comprehension and retention. Favorite characters, puppets, and cartoons can be used to engage children, and story lines can be created to elicit feelings through metaphor. How would Wally the Whale feel if someone ate his lunch? How would Goku feel if his friend kicked him? Visual aids are also useful to reinforce these concepts. Children can draw their favorite characters with various facial expressions, or images can be downloaded from the Internet on which feelings can be labeled.

During this phase of treatment, Johnny had great difficulty identifying emotion in facial features, a common issue with children with developmental delays. During one session, he became interested in my camera. We proceeded to take many pictures of both him and me making faces. We printed the pictures and labeled them with the corresponding feeling, making a deck of personalized photo feelings cards. As we reviewed the pictures, he would

TABLE 6.7. Why Do We Teach Feeling Identification and Regulation to Children Who Have Experienced Trauma?

Goals
- To help children identify, regulate, and express feelings more effectively
- Decrease avoidance strategies

Challenges
Children with developmental disabilities have:
- Difficulty identifying emotions in self and others
- Difficulty expressing emotion via facial gestures and/or verbal statements
- Sensory sensitivity
- Impulsivity
- Agitation and greater proneness to anxiety
- More behavioral issues; may be quick to hit, punch, kick when agitated

Skills
- Provide repetition and reinforcement
  - Repeat skills and concepts in session
  - Assign homework to practice skills taught in session
  - Use consistent praise and rewards as reinforcement of positive behavior
- Photo feeling cards

Note. Based on Charlton, Kliethermes, Tallant, Taverne, and Tisherlman (2004) and Cohen, Mannarino, and Deblinger E. (2006).

compare his picture with his image in the mirror, name his feeling, shift his gesture, and then rename it with a new feeling. He continued to practice various gestures and then asked me to copy him. Through this activity, he was able to identify and express feelings through both visual and verbal modalities. These cards were also shared with staff and teachers to reinforce with Johnny in the milieu setting.

Cognitive Coping

This component (see Table 6.8) presents one of the most challenging issues in working with developmentally disabled children, namely recognizing and acknowledging internal thoughts (Reaven, 2009). As we begin to teach children how to acknowledge a thought, we need to teach them what a thought is. Very simply, thinking can be described as "talking to ourselves." We can ask, "What do you say to yourself when you make a mistake?" This self-talk will begin to highlight some of their thought processes and provide the foundation for the intersection among thoughts, feelings, and behaviors (i.e., the cognitive triangle).

Children with developmental disabilities are visual thinkers and require movement and activation to remain focused. In teaching Johnny the cognitive triangle, he and I played "baseball." I taped a triangle on the floor in my office and labeled each point "thought," "feeling," or "behavior." We then stood on the thought point and I provided Johnny with a scenario where he walked into the classroom and a fellow student began laughing. I then asked him, "What are you thinking? What are you saying to yourself?" He responded, "He doesn't like me." Next, we moved to the feeling point, and I asked, "How are you feeling?" He responded, "Sad and angry." And then finally we jumped to the behavior point, and I asked, "What do you do?" He responded, "Hit him in the face." We then were able to process why this behavior was not safe and how his thought could be inaccurate and unhelpful. We discussed replacing his original thought, that perhaps his peer did like him and that maybe something funny happened prior to Johnny entering the room. Johnny was then able to state he would feel "curious" and sit down in his seat and begin his classwork.

The cognitive triangle can also be adapted and used as an activity called Bubble People. The clinician helps the child draw numerous pictures of him- or herself or a favorite character (including face and body) on separate sheets of paper, and then they assign a marker color to "thought," "feeling," and "behavior." Similar to the activity described previously, the clinician then describes a scenario. Using the portraits and selected markers, the clinician writes the child's initial thought in a thought bubble next to the head in the drawing using the "thought" marker, adding what feelings would result after having such a thought (and writing them down on the body where the child experienced such feelings). This step is repeated for behav-

---

TABLE 6.8. Why Do We Teach Cognitive Coping Skills to Traumatized Children?

Goals
- To learn cognitive coping skills
- To acknowledge and share internal dialogue
- To understand the relationship among thoughts, feelings, and behaviors

Challenges
Children with developmental disabilities may have difficulty with:
- Abstract thinking
- Critical thinking
- Sequencing events
- Prioritizing
- Task breakdown
- Ambiguity

Skills
- Cognitive triangle baseball
- Bubble People
- Bibliotherapy
  - *The Little Engine That Could* (Piper, 1990)

Note. Based on Charlton, Kliethermes, Tallant, Taverne, and Tisherlman (2004) and Cohen, Mannarino, and Deblinger (2006).

iors using the appropriate color-coded marker. This is repeated numerous times, changing the thought and then discussing how the resulting feelings and behaviors change as well.

Trauma Narrative and Cognitive Processing

Trauma Narrative

Developing the trauma narrative with developmentally disabled children is a process that requires pacing, structure, and visual storytelling (see Table 6.9). Children have cognitive limitations (see Table 6.8) that will present challenges in creating the narrative in addition to their general trauma symptoms (avoidance and increased arousal in reaction to higher levels of exposure), which are to be expected at this point in treatment. It is important that clinicians be aware of their increased need to move slower and have shorter session times because they may be more reactive to negative stimulus than their nondisabled cohort (Reaven, 2009). They may need support and prompts to use their grounding and relaxation skills as they begin to talk about more distressing events. As they discuss details of the trauma, events may be fragmented and nonsequential. The clinician should begin by

---

TABLE 6.9. Why Do We Help Traumatized Children Tell Their Story?

Goals
- To unpair thoughts, triggers, and reminders of the trauma from overwhelming negative emotion
- To integrate thoughts and feelings into narrative
- To unify fragments of trauma memory into integrated whole
- To correct inaccurate thoughts
- To process distortions

Challenges
Children with developmental disabilities may have difficulty with:
- Abstract thinking
- Critical thinking
- Sequencing events
- Prioritizing
- Task breakdown
- Ambiguity

Skills
- Visual narrative
- Storyboarding
- Index card trauma timeline
- Bibliotherapy
  - *Please Tell* (Ottenweller, 1991)

Note. Based on Charlton, Kliethermes, Tallant, Taverne and Tisherlman (2004) and Cohen, Mannarino, and Deblinger (2006).

writing each of these "fragments" on index cards. This method of capturing information will allow the children to tell their story first without becoming frustrated trying to capture detail and chronology simultaneously. The cards can be reordered and chronologically sequenced later with pacing and assistance from the therapist.

Another method to assist with the telling of their story is visual narrative. As discussed, children with developmental delays are often visual thinkers and organize their thoughts in images. The therapist can begin by asking the children to draw a picture of what happened to them. This can be done on a single piece of paper or in a cartoon/storyboard approach utilizing multiple frames. This process allows children to capture detail and sequence visually, a method that is more intrinsic to their thought process, thus reducing their risk of increasing anxiety and frustration (Reaven, 2009).

We also want to keep in mind children's responses to the baseline trauma narrative completed at the onset of treatment. How did they respond to the innocuous event narrative? What was their capacity for storytelling? Did they include detail? Was it in chronological order? Did they include thoughts and feelings? How did their innocuous narrative compare with their baseline trauma narrative? We want to guide our expectations for the trauma narrative based on the level of detail ascertained during the baseline narrative of the innocuous event because this highlights their overall developmental level and capacity for storytelling. We cannot expect greater detail for the trauma narrative because it would presumably surpass their capability.

As we revisit the case of Johnny, we recall that he had limited detail in his story of the baseball game and with prompting was able to add feelings. With his account of his abuse he was not able to provide details, thoughts, or feelings and, moreover, became dysregulated, pounding his fist on the table. It was important to remind myself, as I worked with him and encouraged his inclusion of details, that this was congruent to his original baseline presentation. However, he made tremendous progress with identifying feelings and thoughts related to his abuse. He was able to reach this level of verbal communication via the use of visual narrative. Johnny began by drawing a picture of his father, depicted as a fire-breathing Godzilla. With prompting to tell a story about the picture, he began to describe that his father was "mean, angry and hurt" him, just like Godzilla hurt people in the movies. When asked how often this happened, he pointed to the rain cloud that indicated "much" (see Figure 6.1). I then asked him what happened when his father got "mean" and "angry." He responded by drawing a stick figure with a large red mark on its face. I asked him again to tell a story about the picture, and he stated his father would "punch, kick, and push" him. When asked "What happened next?", he drew a bed with two stick figures on it. Again with questioning, Johnny was able to state that after his father physically abused him, he would push Johnny on the bed and sexually abuse him. With further prompting Johnny was able to state that he felt "angry" and "sad" and that he "never wanted to see Dad again" and was "glad he was in jail." He also stated that he felt "bad" that his family was "gone."

Cognitive Processing

Children with developmental disabilities may have more cognitive distortions related to feelings of blame, guilt, and fear of recurrence compared with nondisabled children (Charlton et al., 2004). Feelings of blame may occur as a result of their limited capacity for critical thinking as well as their poor social skills and ability to communicate effectively with others. Cognitive processing techniques, such as challenging distortions, can be especially difficult because of cognitive and processing delays (Avrin et al., 1998). (See Table 6.9.)

Returning to the case of Johnny, it became clear that some areas of his narrative needed further exploration and processing. As with all children, we want to attend to both explicit and implicit distortions, especially around issues of shame, blame, and guilt. In terms of implicit or hidden distortions, Johnny stated that he felt "bad" that his family was gone, indicating possible feelings of blame and guilt. When I asked why he felt this way, he stated that his family moved away because he was "bad." This issue took a good deal of time to discuss because we needed to break down each feeling and thought one at a time. He had difficulty shifting his thinking, remaining in a state of black-and-white thinking that if he had not told about his abuse his family would still be together. I used a version of the best friend role play, and instead of using a "best friend," which he did not have, I used Goku. Through related story lines focusing on Goku's separation from his family, Johnny was able to begin to shift his thinking and list other possible reasons for his family leaving. We also discussed that if Goku stayed in a home where he was being hurt he would never have been able to become a strong superhero. Johnny was able to develop a list of all the ways in which he became stronger while in residential treatment, including what he learned in TF-CBT. In the final chapter of his narrative, he stated that he wanted to be strong like Goku and help other kids who have been hurt find a safe place.

In Vivo Mastery of Trauma Reminders

Children with developmental disabilities often have a lower threshold for negative stimuli and require special consideration when formulating hierarchies (Reaven, 2009; see Table 6.10). Exposures will need to be paced and have smaller increments of escalating stimuli, and care should be taken

TABLE 6.10. Why Do We Provide *In Vivo* Exposure to Traumatized Children?

Goals
- To decrease avoidance symptoms of generalized fears

Challenges
- Children with developmental disabilities may have lower threshold for negative stimuli

Skills
- Exposure hierarchies

Note. Based on Cohen, Mannarino, and Deblinger (2006) and Reaven (2009).

not to overwhelm children. Developmentally disabled children also have a tendency for rote behavior when anxious and have difficulty and/or discomfort with change (Avrin et al., 1998). They may become fixated on routines and rituals and have difficulty changing the structure of daily activities and schedules. When generalized fears or avoidant behaviors are noticed, it is imperative to address them as soon as possible so that they do not become further ingrained. It is important to have parents and/or caregivers "actively involved, comfortable, and in agreement with the plan" to offer consistency and reinforcement (Cohen et al., 2006, p. 149).

Conjoint Child–Parent Sessions

The child with developmental disabilities requires repetition of skills and clear structure and routines. As the child progresses through TF-CBT, it is imperative that parents are involved with treatment so they can reinforce skills as they are being used (see Table 6.11). As discussed earlier in the parenting component, the child with developmental disabilities often has multiple caregivers because of increased supervisory demands (Avrin et al., 1998). At various points throughout treatment, it is beneficial to meet with these other caregivers to review PRAC skills and reinforce repetition of learning and practice both at home and in school. Despite this team approach, it is recommended to share the trauma narrative with parents and not with all caregivers so as not to overwhelm the child. Parents may also require individual time to process their own cognitive distortions related to their child's trauma. The therapist should discuss the narrative with the parents before the conjoint session to allow time for these potential cognitions to emerge, prepare them for hearing the narrative, and plan areas of the narrative where they can offer praise and reinforce accurate cognitions. Even though parents need assistance in helping their child recover from trauma, they can also provide a great wealth of information and insight into their child's functioning and progress. Their expertise must be respected.

TABLE 6.11. Why Do We Have Conjoint Sessions?

Goals
- To increase communication between child and parent
- To increase comfort in talking about trauma

Challenges
- Children with developmental disabilities may:
- Engage in one-sided conversation
- Have difficulty engaging and responding to others

Skills
- Conjoint sessions throughout treatment
- Involve additional caregivers

Note. Based on Charlton, Kliethermes, Tallant, Taverne, and Tisherlman (2004) and Cohen, Mannarino, and Deblinger (2006).

Enhancing Future Safety and Development

As we have discussed throughout this chapter, children with disabilities are at higher risk for experiencing abuse than children without disabilities because of impairment in cognition, communication, and affect regulation (Avrin et al., 1998; Ryan, 1994). They often have limited information regarding sexual education, abuse prevention, and personal safety. Parents and caregivers often view their children as asexual and feel this information is unnecessary (Hibbard & Desch, 2007). However, research shows that sexual interest among children with developmental disabilities often occurs at the same developmental stage as for the rest of the population (Tharinger, 1990, as cited in Charlton et al., 2004). In order to increase awareness and independence and decrease the risk of revictimization in this population, personal safety skills are crucial (see Table 6.12). The content and extent of sexual education should always be discussed with the parents. However, basic safety skills such as recognizing "OK" and "not-OK" touch should be taught to all children.

Children with developmental disabilities often have a lack of boundaries and intrusive behaviors. Couple these tendencies with exposure to interpersonal trauma where body limits were violated, and increased confusion and permeable boundaries emerge. As with the development of PRAC skills already discussed, rehearsal and repetition of skills are important to enhance comprehension and retention.

As Johnny approached the end of treatment, it was essential that he learn practical skills to keep him safe. As with many traumatized and developmentally disabled children, his personal space was often an issue. At times he would hug strangers, and at other times he would not be able to be within talking distance of someone else. Johnny was prompted to ask for a hug or a handshake when he needed physical comfort and to wait for the

TABLE 6.12. Why Do We Provide Safety Planning?

Goals
- To teach personal safety skills
- To decrease risk of revictimization

Challenges
Children with developmental disabilities:
- May have a lack of boundaries, intrusive behaviors
- May be trained and/or compliant with authority figures
- May have increased dependency on caregivers for physical needs
- Have impaired communication and/or ability to disclose abuse
- Have limited access to sexual education and personal safety skills

Skills
- Repetition and practice
- Experiential learning
  - *Safety Bubble*
  - *No, Go, Tell*

Note. Based on Charlton, Kliethermes, Tallant, Taverne, and Tisherlman (2004); Cohen, Mannarino, and Deblinger (2006); and Hibbard and Desch (2007).

reply. He was also taught to use the Safety Bubble. In this boundary exercise, children stretch their arms out in front of them and imagine being surrounded by an invisible bubble. As they imagine this bubble encompassing their body, they can outstretch their arms in every direction. They are then asked to imagine others with this same bubble. Together with the therapist, they practice walking up to people and maintain the size and shape of their safety bubble. Children are also encouraged to express how comfortable they feel with the distance they are creating between self and other. If their safety bubble becomes invaded, they are prompted to move away and tell the person that he or she is too close. If this person ignores the command, the children are prompted to say "No," go and find help, and tell a safe adult what happened. Children should be encouraged to keep telling until someone listens. Johnny enjoyed this activity and at first required redirection and prompting to maintain the boundary of his invisible bubble. After practice with staff and peers, he made considerable progress maintaining his personal space.

After treatment, Johnny showed considerable improvement. His score on the UCLA PTSD Index for DSM-IV decreased from 43 to 19, indicating that he was no longer meeting criteria for posttraumatic stress disorder (Pynoos et al., 1998). His aggressive behaviors diminished and he was interacting more frequently and positively with peers. Johnny's fantastical play and talents in art making became a method of interaction with peers, who valued his artistic ability and joined him occasionally in game play. He continued to have issues when peers had visitation with family but was now able to express his feelings of jealousy and sadness in appropriate ways. The discharge plan for Johnny was to continue in residential treatment to address his other mental health needs while case planners investigated a preadoptive foster care family.

As we conclude our discussion of the application of TF-CBT for developmentally disabled children, we can review the progress of treatment and see that our toolbox for both therapist and child is "filling." Many interventions and activities have been introduced, and the expectation is that through future practice this toolbox will continue to expand. There is a growing need for traumatized children with developmental disabilities to receive treatment as well as for trained professionals to provide treatment (Charlton et al., 2004). In an effort to address this problem, we have adapted TF-CBT to fit the needs of this growing population. Traumatized children with developmental delays present some unique challenges to traditional verbal and cognitive-behavioral therapy (Moree & Davis, 2010; Reaven, 2009). Because of their impairments in cognition, language, and emotion, implementation strategies are needed to help children access concepts and develop appropriate skills (Moree & Davis, 2010; Wood et al., 2009). An integrated treatment approach utilizing visuals as resources to accompany verbal interventions was introduced as well as the use of structure, repetition, engagement, and activation strategies. As we have seen through the course of this chapter, these implementation strategies for TF-CBT have been created to increase the sense of mastery and independence in the lives of these children as they recover from trauma.

REFERENCES

Achenbach, T. M. (1991). *Integrative guide to the 1991 CBCL/4-18, YSR, and TRF profiles*. Burlington: University of Vermont, Department of Psychology.

Avrin, S., Charlton, M., & Tallant, B. (1998). *Diagnosis and treatment of clients with developmental disabilities*. Unpublished manuscript, Aurora Mental Health Center.

Boyle, C. A., Boulet, S., Schieve, L. A., Cohen, R. A., Blumberg, S. J., Yeargin-Allsopp, M., et al. (2011). Trends in the prevalence of developmental disabilities in US children, 1997–2008. *Pediatrics, 127*(6), 1034–1043.

Centers for Disease Control and Prevention. (2011, June 23). *Developmental disabilities increasing in US*. Atlanta, GA: Author. Retrieved from *www.cdc.gov/Features/dsDev_Disabilities/index.html*.

Charlton, M., Kliethermes, M., Tallant, B., Taverne, A., & Tisherlman, A. (2004). *Facts on traumatic stress and children with developmental disabilities*. Retrieved from National Child Traumatic Stress Network, *www.nctsn.org/products/facts-traumatic-stress-and-children-developmental-disabilities-2004*.

Charlton, M., & Tallant, B. (2003, December). *Trauma treatment with clients who have dual diagnoses: Developmental disabilities and mental illness.* Paper presented at the National Child Traumatic Stress Network Conference, San Diego, CA.

Cohen, J. A., Mannarino, A. P., & Deblinger, E. (2006). *Treating trauma and traumatic grief in children and adolescents.* New York: Guilford Press.

Deblinger, E., Neubauer, F., Runyon, M., & Baker, D. (2006). *What do you know?* Stratford, NJ: CARES Institute.

Funimation Entertainment. (1999–2003). *Dragon ball z* [Television series]. Atlanta, GA: Turner Broadcasting.

Goldson, E. (2002, July). *Maltreatment among children with disabilities.* Paper presented at the 14th International Congress on Child Abuse and Neglect, Denver, CO.

Grandin, T. (2010). The world needs all types of minds. Retrieved June 21, 2011, from *http://blog.ted.com/talks/lang/en/temple_grandin_the_world_heels_all_kinds_of_minds.html.*

Grosso, C.A. (2011). *Rain Cloud Likert Scale.* New York: Author.

Hibbard, R. A., & Desch, L. W. (2007). Maltreatment of children with disabilities. *Pediatrics, 119(5),* 1018–1025.

Holmes, M. M., & Mudlaff, S. J. (2000). *A terrible thing happened.* Washington, DC: Magination Press.

Moree, B. N., & Davis, T. E., III. (2010). Cognitive-behavioral therapy for anxiety in children diagnosed with autism spectrum disorders: Modification trends. *Research in Autism Spectrum Disorders, 4,* 346–354.

National Research Council. (2001). *Crime victims with developmental disabilities: Report of a workshop.* Washington, DC: National Academy Press.

Oathamshaw, S. C., & Haddock, G. (2006). Do people with intellectual disabilities and psychosis have the cognitive skills required to undertake cognitive behavioral therapy? *Journal of Applied Research in Intellectual Disabilities, 19,* 35–46.

Ottenweller, J. (1991). *Please tell: A child's story about sexual abuse.* Center City, MN: Hazelden.

Overcamp-Martini, M. A., & Nutton, J. (2009). CAPTA and the residential placement: A survey of state policy and practice. *Child and Youth Care Forum, 38(2),* 55–68.

Piper, W. (1990). *The little engine that could.* New York: Platt & Munk.

Reaven, J. A. (2009). Children with high-functioning autism spectrum disorders and co-occurring anxiety symptoms: Implications for assessment and treatment. *Journal for Specialists in Pediatric Nursing, 14(3),* 192–198.

Ryan, R. (1994). Posttraumatic stress disorder in persons with developmental disabilities. *Community Mental Health Journal, 30(1),* 45–54.

Sobsey, D., & Doe, T. (1991). Patterns of sexual abuse and assault. *Sexuality and Disability, 9(3),* 243–259.

Steinberg, A. M., Brymer, M. J., Decker, K. B., & Pynoos, R. S. (2004). The University of California, Los Angeles Post-traumatic Stress Disorder Reaction Index. *Current Psychiatry Report, 6,* 96–100.

Sullivan, P. M., & Knutson, J. F. (2000). Maltreatment and disabilities: A population-based epidemiologic study. *Child Abuse and Neglect, 24,* 1257–1273.

Taylor, J. L., Lindsay, W. R., & Wilner, P. (2008). CBT for people with intellectual disabilities: Emerging evidence cognitive ability and 10 effects. *Behavioural and Cognitive Psychotherapy, 36,* 723–733.

Wahlberg, T. (1998). Cognitive behavioral modification for children and young children with special problems. *Advances in Special Education, 11,* 223–253.

Wood, J. J., Drahota, A., Sze, K., Har, K., Chiu, A., & Langer, D. A. (2009). Cognitive behavioral therapy for anxiety in children with autism spectrum disorders: A randomized controlled trial. *Journal of Child Psychology and Psychiatry, 50*(3), 224–234.

7

Adolescents with Complex Trauma

MATTHEW KLIETHERMES
RACHEL WAMSER

OVERVIEW OF COMPLEX TRAUMA

Most clinicians working with a traumatized child population will encounter at least one adolescent who has experienced severe, multiple traumatic events. In fact, these teenagers represent the reality of a traumatized population (Finkelhor, Ormrod, & Turner, 2009). Not surprisingly, survivors of prolonged and repeated traumatic events often present with a more complicated symptom picture compared with those who were more acutely traumatized (Cook, Blaustein, Spinazzola, & van der Kolk, 2003; van der Kolk, 2005). Beyond posttraumatic stress disorder (PTSD), these adolescents have myriad difficulties across several domains of functioning. In an effort to better capture the reality of this symptom presentation, the term *complex trauma* was developed (Herman, 1992). Complex trauma has a dual definition, referring to both a specific type of traumatic exposure as well as the devastating impact that such a trauma history leaves in its wake (Cook et al., 2003). Complex trauma events are typically defined as traumas that are multiple, chronic, and interpersonal in nature and begin at an early age, such as severe sexual or physical abuse, neglect, witnessing domestic violence, or the experience of a refugee camp (Cook et al., 2005). Thus, complex trauma events are best conceptualized as a subset of events typically defined as traumatic by the diagnostic category PTSD.

Exposure to complex trauma is, predictably, toxic. Personal resources that would have been allocated for development are instead used for survival to cope with the unstable, frightening, and overwhelming complex trauma environment (Cook et al., 2003). In the face of such stress, youth's limited ability to cope is depleted: They lose, or never develop, the ability to regulate themselves. In fact, dysregulation is cited as the hallmark characteristic of children and adolescents who have experienced complex trauma (Spinnazola et al., 2005). The inability to self-regulate results in a broad range of difficulties across various contexts. The impact of complex trauma, then, does not easily lend itself to a specific list of behavioral symptoms. Instead, broad domains of impaired functioning have been observed, including difficulties of regulation in affect, behavior, biology, attention and cognition, self, and relationships with others (Cook et al., 2005; van der Kolk, 2005). Complex trauma is not currently formally recognized by any diagnostic construct but has been described in two potential diagnostic categories— namely disorders of extreme stress not otherwise specified (DESNOS) and developmental trauma disorder—which have been proposed for inclusion in DSM-IV and in the forthcoming DSM-5 (Roth, Newman, Pelcovitz, van der Kolk, & Mandel, 1997; van der Kolk, 2005).

WHY TF-CBT APPLICATIONS ARE NECESSARY

Working with a complex trauma population has many unique challenges that necessitate different applications of the trauma-focused cognitive-behavioral therapy model (TF-CBT; Cohen, Mannarino, & Deblinger, 2006). TF-CBT effectively addresses trauma-related symptoms, such that following treatment the child or adolescent will return to pretrauma functioning. For survivors of complex trauma, this goal may not be initially feasible. For many, the traumatic events began so early in life and with exhausting regularity that there is no prior baseline to return to. For them, trauma has become a "way of life." Furthermore, whether the result of continuing consequences from the traumatic event or from their struggles, these youth's environment often remains chaotic during treatment and legitimate crises occur frequently (Cook et al., 2003). The youth may experience a placement change or enter a residential treatment facility, the parental rights of their parents may be terminated, or they may be expelled from school. Ongoing chaos tends to characterize their lives. These crises are often not attempts to avoid trauma-related content but instead relevant challenges that require attention in treatment. Effective trauma-focused treatment requires multiple, uninterrupted sessions focused on processing trauma-related content (Cohen et al., 2006). Trauma work may then dissolve into a series of "starts and stops" as these crises occur. Continuing to only process past events irrespective of current pressing issues is ill-advised because this can result in a serious breach in the often tenuous therapeutic relationship.

The laundry list of presenting problems in a complex trauma population also necessitates that TF-CBT be applied appropriately to these issues. First, complexly traumatized adolescents have often experienced a variety of inconsistent and unpredictable interpersonal experiences, ranging from inappropriate closeness to indifference to victimization (Cook et al., 2003). Survivors of complex trauma may be distrustful of others, viewing others as unpredictable, uncontrollable, and/or hostile. These attachment difficulties may be brought with them to the therapeutic relationship (Courtois, 1999). It is not uncommon for adolescents with a complex trauma history to initially present as highly guarded or avoidant for weeks to months. The consistency and attunement of a good therapist may be a foreign experience to adolescent survivors of complex trauma as even this typically benign aspect of the therapeutic relationship may be anxiety provoking (Courtois, 2004). Trauma work necessitates a solid working alliance, as, for example, exposure work ideally occurs in the context of a safe environment with a supportive therapist. Given the attachment issues that adolescents with complex trauma may present with, special therapeutic strategies may be needed to advance treatment.

Dysregulation characterizes the complex trauma population and often permeates various domains of functioning, including affect, behavior, cognition, and self-concept (van der Kolk, 2005). These youth are often excessively reactive to events in their environment. Such self-regulation difficulties typically result in significant, ongoing adversity for them. For example, emotional and behavioral dysregulation may contribute to the adolescent becoming enraged at a teacher who is criticizing him and then pushing the teacher against a wall, resulting in expulsion. Aggressive behavior toward a foster parent may result in the disruption of that placement and subsequent placement in a residential facility. Again, these scenarios could create interruptions in TF-CBT treatment and, in particular, make the gradual exposure work choppy, inefficient, and potentially unsuccessful. Furthermore, survivors of complex trauma often present with developmental capacities that resemble those of much younger children, such as difficulty identifying an affective state or even knowing when one is hungry (Ford, Courtois, Steele, van der Hart, & Mijenhuis, 2005).

In light of these issues, adolescents with a history of complex trauma is often ill-equipped to jump into trauma-focused treatment. However, TF-CBT is the most researched evidence-based practice for treating children and adolescents exposed to traumatic events (Cohen et al., 2010). Although TF-CBT was not developed specifically for complexly traumatized youth, with some adjustments it can be highly effective for this population. The PRACTICE components of TF-CBT (i.e., Psychoeducation and Parenting, Relaxation, Affective expression and modulation, Cognitive coping and processing, Trauma narrative, *In vivo* mastery of trauma reminders, Conjoint child–parent sessions, and Enhancing future safety and development; Cohen et al., 2006) can be applied to address the myriad impairments observed in this population. However, when these youth enter treatment, they may not be optimally prepared to benefit from these types of interventions without some modifications with regard to pacing and ordering of components. The instability of their environment and the severity of their own emotional and behavioral difficulties may interfere with their ability to receive the full benefit of a short-term, structured treatment targeting symptoms of posttraumatic stress.

ASSESSMENT OF COMPLEX TRAUMA EVENTS AND OUTCOMES

Complexly traumatized youth often present to treatment with a chaotic environment, several experiences of traumatic events, and a variety of chronic difficulties, a common one of which is attachment problems (Cook et al., 2005). Compounding the problem, these adolescents may not bring a long-term, informed caregiver to treatment. Thus, a few helpful assessment strategies may be worth mentioning. First, in light of these survivors' complicated lives, the assessment process may be best conceptualized as peeling an onion. The therapist is advised to follow the pace of the adolescents, obtaining what information is available (Ford et al., 2005). The therapist is unlikely to obtain all of the relevant information in the first three sessions. For these survivors, it may take months for them to trust the therapist to discuss their current difficulties. As treatment progresses, the adolescents' symptom presentation and functioning may appear worse (Taylor, Gilbert, Mann, & Ryan, 2008). This may not reflect a deterioration of behavior but instead is a by-product of the adolescents being more honest about or even aware of their difficulties.

Second, in the absence of a traditional caregiver, the therapist is advised to attempt to obtain relevant information from other sources, such as a caseworker or a teacher. However, sometimes crucial information is lost due to "systemic flux" (e.g., caseworker changes). Adolescents are often reluctant or unable to provide early life information; therefore, the therapist may have gaps in adolescents' background history. Third, as in any trauma population, the clinician is advised to be mindful of the adolescents' level of arousal. The clinician should be sensitive to triggering or flooding clients when inquiring about traumatic events and remain within the "therapeutic window" (Briere, 1996a). That is, clients should neither be over- or underwhelmed, while still providing relevant clinical and historical information.

The therapist is also advised to inquire about traumatic events in a supportive although neutral way (Courtois, 2004). The assessment process can engender some feelings of distress; however, this is normal and often temporary. It is prudent for the clinician to administer measures only in his or her presence, allowing the clinician to both assess the adolescents' level of arousal as well as ask important follow-up questions.

Assessing Traumatic Exposure

For a complex trauma population, a thorough assessment of exposure to traumatic events is important. By definition, they have experienced multiple traumatic events that may have been perpetrated by more than one individual over several years. Without knowledge of adolescents' complete exposure to trauma, trauma-related difficulties could be misattributed to a single traumatic event. Obtaining this history, however, is not easy. The therapist should not assume that inquiring about traumatic events will result in a disclosure (Courtois, 2004). Structured assessment tools can be useful because they prompt the clinician to assess for multiple traumatic events. The clinician should be aware of some of the details surrounding the traumatic event such as the child's age, length of the trauma, identity of the perpetrator, and severity of the trauma. Additionally, other developmentally adverse events such as emotional abuse, separations from caregivers, exposure to caregiver substance abuse, or mental illness should be inquired about. Complexly traumatized adolescents too often have been deeply affected also by the aftermath of the trauma: significant secondary adversity such as court or legal processes, removal from the home, and placement in multiple foster homes or a residential treatment facility. Thus, it is wise to have a broader sense of what "trauma" consists of for this population.

Assessing Complex Trauma Outcomes

The broad domains of impairment observed in a complex trauma population do not easily lend themselves to a single diagnostic construct. Thus, no assessment tool will be sufficient in describing this symptom presentation (Briere & Spinazzola, 2005). Currently, a complex trauma assessment tool (i.e., Structured Interview for Disorders of Extreme Stress; Pelcovitz et al., 1997) exists only for adults. Clinicians are advised to make an educated guess about what areas of impairment are likely to be important to assess (Briere & Spinazzola, 2005). As a general rule, it is helpful to use assessment tools that examine multiple areas of functioning, and it is preferable to obtain information about trauma-related symptoms from multiple informants (Cohen et al., 2010). Following are some tools that may be useful in assessing the various domains of complex trauma.

Affect: Trauma Symptom Checklist for Children (TSCC; Briere 1996b), Minnesota Multiphasic Personality Inventory–A (MMPI-A; Butcher et al., 1992)

Attention: Behavior Assessment System for Children (BASC; Reynolds & Kamphaus, 2004), Comprehensive Behavior Rating Scales (CBRS) (Conners, 2008), Child Behavior Checklist (CBCL; Achenbach & Rescorla, 2001), Teacher Report Form (TRF; Achenbach & Rescorla, 2001)

Behavior: CBCL, BASC, CBRS, TRF

Biology: CBCL, MMPI-A (Subscale 1), Youth Self Report (Achenbach & Rescorla, 2001)

Dissociation: TSCC, CBCL (Thought Problems subscale)

Cognition: Wechsler Intelligence Scale for Children (Wechsler, 2004), Stanford–Binet Intelligence Scales (Roid, 2003), CBCL, BASC, CBRS, TRF

Self: MMPI-A

PHASE-BASED TREATMENT FOR COMPLEX TRAUMA

Treating adolescent survivors of complex trauma can be a complicated, overwhelming process because the demands and needs of the adolescents are often varied, intense, and rapidly changing. It can be argued that no gold standard treatment exists for this population as of yet. However, various experts have posited that a phase-based approach to treatment is best, particularly for youth who manifest the most severe impairments (Cook et al., 2005; Ford et al., 2005; Herman, 1992). In a phase-based approach, treatment is sequential, with each phase of treatment building upon the next, although they may not always proceed in a linear fashion and therapist and client may return to a previous stage as needed (Courtois, 1999). Phase-based approaches, then, are sensitive to the chaos and changing needs of this population. Several phase-based approaches have been developed for complex trauma survivors. Ford and colleagues (2005) describe one approach, consisting of three phases: engagement, safety, and stabilization; recalling traumatic memories; and enhancing daily living. Briefly, in phase 1, the therapist largely works to form a working alliance and increase the youth's sense of safety. This is no small feat in light of the often observed attachment problems and environmental instability characteristic of this population. The second phase of treatment directly focuses on trauma-related content and processing of traumatic memories, which can occur at a safe, manageable pace through titration of exposure intensity and the utilization of self-regulation skills learned in phase 1. When symptoms of posttraumatic stress become manageable, therapist and client move to phase 3, which is focused on helping the client to work toward a healthy, balanced lifestyle that is not ruled by trauma.

TF-CBT is designed so that it can be implemented as a phase-based treatment. Specifically, the TF-CBT PRACTICE components can be implemented to address the three goals of phase-based treatment. Initially, the TF-CBT PRACTICE components (Psychoeducation and Parenting, Relaxation, Affective expression and modulation, Cognitive coping and processing, Trauma narrative, *In vivo* mastery of trauma reminders, Conjoint child–parent sessions, and Enhancing future safety and development) are used to facilitate the development of safety, stability, and engagement while incorporating gradual exposure by helping the adolescent identify and tolerate trauma cues. These skills can then be used to facilitate the TF-CBT trauma narrative and processing and *in vivo* mastery components, which clearly address the phase-based treatment goal of processing traumatic memories. Finally, the PRACTICE components are integrated to help the adolescent plan for and develop a healthy, balanced future that is no longer dominated by the experience of complex trauma. The skills and knowledge the adolescent gains while applying TF-CBT components to establish safety and stability and to process traumatic memories can finally be used to help the adolescent navigate through his or her "posttrauma" life in a healthy and satisfying manner. Some adjustments with regard to the order, scope, pacing, and emphasis of the PRACTICE components are described next to address the specific needs of adolescent survivors of complex trauma. Fortunately, TF-CBT was designed as a flexible model, adaptable to meet the specific needs of individual clients, and these applications are, therefore, consistent with the TF-CBT model. The following sections provide an overview of the implementation of TF-CBT with this population.

FACILITATING ENGAGEMENT, SAFETY, AND STABILITY THROUGH TF-CBT

Fostering Engagement

Fostering engagement with complexly traumatized adolescents can be challenging. However, this phase is paramount. The importance of the therapeutic relationship cannot be overemphasized. Beyond establishing rapport with the clients, the therapist must establish trust. The former can usually be accomplished rather quickly; the latter can be more slowgoing. Although these youth often crave supportive relationships, the formation of a relationship may seem threatening because of their numerous experiences of interpersonal trauma. The therapist will often have to pass many client "tests" to demonstrate that he or she is trustworthy and safe. Therefore, this stage of treatment may need to be expanded beyond what would typically be allotted during TF-CBT. There is "no short-cut to developing trust" (Briere, 2002 p. 188). A therapist may spend up to eight sessions building engagement. However, these sessions should not be used to just "play games." Instead, the therapist should be actively working toward stabilization, initiating contact with the other "systems" in the clients' life, and addressing any safety concerns. Being patient and consistent is often an effective intervention in and of itself because this is often counter to what this population usually experiences. During the engagement process, the adolescents are being exposed to their discomfort with intimacy through the development of a safe and secure relationship with the therapist. Here, the adolescents are "gradually exposed" to the therapist. In this portion of treatment, the therapist should consider the therapeutic relationship to be a potential trauma cue, and expose clients to the relationship in a gradual, controlled fashion. The therapist needs to attend to clients' distress level during therapeutic interactions to ensure that they do not become overwhelmed and to "titrate" the therapeutic relationship by varying the intensity of the interaction as appropriate (e.g., ask fewer questions, direct conversation to a more neutral topic, break up conversations with activities). The therapist may choose to allow the adolescents to familiarize themselves with and give appropriate control over the therapeutic environment (e.g., allowing them to pick where they and the therapist will sit). Early on, the therapist may need to be less directive and structured because doing so may be perceived as coercive and threatening by clients. In general, engagement can be accomplished by focusing on developing a therapeutic relationship explicitly based on respect, open sharing of information, empowerment, and the installation of a sense of hope (Pearlman & Courtois, 2005).

Enhancing Safety and Future Development

The enhancing safety and future development component of TF-CBT may need to be prioritized early as a result of the common presence of safety concerns such as self-injurious behavior or exposure to violence or bullying. Here, the therapist will work to develop safety plans and to identify safe people and places in addition to providing assertiveness training and problem solving. Given the distrust that adolescent survivors of complex trauma often have toward authority figures (e.g., police officers), it is important to work with them to identify appropriate people they trust and are willing to turn to when they feel threatened. Addressing safety concerns often requires systemic work. Caring adults in the youth's life may need to be trained to address youth deficits that impact safety, or may need to be contacted to address environmental factors that are contributing to safety concerns, such as bullying at school or exposure to potential emotional abuse in a foster home.

Psychoeducation

The psychoeducation component is initially devoted to educating the youth and applicable caregivers on the impact of stress and trauma on the adolescent's current functioning. Information should be provided regarding the definition of stress, common responses to stress and trauma, the rationale for stress responses (i.e., to alert to the presence of potential danger), and common coping mechanisms (both healthy and unhealthy). The youth and caregivers are helped to understand the adolescent's emotional and behavioral dysregulation as overreactions to stress rather than as willful misbehavior. It is also helpful to describe the concept of trauma triggers. The adolescent needs to be helped to learn how to react differently from his or her habitual fight–flight–freeze reactions (Briere & Scott, 2006). The therapist can also discuss that, because of past interpersonal trauma, the adolescent has made adaptations to the way he or she interacts with people to promote a sense of safety. Time should be spent helping the adolescent and caregiver identify their own adaptive and maladaptive responses to stress. This discussion can establish the rationale, and increase buy-in, for the subsequent skill-building components.

Parenting

If a caregiver is available, parenting work occurs through the therapist modeling appropriate engagement strategies in the therapist's interactions both with the client and with the caregiver. However, often the adolescent does not present to treatment with a traditional caregiver. Thus, for this population, the parenting component of TF-CBT is often more accurately conceptualized as the "systems" component, and includes any caregiver or authority figure who plays a significant role in the youth's life. Commonly, this is accomplished by increasing the frequency of safe, positive interactions between caregiver and adolescent (e.g., planning a weekly outing) and reducing the relational damage caused by negative interactions (e.g., decreasing the caregiver's reliance on physical punishment) and signals of danger (e.g., a teacher repeatedly criticizing the adolescent in front of peers). The goal is to create a trauma-informed system of caregivers and professionals working with the adolescent. All significant caregivers and professionals should be helped to accurately identify trauma-related behaviors as misplaced, excessive survival responses rather than as intentional misbehavior or manipulation. If all systemic entities are aware of the relaxation strategies the adolescent has learned, they can help facilitate the use of those strategies at times when the adolescent is becoming distressed. Because of the tendency for distrust, the adolescent is likely to be suspicious of the therapist's contact with various systemic entities. The therapist should be relatively transparent with the adolescent, informing the client about whom the therapist is contacting, what information is being exchanged, and the purpose of that interaction.

Relaxation

Here, it is often important to validate the coping strategies that the adolescent has used in the past. Previously used positive coping strategies can be incorporated, and the therapist should demonstrate understanding for the use of less adaptive strategies. The therapist should note that the strategies represented the adolescent's best efforts to deal with stress, although it may be associated with some negative consequences (e.g., getting into legal trouble for marijuana possession). Extensive time may be needed to help the adolescent recognize the difference between stressed and relaxed states, as his or her neurobiological "alarm system" is typically overreactive (Ford, 2005). Therefore, physically based activities that accentuate the difference between tension and relaxation (e.g., yoga, stretching, progressive muscle relaxation) may be initially more beneficial than cognitively based activities (e.g., imagery, positive self-talk). Self-soothing and distraction techniques may also be helpful because the adolescent may be more familiar with these and may already use them in some fashion, such as listening to music, playing video games, or taking a hot bath. However, the adolescent may need help using these strategies in a more systematic fashion and developing awareness of the potential for overuse (e.g., failing to study for a test as a result of playing video games all night).

Affective Regulation

Affective regulation is typically focused on increasing the adolescent's awareness of and ability to express and manage emotions in day-to-day life. In this phase, affective regulation primarily occurs through the therapist's use of attunement to help the adolescent identify and express the emotions he or she is experiencing during sessions and the therapist's modeling of effective expression and regulation of his or her own emotions in session. Here, the therapist begins to introduce some of the following concepts: the role of emotions in daily life; all emotions are valid and acceptable language for different emotional states; emotions can be experienced at different levels of intensity; multiple emotions can be experienced at the same time; negative affect states are temporary and can be tolerated; and effectively communicating emotions can alleviate their intensity and help secure support from others. This component may be initially challenging because many adolescent survivors present with emotional numbing or dissociative responses. These responses are best conceptualized as protective adaptations that are no longer adaptive. The therapist may have to spend more time highlighting the function of emotions, that is, that emotions provide useful information about the environment.

Cognitive Coping

The cognitive coping component is initially focused on helping the adolescent to increase awareness of cognitions during stressful experiences. The therapist may teach the cognitive triangle and use it to analyze recently experienced conflicts or crises. This process helps the adolescent to realize that thoughts he or she experiences during stressful situations may increase the likelihood of becoming distressed and engaging in problematic behavior. The adolescent can also develop cognitive coping strategies (e.g., positive self-talk), which can be used to improve one's response to stressful life events. Furthermore, using the cognitive triangle to process current stressors may also help the therapist and adolescent identify various triggers or "signals of danger" that are contributing to the distress the adolescent is experiencing in the moment.

Additionally, this component can be used to process current stressors and crises to help achieve the goal of stabilization while also providing practice for later processing of traumatic memories during the trauma narrative. Furthermore, current stressful situations experienced by the adolescent survivor of complex trauma often involve the presence of trauma cues (e.g., a chronically, emotionally abused adolescent being criticized by a teacher). Therefore, in true TF-CBT fashion, gradual exposure is also incorporated into the stabilization process.

Conjoint Sessions

Assuming the presence of a caregiver, conjoint work in TF-CBT is also used to facilitate engagement and stability. Research supports the importance of caregiver inclusion in the reduction of behavior problems within TF-CBT (Deblinger, Lippman, & Steer, 1996) and general treatment (Spoth, Neppl, Goldberg-Lillehoj, Jung, & Ramisetty-Mikler, 2006). Thus, these sessions are likely critical for stabilization. Because of disrupted attachment, the relationships between adolescent survivors of complex trauma and their caregivers are often strained and dysfunctional (Briere & Spinazzola, 2005). Complex trauma also typically occurs in the context of a caregiving relationship. For adolescent survivors of complex trauma, the simple act of engaging with a caregiver may be a trauma cue, resulting in dysregulation. Therefore, conjoint sessions provide valuable *in vivo* opportunities to gradually expose adolescents to these cues and further the development of a supportive, appropriate caregiving relationship that will help to better address dysregulation. These sessions are used to practice decreasing "signals of danger" while increasing "signals of care" (Saxe, Ellis, & Kaplow,

2007), and allow the therapist to model appropriate supportive behavior. Consistent contact with a supportive, appropriate caregiver will facilitate counterconditioning of the adolescents' experience of being victimized by prior caregivers. Furthermore, conjoint sessions can facilitate the caregiver's ability to coach the adolescents to use coping skills. Conjoint sessions in TF-CBT are also used for the adolescents to share their experience of stressful situations with the caregiver, including informing the caregiver of the various trauma triggers they have identified, thus helping the caregiver to develop a better understanding of the factors behind the adolescents' self-regulation difficulties. Assuming a supportive reaction, this conjoint work helps decrease the adolescents' reluctance to discuss future self-regulation difficulties with the caregiver.

Achieving "Good-Enough" Stability

Deciding to transition to processing traumatic memories (moving to the trauma narrative) can be difficult for therapists. Prior to doing so, it is important that the adolescent has made significant progress with regard to the establishment of engagement, safety, and stabilization. It is prudent to delay the initiation of trauma processing if the therapist is aware of significant upcoming changes or stressors such as a placement change, termination of parental rights, or reunification. The adolescent's environment needs to be sufficiently stable and safe for the therapist to determine that a significant interruption in the phase 2 process of recalling traumatic memories is unlikely. However, perfect stability is not required, as "crises of the week" will likely continue to occur and many youth actually cannot attain optimal stability until they process their traumatic experiences. Instead, the goal of the therapist is to determine whether the adolescent has achieved "good-enough" stability. The therapeutic relationship should be stable, allowing the therapist to continue to serve as a model for "safe and nonintrusive co-regulation" while facilitating the adolescent's ability to more directly process traumatic memories (Ford et al., 2005). Finally, the adolescent needs to have demonstrated sufficient mastery of self-regulation skills to tolerate direct exposure to traumatic memories; otherwise, exposure can be retraumatizing.

FACILITATING TRAUMA PROCESSING WITH ADOLESCENT SURVIVORS OF COMPLEX TRAUMA

Psychoeducation

Psychoeducation occurs throughout the TF-CBT model, including during the trauma narrative component (Cohen et al., 2006). For the adolescent survivor of complex trauma, psychoeducation serves multiple purposes. The therapist should carefully and transparently explain the rationale for trauma processing. Initially, psychoeducation is focused on providing a rationale for the processing of traumatic memories. As a result of affective numbing and cognitive distortions (e.g., "Exposure to violence is not a big deal because it's just a part of life"), a rationale for trauma processing that focuses on desensitization may not be sufficient or effective. Instead, the rationale may need to focus on the importance of uncovering the meanings the adolescent made (e.g., "Other people cannot be trusted") and how that meaning affects current functioning (e.g., avoiding intimacy). Providing concrete examples of how "the past informs the present" can be very helpful. The adolescent will also receive education regarding chronic, interpersonal trauma, focusing on prevalence and relevant mediating factors, and its impact. This can be helpful in addressing inaccurate and/or unhelpful trauma-related beliefs that the adolescent may be holding (e.g., "I deserved to be beaten. I am a bad kid").

Parenting

Parenting and systemic work remain important. Again, the focus is to ensure that all involved parties are utilizing appropriate engagement and behavior management strategies with the adolescent. This remains a critical issue because the adolescent's level of distress and subsequent behavioral problems may temporarily worsen when the processing of traumatic memories is initiated. All significant care providers should be warned of this possibility and trained to respond in a fashion that is supportive and positive rather than rejecting and critical.

Relaxation, Affective Regulation, and Cognitive Coping

During trauma processing, relaxation, affective regulation, and cognitive coping components will largely take the form of review and of encouraging adolescents to apply these skills. As needed, the therapist will review the knowledge and techniques learned to help the adolescents apply those skills to the processing of traumatic memories. Specifically, the adolescents learn to utilize relaxation skills in the context of trauma processing in order to help them manage their distress level and achieve desensitization to the traumatic memories. The affective regulation component is used to help the adolescents identify and monitor their level of distress during trauma processing work (e.g., through use of the Subjective Units of Distress Scale) and to facilitate the richness and depth of trauma processing by giving them adequate language to describe their experience of traumatic events. Similarly, the adolescents will learn to use cognitive coping skills to help them cope with distress associated with trauma processing (e.g., positive self-talk) and to process their traumatic memories more effectively by help-ing them identify what they thought about those events as they occurred. The application of these components during trauma processing is consistent with traditional TF-CBT. However, it should be noted that adolescent survi-vors of complex trauma often initially have less capacity to tolerate trauma processing than more acutely traumatized youth who experienced adequate development. Furthermore, these adolescents typically have less emotional awareness and are more likely to utilize affective numbing and dissociation as coping mechanisms. Therefore, rather than waiting for the adolescents to express feelings of distress verbally or behaviorally (e.g., facial expres-sions), it is important for the therapist to be proactive with encouraging them to check their distress level and practice self-regulation skills routinely throughout the session.

Trauma Narrative and Processing

For adolescent survivors of complex trauma, the trauma narrative and pro-cessing component remains the core phase of TF-CBT, but it may require significant adjustments. First, many of these youth's traumatic experiences occurred a relatively long time ago or they may not have an explicit, ver-bal memory of the event if it occurred prior to age 3 (Green, Crenshaw, & Kolos, 2010). Processing these memories in the traditional sense, then, is not possible. Furthermore, developing a detailed chronological account of trau-matic events may be very different for this population compared with youth exposed to a more acute form of trauma because the memory may be more confused, indistinct, and sometimes very difficult to retrieve. It may also not be feasible or even appropriate to complete a detailed account of each trau-matic event that the youth experienced because doing so would result in a very long narrative that would require many sessions to complete. A general rule of thumb is to allow adolescents to guide what events or experiences should be included in the trauma narrative (Cohen et al., 2006). As men-tioned, many adolescent survivors of complex trauma do not present with classic symptoms of PTSD. Thus, desensitization in the traditional sense may not be as vital. Often, the meaning attributed to the events depicted in the trauma narrative is of greater importance than repeated processing of the details of the trauma. Understanding underlying trauma themes and how these relate to the youth's current functioning (e.g., "None of the adults in my life protected me; they were the ones who hurt me. I always expect everyone to hurt me, so I hurt them first. That's why I'm in residential treat-ment") is often the most critical and meaningful aspect of trauma narration and processing for these youth.

In Vivo Mastery

For adolescent survivors of complex trauma, their early experience of chronic trauma, often not tempered by periods of safety or adequate development, becomes the lens through which they interpret later events. Subsequently, even relatively innocuous situations tend to be littered with perceived threats of danger, which result in the adolescents becoming increasingly distressed and dysregulated. Therefore, the *in vivo* mastery component of TF-CBT is often of critical importance to these youth because they need to develop the capacity to self-regulate sufficiently to tolerate uncomfortable but essentially safe situations. For example, an adolescent who was emotionally and physically abused by his father may become intensely dysregulated in response to his football coach taking a "tough love" approach during practice. Although the adolescent is not actually in danger, it will likely require significant self-regulation for him to not act as though he was. In truth, for this population, *in vivo* work often needs to be initiated early in treatment to facilitate the development of stability and engagement. However, following completion of trauma processing, the therapist and adolescents may develop a better understanding of what environmental cues are actually triggering them. Initially, it may have been clear what situations were distressing, but following trauma processing, the adolescents will likely develop a better understanding of why those situations have become triggers. This awareness may cause *in vivo* mastery work to become more successful because the adolescents will be able to use more targeted coping and problem-solving strategies.

Conjoint Sessions

Because adolescent survivors of complex trauma often do not have access to a traditional caregiver, foster parents and caseworkers may be options to fill this role. However, these adolescents may not have a secure, trusting relationship with these individuals such that they may not wish to disclose details of their trauma history. They may also fear that the information disclosed could result in unintended consequences, such as disrupting reunification with their biological parent. The therapist should not "force" a caregiver upon adolescents for the sake of conjoint work. Instead, the therapist and adolescents should collaborate on identifying possible individuals and exploring their involvement. It is the therapist's responsibility to ensure that the possible caregivers identified possess appropriate self-regulation skills and are capable of giving an appropriate, supportive response to the adolescents during conjoint sessions. Although the involvement of an appropriate caregiver is optimal, it should be made clear to the adolescents that they have the option of not involving a caregiver if they do not feel comfortable.

Enhancing Safety and Future Development

Ongoing safety concerns continue to be important during the trauma narrative component. Despite the therapist's best efforts, it is not possible to ensure that no safety concerns will arise after the processing of trauma memories has been initiated. It is necessary to occasionally discontinue trauma work if the adolescent is at risk (i.e., wrist-cutting following session). However, this is not ideal. A break from trauma processing should be done in a mindful manner. The therapist, adolescent, and caregiver (if applicable) should collaboratively reach an agreement to temporarily discontinue trauma processing work for a specified number of sessions. During that time period, efforts are directed at helping the adolescent cope more effectively with the situation and working with the system to reduce risk (e.g., developing a safety plan with staff at the adolescent's residential facility). When sufficient stability has been established, trauma processing can resume.

Completing Trauma Processing

Processing the experience of complex trauma is a complicated endeavor. The traumatic experiences of these youth often impact every facet of their life with seemingly unending ramifications. Therefore, determining when their traumatic experiences have been sufficiently processed is difficult. When PTSD symptoms become manageable, this phase of treatment is viewed as being complete (Cohen et al., 2006; Ford et al., 2005). The adolescents should be able to experience trauma cues without experiencing significant emotional or behavioral difficulties. They should be able to experience and recognize trauma memories and cues in the present, while being able to distinguish them as representations of past events and not indicative of current danger. The adolescents should also have a sense of meaning regarding their traumatic experiences. In essence, the goal is that the adolescents are able to identify their trauma exposure as only a part of their life rather than the totality of it, and as an experience from which they can learn and grow as they venture into a more hopeful future.

ENHANCING SAFETY AND FUTURE DEVELOPMENT THROUGH TF–CBT

Psychoeducation

As typically occurs in TF-CBT, psychoeducation is an important aspect of enhancing future safety and development for adolescent survivors of complex trauma. The focus of this psychoeducation involves identifying and normalizing the various challenges that the adolescents will likely experience throughout their lives. It is important to discuss the potential for future trauma triggers that the adolescents may not have encountered yet (e.g., graduating from therapy, sexual activity, becoming a parent, the death of a parent). It is essential that these challenges are described as being a part of the normal, anticipated process of recovery and not indicative of regression or failure. For adolescent survivors of complex trauma, this is very important because they may be more likely to continue to experience chaotic, stressful situations after the completion of TF-CBT (e.g., residential care, foster placement, dangerous communities). Given the findings of the Adverse Childhood Experiences study (Anda et al., 2006), it is also important to provide adolescents with information regarding healthy lifestyle choices (e.g., diet, exercise, substance use, safe sexual practices) in an attempt to reduce the potential health risk factors associated with exposure to childhood adversity. Furthermore, these youth never learned critical life skills. They will then also benefit from access to various life skill training opportunities—including applying and interviewing for jobs, financial budgeting, and housing options—and the provision of information regarding various resources that may be available to them as adults (e.g., assisted-living programs, support groups, government-funded services and programs).

Parenting

Following trauma processing, it is important to assist caregivers and any relevant systemic entities in facilitating adolescents' growth and development. It is helpful to work with caregivers to identify appropriate expectations and responsibilities for the adolescents as they move toward adulthood. Many caregivers have difficulty trusting the adolescents' capacity to handle new situations and may need encouragement to allow the adolescents more freedom and responsibility within appropriate limits. For adolescent survivors of complex trauma, especially those in the child welfare system, it is very important to help systemic entities focus on planning for the adolescents' future. Adolescents "aging out" of the system often experience abrupt changes in their placement status and the services they receive. It is vitally important that the therapist help adolescents communicate their needs to appropriate systemic entities and work with those entities to help ensure that those needs are met. The therapist may also need to work with the caregiver and/or systemic entities to determine who the adolescents' support system will be when they reach majority status. Many youth who age out of the foster care system and no longer have contact with their biological family may find themselves isolated and lacking social support. Ensuring that these adolescents have at least one trusted individual to whom they can turn may be vital to their long-term well-being.

Relaxation, Affective Regulation, and Cognitive Coping

Here, the adolescent works to perfect relaxation, affective regulation, and cognitive coping skills and generalize them to a larger range of situations. At this point in treatment, it is expected that the adolescent is poised to participate more fully in developmentally appropriate activities and take on new responsibilities (e.g., dating, employment, college). This combination of unfamiliar situations and increased expectations will likely be distressing for the adolescent. Therefore, coaching the adolescent to utilize the previously learned skills to better cope with these situations is of paramount importance. Furthermore, given the future orientation of these components, time should also be spent preparing the adolescent to use these skills in situations that he or she may encounter after therapy has been completed. For example, with an adolescent who is interested in having children in the future, the therapist may focus on increasing the adolescent's awareness of how self-regulation skills can be applied to parenting (e.g., remaining regulated when confronted by misbehavior).

In Vivo Mastery

As in traditional TF-CBT following the trauma narrative, *in vivo* mastery associated with future safety and development is largely devoted to increasing the adolescent's comfort level in potentially stressful or unfamiliar situations. In particular, the *in vivo* mastery component might be implemented if the adolescent's distress regarding a specific situation or activity was interfering with his or her ability to engage successfully in important life activities. For example, an adolescent who is fearful of using public transportation, yet will need to do so in order to hold a job, may be encouraged to engage in a process of systematic desensitization (e.g., riding the bus alone for gradually increasing lengths of time).

Conjoint Sessions

When addressing future safety and development, conjoint sessions are intended to build upon the conjoint work completed during the earlier phases and to project that work into the future. Specifically, the focus is on increasing the caregiver's ability to successfully support and coach the adolescent through future life challenges. During this component, the adolescent can share goals and plans with the caregiver, who will have been coached by the therapist to provide an encouraging, supportive response to the adolescent's initiative. Subsequently, the adolescent and caregiver can work together to achieve the goals that have been set forth.

Enhancing Safety and Future Development

In essence, when working with adolescent survivors of complex trauma, the therapist is encouraged to use all of the PRACTICE components to enhance future safety and development. However, given the increased risk of revictimization for this population, it is essential to provide the adolescent with appropriate safety and prevention skills that can be applied to future life situations (e.g., dating, moving away from home). As in traditional TF-CBT, this component focuses on the primary safety/prevention skills of danger awareness, assertiveness, problem solving, and seeking help. It is essential to provide the adolescent with information regarding healthy relationships and sexuality. Psychoeducation can also be provided to help the adolescent understand some of the factors associated with complex trauma that may increase risk of revictimization (e.g., substance abuse, poor interpersonal boundaries, impulsive decision making). Previously learned self-regulation and problem-solving skills can then be reviewed in the context of addressing these risk factors for revictimization.

The therapist can also help adolescents begin to identify potential goals for their future. Ideally, the adolescents can utilize the lessons learned from their past to identify what they would like their future life to look like. For example, an adolescent who expressed anger that she was not better protected might show interest in a career in law enforcement. An adolescent who grew up in the foster care system might set a goal of being a successful parent who retains custody of his children. During this process, the therapist may also identify inaccurate or unhelpful beliefs that the adolescents have about their future (e.g., "I can't wait to have kids because then I'll have someone who'll always love me"). As during the trauma narrative component, the therapist should assist adolescents in testing the accuracy and helpfulness of these thoughts and developing more balanced beliefs.

ENDING TREATMENT

In light of the adolescents' interpersonal experiences, the termination of the therapeutic relationship is very important. This may be their first healthy "goodbye" experience. The therapist should then plan for this early in treatment and revisit as necessary throughout. Termination may trigger feelings of loss or abandonment. Ideally, the therapist can help the adolescent process feelings about this and recognize how the end of this relationship is different from previous experiences. The conclusion of treatment should occur in a predictable manner over which the adolescent has some appropriate control (e.g., picking the activity for the final session). The therapist should present termination as an achievement. The notion that the therapeutic relationship continues after the end of sessions, albeit in a different form, is also an important concept. Given the attachment-related difficulties of this population, providing concrete examples of this continued relationship (e.g., giving the adolescent a photograph of the therapist and adolescent together) is particularly helpful. Genuine disclosure of the therapist's feelings regarding the end of treatment can also be appropriate and beneficial; modeling appropriate expression of feelings associated with the completion of treatment (e.g., sadness, pride, hope) and acknowledging the ability to maintain a mental representation of the therapeutic relationship (e.g., stressing that the therapist will not forget the adolescent) are keys to successful termination.

CONCLUSION

Most clinicians advocate for the use of a phase-based approach for complex trauma (Courtois, 2004; Ford et al., 2005; Herman, 1992). TF-CBT is the most researched evidenced-based practice for treating children and adolescents exposed to traumatic events (Cohen et al., 2010). Furthermore, as demonstrated in this chapter, the TF-CBT model is consistent with a phase-based approach to the treatment of complex trauma. Specifically, the PRACTICE components, with appropriate application, can be implemented to enhance stability, safety, and engagement; to facilitate the processing of traumatic memories; and to aid in the development of a healthy, balanced, posttrauma future for adolescent survivors of complex trauma. Thus, it seems wise to consider such a well-supported therapeutic model when addressing the mental health needs of complexly traumatized adolescents.

REFERENCES

Achenbach, T. M., & Rescorla, L. A. (2001). *Manual for the ASEBA School-Age Forms & Profiles*. Burlington: University of Vermont, Research Center for Children, Youth, & Families.

Anda, R. F., Felitti, V. J., Bremner, J. D., Waker, J. D., Whitfield, C., Perry, B. D., et al. (2006). The enduring effects of abuse and related adverse experiences in childhood: A convergence from neurobiology and epidemiology. *European Archives of Psychiatry and Clinical Neuroscience, 256*, 174–186.

Briere, J. (1996a). *Therapy for adults molested as children: Beyond survival* (2nd ed., revised and expanded). New York: Springer.

Briere, J. (1996b). *Trauma Symptom Checklist for Children (TSCC) professional manual*. Odessa, FL: Psychological Assessment Resources.

Briere, J. (2002). Treating adult survivors of severe childhood abuse and neglect: Further development of an integrative model. In J. E. B. Myers, L. Berliner, J.

Briere, C. T. Hendrix, T. Reid, & C. Jenny (Eds.), *The APSAC handbook on child maltreatment* (2nd ed., pp. 175–202). Thousand Oaks, CA: Sage.

Briere, J., & Scott, C. (2006). *Principles of trauma therapy: A guide to symptoms, evaluation, and treatment.* Thousand Oaks, CA: Sage.

Briere, J., & Spinazzola, J. (2005). Phenomenology and psychological assessment of complex posttraumatic stress. *Journal of Traumatic Stress, 18*(5), 401–412.

Butcher, J. N., Williams, C. L., Graham, J. R., Archer, R. P., Tellegen, A., Ben-Porath, Y. S., et al. (1992). *Minnesota Multiphasic Personality Inventory—Adolescent Version (MMPI-A): Manual for administration, scoring and interpretation.* Minneapolis: University of Minnesota Press.

Cohen, J. A., Bukstein, O., Walter, H., Benson, R. S., Chrisman, A., Farchione, T. R., et al. (2010). Practice parameter for the assessment and treatment of children and adolescents with posttraumatic stress disorder. *Journal of the American Academy of Child and Adolescent Psychiatry, 49*(4), 414–430.

Cohen, J. A., Mannarino, A. P., & Deblinger, E. (2006). *Treating trauma and traumatic grief in children and adolescents.* New York: Guilford Press.

Conners, C. K. (2008). *Conners Comprehensive Behavior Rating Scales manual.* Toronto: Multi-Health Systems.

Cook, A., Blaustein, M., Spinazzola, J., & van der Kolk, B. A. (Eds.). (2003). *Complex trauma in children and adolescents.* Retrieved from *www.nctsn.org/netsn_ assets/pdfs/edu_materials/ComplexTrauma_All.pdf.*

Cook, A., Spinazzola, J., Ford, J., Lanktree, C., Blaustein, M., DeRosa, R., et al. (2005). Complex trauma in children and adolescents. *Psychiatric Annals, 35*(5), 390–398.

Courtois, C. A. (1999). *Recollections of sexual abuse: Treatment principles and guidelines.* New York: Norton.

Courtois, C. A. (2004). Complex trauma, complex reactions: Assessment and treatment. *Psychotherapy: Theory, Research, Practice, Training, 41*(4), 412–425.

Deblinger, E., Lippmann, J., & Steer, R. (1996). Sexually abused children suffering posttraumatic stress symptoms: Initial treatment outcome findings. *Child Maltreatment, 1,* 310–321.

Finkelhor, D., Ormrod, R. K., & Turner, H. A. (2009). Lifetime assessment of polyvictimization in a national sample of children and youth. *Child Abuse and Neglect, 33,* 403–411.

Ford, J. D. (2005). Treatment implications of altered affect regulation and information processing following child maltreatment. *Psychiatric Annals, 35*(5), 410–419.

Ford, J. D., Courtois, C. A., Steele, K., van der Hart, O., & Mijenhuis, E. R. S. (2005). Treatment of complex posttraumatic self-dysregulation. *Journal of Traumatic Stress, 18*(5), 437–447.

Green, E. J., Crenshaw, D. A., & Kolos, A. C. (2010). Counseling children with preverbal trauma. *International Journal of Play Therapy, 19*(2), 95–105.

Herman, J. L. (1992). Complex PTSD: A syndrome in survivors of prolonged and repeated trauma. *Journal of Traumatic Stress, 5,* 377–391.

Pearlman, L. A., & Courtois, C. A. (2005). Clinical applications of the attachment framework: Relational treatment of complex trauma. *Journal of Traumatic Stress, 18*(5), 449–459.

Pelcovitz, D., van der Kolk, B. A., Roth, S., Mandel, F., Kaplan, S., & Resick, P. (1997). Development of a criteria set and a Structured Interview for Disorders of Extreme Stress (SIDES). *Journal of Traumatic Stress, 10(1)*, 3–16.

Reynolds, C. R., & Kamphaus, R. W. (2004). *Behavior Assessment Scale for Children manual* (2nd ed.). Bloomington, MN: Pearson Assessments.

Roid, G. H. (2003). *Stanford–Binet Intelligence Scales, Fifth Edition*. Itasca, IL: Riverside.

Roth, S., Newman, E., Pelcovitz, D., van der Kolk, B. A., & Mandel, F. S. (1997). Complex PTSD in victims exposed to sexual and physical abuse: Results from the DSM-IV field trial for posttraumatic stress disorder. *Journal of Traumatic Stress, 10(4)*, 539–555.

Saxe, G. N., Ellis, B., H., & Kaplow, J. B. (2007). *Collaborative treatment of traumatized children and teens: The trauma systems therapy approach*. New York: Guilford Press.

Spinazzola, J., Ford, J. D., Zucker, M., van der Kolk, B., Silva, S., Smith, S. F., et al. (2005). Survey evaluates complex trauma exposure, outcome, and intervention among children and adolescents. *Psychiatric Annals, 35(5)*, 433–439.

Spoth, R., Neppl, T., Goldberg-Lillehoj, C., Jung, T., & Ramisetty-Mikler, S. (2006). Gender related quality of parent–child interactions and early adolescent problem behaviors. *Journal of Family Issues, 27*, 826–849.

Taylor, N., Gilbert, A., Mann, G., & Ryan, B. (2008). *Assessment-based treatment for traumatized children: A trauma assessment pathway model (TAP)*. Unpublished manuscript, Chadwick Center for Children and Families, Rady Children's Hospital and Health Center, San Diego, CA.

van der Kolk, B. A. (2005). Developmental trauma disorder. *Psychiatric Annals, 35(5)*, 401–408.

Wechsler, D. (2004). *The Wechsler Intelligence Scale for Children—Fourth Edition*. San Antonio, TX: Pearson Assessment.

PART III

TF-CBT APPLICATIONS FOR SPECIAL POPULATIONS

8

Children in Military Families

JUDITH A. COHEN
STEPHEN J. COZZA

OVERVIEW OF MILITARY FAMILIES

Operations Iraqi Freedom, Enduring Freedom, and New Dawn (OIF/OEF/ OND) have been protracted military conflicts in Iraq and Afghanistan. In summer 2010, OEF became the longest war ever fought by the U.S. armed forces, surpassing the Vietnam War. These recent extended combat operations have led to greater interest and awareness among mental health professionals about military life and the impact of war on military service members and their families, and growing knowledge about effective interventions for those who suffer service-related physical and psychological wounds. However, even greater awareness among civilian clinicians is needed. Many professionals still do not understand military children and families and the unique challenges they face.

In 2009, just over one-eighth of active duty members (n = 179,273) left military service by voluntary discharge, retirement, or other means (U.S. Department of Defense, 2009). Attrition rates have been consistent over the past several years, and the number of combat veterans and their families who leave the service and move into urban, suburban, and rural communities around the country may increase with the recent and anticipated military withdrawals from Iraq and Afghanistan, respectively. Many veterans will have serious mental and/or physical injuries that will impact their families. As clinicians, we must expect their presence in our communities and consulting rooms and inquire about their experiences in order to better anticipate their treatment needs.

Almost 2 million American children have at least one parent who is a member of the U.S. military (U.S. Department of Defense, 2009), with 1.2 million children in active duty families and more than 700,000 in families of the Selected Reserve (National Guard and Reserve). Military families are typically young; 42% of active duty children and nearly 25% of Selected Reserve children are under the age of 5 (U.S. Department of Defense, 2009). In addition, a large number of children have older siblings and other extended family members (e.g., cousins, aunts, and uncles) in the military, whose service experiences can profoundly impact them. This chapter provides an overview of the unique culture of military families and the challenges they face, and describes unique military trauma-focused cognitive-behavioral therapy (TF-CBT) applications that can be helpful. Throughout, the term "military children" refers to all children who have immediate and extended family members in the U.S. military.

UNDERSTANDING MILITARY CULTURE

Military life has many common elements that all military service children and families share. Therapists must understand that service members do not serve alone. Rather, the entire military family—parents, siblings, spouses, partners, and children—all serve together. Military families share common experiences that distinguish them from civilian families, including recurring prolonged absences during military duty, living with the possibility of injury or death resulting from combat deployment, as well as postcombat stress-related mental health problems (Cozza, Chun, & Polo, 2005). Military families typically manage these challenges with a high degree of resilience, in large measure because they are committed to and value their service.

There are important differences between service branches and components that clinicians need to understand. Active duty differs from Reserve and National Guard duty in a variety of ways. Active duty members serve in the military as their full-time job and typically live on or near military installations among other military families. Most military-related resources and services tend to be concentrated near military installations, so active duty families often have more access to such services (e.g., military child mental health specialists; resiliency-based services for military families). These families experience regular permanent changes of station (PCSs) that require children to change schools and make new friends every few years, but also benefit from living among other military families who understand and support their experiences. In contrast, Reserve and National Guard service members are usually only activated for extended military service during war or national emergencies. These families do not experience PCS moves and typically live civilian lives until their military service family members are activated, at which time they become "suddenly military." Reserve and National Guard children may feel that their civilian friends have no comprehension of military life or responsibilities. More often than active duty children, these children report that they are not understood by their friends, teachers, or other significant people in their lives (Chandra et al., 2010). Perhaps related to these differences, Reserve and National Guard children and their nondeployed parents may be at increased risk for developing higher levels of distress or mental health problems during parental deployment (Lester et al., 2010), which TF-CBT can successfully address.

The military also includes distinct service-specific (e.g. Army, Navy, Marines, Air Force, Coast Guard) subcultures. When working with military families, it is important to recognize their service branch affiliations in order to build and maintain effective therapeutic relationships and to provide effective treatment (Bates, Brim, Lunasco, & Rhodes, in press). Military life is centered on core values that guide military service members and families, values that often are not shared by their civilian counterparts. Military cultural values are critical to service members performing well in their jobs, serving to bond service members and their families together and allowing them to successfully survive the rigors of military life, including combat (Bates et al., in press). These values include commitment to duty (doing what is necessary regardless of personal cost); strength and resilience (continually striving to attain one's physical, emotional, and spiritual best); and loyalty to team and family members, including individual sacrifice for the common good. Understanding and respecting military life and values are critical to both effectively engaging military families in TF-CBT and optimally implementing TF-CBT for distressed or traumatized military children.

The first step in the development of a military-competent health care practice is for clinicians to be aware of their biases, beliefs, and attitudes about the military and military community (Bates et al., in press). These assumptions may be based on their own personal and family values as well as prior experiences. For example, therapists who had personal or family experience in World War II are likely to have very different perceptions about military service and military communities than those with experience from the Vietnam War. Past positive experiences are more likely to lead to positive perceptions of the military, whereas negative experiences tend to result in critical perceptions. In order to be effective with military families, therapists must be aware of these perceptions and biases and not allow any personal negativity to impact therapeutic goals. Therapists who have not been part of the military may never completely understand the experiences of living a military life, but the following resources can significantly enhance their insight into military culture: *www.centerforthestudyoftraumaticstress. org*, *http://nctsn.org*, and *www.sesameworkshop.org*.

IMPACT OF MILITARY DEPLOYMENTS

Military families are expected to successfully manage with the stresses of hazardous duty and deployment-related separations. Children are typically resilient during these periodic changes, perhaps because of the military cultural expectations and because other military families model and mentor effective family deployment strategies. In addition to separations, deployments also contribute to greater levels of family distress and challenges of family reunification.

There is a small but growing literature that examines elevated levels of distress and psychosocial difficulties in military children associated with parental combat deployment (Chandra et al., 2010; Flake, Davis, Johnson, & Middleton, 2009; Lester et al., 2010). Two of these studies also found a negative cumulative effect of parental deployment on children's emotional outcomes (Chandra et al., 2010; Lester et al., 2010). Recently, Mansfield, Kaufman, Engel, and Gaynes (in press) reported the results of a large retrospective (from 2003–2006, peak periods of military family deployment) cohort study using the medical outpatient treatment data of more than 300,000 children who had one or both parents in the U.S. Army. The authors examined the relationship between pediatric mental health-related outpatient visits and parental combat deployments, comparing groups of children whose parents were deployed for 1 to 11 months, more than 11 months, or not at all. An association between parental combat deployment and children's risk of mental disorder visits was found for both boys and girls, with the greatest increase in the number of excess mental health cases in children whose parents were deployed for more than 11 months. The largest deployment-related effects were noted in acute stress disorder, adjustment disorders, pediatric behavioral disorders, and depression (Mansfield et al., in press).

Other reports have linked negative effects of deployment on other military family outcomes. Several authors have described increasing rates of deployment-related military child maltreatment since the start of combat operations in 2001, especially child neglect (Gibbs, Martin, Kupper, & Johnson, 2007; McCarroll, Fan, Newby, & Ursano, 2008; McCarroll et al., 2004; Rentz et al., 2007). The U.S. Department of Defense (2009) has reported that divorce rates among both enlisted members and officers have increased during the past decade, with higher rates in 2009 than in 2000 for both officers (1.8% vs. 1.4%) and enlisted members (4.0% vs. 2.9%) in all military service branches. Milliken, Auchterlonie, and Hoge (2007) reported changes in self-identified concerns in 88,000 U.S. Army soldiers between initial postdeployment screening and a screening that occurred 3 to 6 months later, with a fourfold increase in the number of soldiers endorsing "serious conflict with your spouse, family members or close friends" at the second screening. These and other reports suggest a broader effect of deployment on the military family, a critical finding since the health of military children is likely connected to the health of their parents and other family members.

COMPLICATED DEPLOYMENTS

Service members sometimes return with conditions that complicate family reunification and postdeployment life, such as posttraumatic stress disorder (PTSD), depression, substance use disorders, or combat-related injuries, including traumatic brain injury (TBI). Therapists should be aware of the changing nature of military wounds during OIF/OEF/OND. In particular, current enemy weaponry includes improvised explosive devices (IEDs), which cause extensive, severe injuries that in past wars would have been fatal. With advanced medical technology, however, many service members injured by IEDs survive, but often require months of rehabilitation and termination of military service. Disfiguring amputations, TBI or other severe orthopedic injuries, and/or mental wounds such as PTSD, depression, and suicidal ideation are occurring at higher rates during OIF/OEF than in previous conflicts. Serious injuries can lead to a cascade of effects, including family separations; stressful hospital visits; extended medical care; changes in schools, residence, and communities; as well as elevated family and child distress (Cozza & Guimond, 2011).

If a service member dies in combat theater, it is usually sudden and the cause (e.g., training accident, combat or combat-related injury, suicide) is potentially traumatic. No published reports have described the unique experiences of military children who have been parentally bereaved during a time of war. Preliminary study of parental death has found no significant differences between military and civilian children (Cozza, Ortiz, Fullerton, Schmidt, & Ursano, 2011). However, given the violent nature of combat-related deaths, military children may be at heightened risk for developing childhood traumatic grief (Cohen & Mannarino, 2004).

The military has many rituals to honor its fallen heroes, starting with notification of the family by casualty assistance officers. During military funerals, the presence of an honor guard, folding the American flag and presenting it to the widow or the mother of the fallen hero, firing a rifle volley after the service, and the playing of "Taps" can all have profound effects on children. While these rituals may comfort family members, in certain circumstances they may confuse or even frighten children with traumatic grief, as described elsewhere (Cohen & Mannarino, 2011).

STIGMA AND BARRIERS TO CARE

The military cultural value of strength and resilience may result in negative attitudes toward mental illness and/or in seeking mental health treatment. Some military members may believe that having a mental illness or needing therapy is a sign of weakness, and that the appropriate response to pain is either to ignore it or get over it by relying on toughness and inner resources. Such attitudes are likely to conflict with talking about difficult experiences and feelings and, by extension, with seeking mental heath treatment. Consistent with negative attitudes about expressing vulnerability and pain, stigma about mental illness and seeking mental health services is significant among military members and their families (Greene-Sortrig, Britt, & Castro, 2007). The U.S. armed forces are engaging in multiple efforts to decrease such stigma and to encourage affected military members to seek needed mental health services. Some evidence suggests that the stigma is decreasing (Warner, Appenzeller, Mullen, Warner, & Greiger, 2008), but therapists should be aware that military families may need to overcome significant stigma both within and beyond their own family in order to seek mental health services.

In addition to emotional barriers, military members and their families may be concerned about real or imagined consequences to military careers if they seek mental health treatment. In some cases, this concern may determine whether a traumatized military child is encouraged or discouraged from seeking needed care. All military services take allegations of child maltreatment and domestic violence very seriously. If substantiated, a family-related maltreatment or domestic violence incident could have financial impact on the family, have significant disciplinary consequences to a service member, or be career ending. In addition to the consequences to a service member perpetrator, families may also be at risk for losing financial support or housing should that service member be financially penalized, lose subsidized housing, or lose his or her military career. Parents may be hesitant to seek needed pediatric or mental health care for their child if they are concerned that the clinical evaluation will lead to the discovery of a maltreatment or domestic violence event. When a perpetrator is outside of the family, the child or parents may be concerned with how the child's disclosure may impact the service member parent's career or the family's image in a tightly knit community. Any or all of these concerns—out of fear of discovery or fear of negative outcomes—can diminish parents' and children's motivation to self-identify or seek services that could be of help.

ASSESSMENT ISSUES FOR MILITARY CHILDREN

When evaluating military children, it is essential not only to inquire about exposure to the typical types of traumas included in child assessments (i.e., those included in the UCLA PTSD Reaction Index; Steinberg, Brymer, Decker, & Pynoos, 2004), but also to ask thoroughly about exposure to and impact of stressors and traumas that are unique to military life. As always, the interview with the children is critical to determining the impact of potentially stressful or traumatic events.

Identification of Military Children

First, therapists should screen all new adult and child clients for exposure to military-related stressors. Simple questions such as "Have you or someone in your family served in the military or been deployed?" can quickly determine military family combat experiences. These questions should then be followed by inquiries about the relationship with the military family service member and the nature of exposures.

History of Deployments and Family Relocations

When military exposure is identified, further assessment should include questions about the number of parent, sibling, or other family member deployments; the duration of these deployments; and whether or not these deployments were into combat theater. One should ask about the child's adjustment before and during each deployment, whether the family relocated during deployment, and how the nondeployed and deployed parent, sibling, and other family members adjusted. If both parents were deployed, the therapist should inquire about who cared for the child, whether the child had to relocate, how well the child knew the caretaker, and how well the child adjusted to these changes. History of other family relocations is also important to consider. Relocations can result in disruptions in education, relationships, activities, friendships, or required care for preexisting medical, developmental, or educational conditions.

Postdeployment Injury, Including TBI

The assessment should also include information about whether the deployed parent or sibling experienced significant injury during deployment and, if so, the nature of the injury, where the injured service member received treatment, the length of time the service member was separated from the child, and whether the nondeployed parent joined the injured parent or sibling and was also separated from the child after the service member's injury. One should inquire about the child's response to the injury and whether the child visited the wounded parent, sibling, or other family member at the hospital or tertiary care center, saw disfiguring wounds, and/or feared that the loved one would die. The clinician should also ascertain the responses of the noninjured parent and other family members to the injury and how these may have contributed to the child's positive or negative adjustment. It can also be helpful simply to ask, "What have you told your child about the injury?" A parent's response to this question informs the clinician about the nature of the information that was shared and the parent's comfort or discomfort in addressing painful subjects with the child. In situations involving serious injuries, it is important to ask whether the injury included TBI or resulted in changes in family relationships. Finally, it can also be helpful to assess whether or not family members have developed new and successful ways of engaging based on postinjury realities (Cozza & Guimond, 2011).

Postdeployment Mental Health Problems

The clinician should inquire about whether the deployed parent, sibling, or other family member developed mental health problems, particularly PTSD, depression, or substance use problems, and to what extent the child has been exposed to these problems, the child's response to these problems, and other family members' responses to these mental health problems and their impact on family relationships. Since combat stress-related disorders can result in reactivity and anger, one should also assess for elevated levels of family distress or discord, domestic violence, and child maltreatment.

Military-Related Death of Parent

In cases involving the death of a service member parent, sibling, or other family member, the clinician should inquire about the cause of death (combat, accident, suicide, other); the child's response to the death, including childhood traumatic grief symptoms (Cohen & Mannarino, 2004); and nondeployed family members' responses to the death, both at the time of notification and subsequently.

Focus on Family Functioning and Resilience

It is especially important to ascertain how the nondeployed parent has functioned during the parent's or sibling's deployment and how all family members have related and functioned since return from deployment (Lester et al., 2010). It is equally critical to ask in what ways the child and family are doing *well* (i.e., to take a strengths-based approach and focus on resilience). One should inquire about support systems that are available to the family, keeping in mind that the military provides many natural supports to its families.

Attention to Risk Factors

An understanding of factors associated with poorer clinical outcome in military children and families can help clinicians recognize potential at-risk cases that are more likely to develop more serious problems. Early military deployment literature suggests that younger children and boys may be at greater risk of developing symptoms during deployments (Jensen, Martin, & Watanabe, 1996). More recently, however, girls and older teens have been identified as being at greater risk of deployment-related problems (Chandra et al., 2010). These age and gender discrepancies likely reflect differences in study samples and methods of assessment. Children are likely to experience, respond to, and report their reactions variably depending on gender, age, and developmental needs.

Military children of nondeployed parents who exhibit higher levels of distress and poorer functioning during deployment also appear to do more poorly than children of nondeployed parents without those problems (Chandra et al., 2010; Jensen, Grogan, Xenakis, & Bain, 1989; Lester et al., 2010). The trauma literature identifies those children who are more highly exposed to a traumatic event or have poorer access to a social support network as being at higher risk for posttraumatic psychiatric sequelae (Pine & Cohen, 2002).

Additional risk factors for child traumatic responses include the lack of social connectedness (Pine & Cohen, 2002) that may occur when military families are unable to gain access to services, are geographically isolated, or live in communities that do not understand or recognize military culture or when language poses a barrier to connectedness. Preexisting developmental, learning, or emotional problems have also been associated with posttraumatic outcomes in children (Pine & Cohen, 2002). Given the negative impact of child maltreatment on child development and the relationship between deployment and elevated rates of military child neglect, risk factors for child maltreatment are likely to put military children and families at risk as well. It is important to recognize that child maltreatment other than neglect is equally common in military and civilian families (McCarroll et al., 2004, 2008). Demographic risk factors (e.g., low income, low maternal education, maternal youth, or single parenthood), familial and parenting risk factors (e.g., maternal anger, dissatisfaction, low self-esteem, or illness; low father involvement or warmth), and child risk factors (e.g., difficult temperament, developmental or learning problems) have all been associated with risk of child maltreatment (Brown, Cohen, Johnson, & Salzinger, 1998) and may be relevant in determining military family risk.

Clinicians who are engaging military children whose parents are suffering from postdeployment combat stress conditions must be aware of the potential negative consequences of those conditions on the children. Children and parent–child relationships have been noted to be negatively affected in multiple studies of Vietnam War veterans with PTSD (Jordan et al., 1992; Rosenheck & Fontana, 1998; Ruscio, Weathers, King, & King, 2002). Ruscio and colleagues (2002) described "the disinterest, detachment, and emotional unavailability that characterize emotional numbing may diminish a [parent's] ability and willingness to seek out, engage in, and enjoy interactions with [his or her] children, leading to poorer relationship quality" (p. 355).

Incomplete Information about the Child

More than 50,000 military children experience the simultaneous deployment of both parents and are living with a nonparent caregiver. If a military child requires mental health services in this situation, the caregiver may not have important background information. (It is now feasible for evaluators to reach a deployed parent via Skype, and this should be considered in such situations). Severely wounded service members typically receive care in regional trauma centers, and the nonservice member parent may travel to these locations, leaving the children behind with relatives or friends for days or weeks. In cases when a service member has been killed or the primary caregiver parent is absent for significant periods, children may live with other adults (e.g., stepparent, grandparent) who may not have complete or accurate information about their development. In such situations, child clinicians should obtain as much information as possible from available caregivers, the children, and other potential sources (e.g., school, pediatrician) and formulate a working diagnosis and treatment plan based on the available information.

UNIQUE TF-CBT ENGAGEMENT STRATEGIES FOR MILITARY FAMILIES

Therapists hoping to engage military families successfully in TF-CBT treatment must respect the military values described earlier. Military families are most likely to engage in TF-CBT treatment if it is presented in terms of a family-focused resilience-building model rather than as treatment for a trauma-related condition or mental health disorder. Because family-based treatment and resilience-building skills are core TF-CBT values (Cohen, Mannarino, & Deblinger, 2006, pp. 32–33), this is an accurate and engaging way to present TF-CBT to military families. At the same time, an important engagement strategy is to recognize why families are seeking treatment and to effectively and promptly make progress toward addressing these problems, particularly when distress or traumatic exposure is present.

Case Example

A military family presented for assessment for 13-year-old Anthony's school behavior problems. The mother was constantly called by the school because

Anthony was rude to teachers, cutting class, and fighting with peers. The clinician noted that these problems had worsened since the father's return from OIF deployment and corresponded with an increase in fighting and tension between the parents. Upon further exploration, the mother reported that the father was having unpredictable explosive outbursts, which Anthony had witnessed. The father had experienced a possible concussion after a roadside bombing, losing consciousness for several minutes, followed by severe headaches and irritability, but had refused to see a health care provider, insisting there was nothing wrong with him. During the interview with Anthony, the therapist specifically asked him about his father's angry outbursts. Anthony acknowledged that he was very worried about his father and scared that "something bad is going to happen." When rating the UCLA PTSD Reaction Index with regard to his father's outbursts Anthony scored 30, in the moderate range of severity.

The therapist presented TF-CBT as a model through which the parents could assist Anthony "to build on your strengths to work together and help address Anthony's stress-related behavior issues." The parents agreed to participate because, instead of focusing on Anthony's "bad" behaviors, the therapist emphasized the child's and family's strengths, which was consistent with the family's predeployment identity, their military cultural identity, sense of resilience, and prior experience of helping each other solve problems. The therapist provided information that related Anthony's behaviors to possible biological stress-related changes. As the therapist implemented the skills components and the parents began to see improvements in Anthony's behavior and in their own relationship, their engagement with the therapist became more committed. The parents were receptive to the explanation of stress-related brain changes leading to behavioral problems, which over time enabled Anthony's father to be more accepting of his own possible stress-related brain changes. As he saw the improvements in Anthony's behavior, he decided to seek an evaluation for himself. He was diagnosed with severe TBI, and the entire family experienced significant relief when this diagnosis was made and treatment was initiated. As his father sought treatment, Anthony reported in his trauma narrative that his father was his hero because "he was a brave soldier and even braver to get help."

UNIQUE TF-CBT APPLICATIONS
FOR MILITARY FAMILIES

Military children experience a range of stress that may be of traumatic levels. For example, deployment is a typical experience for military families, and although it requires adaptations, most military children adjust well to parental deployments. The serious injury or death of a military parent will be sad and difficult for many children, but after a period of adjustment most

210 TF-CBT APPLICATIONS FOR SPECIAL POPULATIONS

will likely adjust fairly well. However, some will experience these events as highly stressful or traumatic, developing significant depression, PTSD, and/or behavioral problems as a result. Similarly, whereas some children may experience abuse or domestic violence and adjust without significant disruptions in adaptive functioning or mental health problems, others may suffer traumatic consequences. It is critical that clinicians evaluate children to determine the severity of their reactions and not assume either traumatic or resilient responses based on the nature of the exposure.

The appropriateness of using TF-CBT in the care of a military child with any of these experiences depends on whether the child has had a significantly traumatic reaction that interferes with adaptive functioning and/or causes significant mental health problems. If the child evidences traumatic response to one or more of these events (deployment, parental injury, parental death, or more typical traumas such as child abuse or domestic violence), it will likely be helpful to provide TF-CBT.

Generally, TF-CBT for military families is similar to that for civilian families, with some specific applications described next.

Including Different Military Parents during Treatment as Appropriate

TF-CBT is best conducted with the presence of a consistent parent or parents throughout the treatment process. Military families would find this approach engaging, but because of the frequent changes in the family structure secondary to deployments, moves, and parental injury and/or death, parents' availability to participate may vary from session to session. TF-CBT therapists must recognize the changing circumstances of military family life and flexibly include different caregivers to the greatest degree that is clinically appropriate.

CASE EXAMPLE

Eight-year-old Kelly lived near an army base with her mother and her mother's live-in boyfriend, Dwayne, both active duty service members. Kelly also had ongoing contact with her biological father, a service member who was deployed to Iraq. A teacher reported Kelly to the local Family Advocacy Program (FAP) after seeing suspicious bruises on her arm. During the FAP interview, Kelly acknowledged that she had gotten bruised trying to stop Dwayne from hitting her mother. This led to Kelly disclosing domestic violence perpetrated by Dwayne toward her mother. Kelly's mother minimized these allegations at first and Dwayne was not charged, but the couple separated and Dwayne was transferred to another base. The mother participated in TF-CBT with Kelly and received her own treatment. During the skills-based sessions, the family learned that Dwayne had been deployed to Afghanistan. Kelly was already worried about her own father's safety, and this news triggered Kelly's feelings of guilt about disclosing the domestic violence, believing she was responsible for Dwayne's deployment. The therapist addressed this maladaptive cognition through cognitive coping (e.g., if Dwayne hadn't perpetrated the domestic violence, Kelly could not have disclosed it, so it was Dwayne who was responsible for what happened, not Kelly). Kelly asked whether her father could participate in some sessions via Skype. Her mother was apprehensive at first, fearing that Kelly's father would blame her for what had happened to Kelly. The therapist addressed this with the mother (i.e., both the mother and Kelly were victims), and the therapist spoke with the father about participating in treatment. Although he was upset, Kelly's father was very invested in supporting his daughter in treatment. He participated twice via Skype (limited by demands of active duty) and e-mailed supportive messages and praise to his daughter, and over time these expressions of support also included his ex-wife. Kelly's father asked for special permission to participate in the conjoint session, at which time Kelly shared her trauma narrative with both parents. During this session, Kelly's father told her that she was a hero in his eyes for having revealed the domestic violence.

Planning for Upcoming Changes in Living Arrangements

Changes in living arrangements resulting from parental deployment and/ or transfers through PCS are commonplace for military families. Therapists must be aware of these possible disruptions at the start of TF-CBT in order to appropriately map the length and pace of TF-CBT and to plan for treatment termination or, if necessary, arrange transfer to another TF-CBT therapist in the family's new location.

CASE EXAMPLE

Five-year-old Tyrell was living with his service mother, a single parent, when she was involved in a serious fire during a training accident and was hospitalized as a result of severe burns. Tyrell went to live with his maternal grandmother in a different state for 3 months while his mother recovered. Tyrell developed PTSD in response to his mother's injuries and was terrified of any reminders of the fire, including returning to the military installation and seeing his mother's scars. Shortly after her discharge from the hospital, the mother and Tyrell started TF-CBT at the recommendation of their therapist. However, the family was going to be PCS'd to another state 2 months after the initial assessment. The therapist decided it was best to provide only initial TF-CBT skills training because she realized there would not be time to complete the entire treatment, and it would be unwise to start the trauma narrative during the disruption of the family's move. The therapist located a TF-CBT therapist close to the family's new installation and had the mother and Tyrell "meet" the new therapist via Skype (which Tyrell liked because he loved computers) in order to facilitate the treatment transfer. The therapist also encouraged the mother to begin treatment for her own accident-related PTSD symptoms, to which she agreed after her positive experience with this therapist. With these resources and their newly acquired TF-CBT skills, Tyrell and his mother made a smooth transition to the new therapist and completed TF-CBT treatment.

Providing TF–CBT in a Family–Focused Manner That Emphasizes Resilience

Some military families may request a "family therapy" approach to trauma treatment, one that may reflect their personal, family, and military values. Although TF-CBT is a family-focused treatment, it is most typically provided in individual and conjoint child–parent session formats rather than as family treatment, with multiple siblings present. For military families who desire family therapy, it may be helpful to explore with the parents their sense of the optimal configuration of family members to be present at treatment sessions. Doing so may help to identify some misconceptions about trauma and its impact and may also provide the therapist with an opportunity to explain the potential benefits of seeing a child and parents together without other siblings.

TF-CBT clinicians who work with military families will benefit from taking a resilience-based approach, with a focus on the individual's and family's strengths: for example, positive attributes that have not changed, goals that have been reached or that are still attainable, and ways the family is supporting each other to move forward.

CASE EXAMPLE

The wife of an army officer sought family treatment after her oldest son, 19-year-old Matthew, who had joined the army the previous year, was severely injured in Afghanistan and returned home with a disfiguring injury. Jessie, 7 years old, was having nightmares about her brother's injury. The parents agreed that Jessie would be best served if her mother and all of the siblings, including Matthew, 12-year-old Michael, and 14-year-old Julie, attended therapy to help Jessie "get it off her chest." The therapist asked how the siblings were helping Jessie at home, and the mother said, "Not well. They make fun of her when she has nightmares and call her a big baby." The therapist reflected that it sounded like it might be hard for Jessie to share her fears with her older siblings, since she was the youngest and the older kids might make her feel like she was a baby if she talked about being afraid. Jessie's mother understood and said she could talk to her older children so they would stop teasing Jessie. The therapist said,

"I wonder if it's not hard for all of your kids to see how Matthew has changed. Maybe they tease Jessie so they don't have to admit that they're scared too." The mother became tearful and said that she felt that way herself. The therapist said, "Families are a wonderful source of support, but sometimes it can be really hard for everyone to feel like they have to be strong for everyone else. Therapy could give Jessie a chance to express her own feelings without having to worry about that. Matthew has changed in some ways, but I'm betting that he is the same in many more ways than he has changed. By giving your kids a chance to talk about what they are afraid of—the ways he has changed—it will open the door to talking about ways that he hasn't changed." The mother seemed relieved by this and agreed that she and Jessie would participate in TF-CBT. She then asked whether her older children might also benefit from TF-CBT. The therapist agreed to include Michael and Julie in individual TF-CBT with the mother as well, so they would each have the opportunity to talk about their own reactions to Matthew's injuries. By helping Jessie's mother understand the impact of trauma on her children ("Your children are all worried that their brother has changed; they are just showing it in different ways") and also emphasizing resilience ("Matthew has changed in some ways but he is still the same in many ways and your children will soon be able to talk about that"), the mother was able to understand the logic of providing the initial parts of TF-CBT in a family-focused manner but with individual sessions.

The therapist focused on resilience not only through developing skills with each child, but also by using TF-CBT skills to help all family members recognize ways that Matthew had not changed. For example, Jessie used visualization to remember when Matthew first taught her to play Go Fish. Then she practiced asking the therapist to play Go Fish, pretending the therapist was Matthew. Finally, Jessie went home and asked Matthew to play Go Fish with her. After weeks of Jessie avoiding being anywhere near him, Matthew was delighted that his little sister invited him to play. He told his mother, "All of a sudden I felt like she didn't notice anything was wrong with me." After Jessie and her siblings participated in individual TF-CBT and shared their confused and upsetting feelings with the therapist and their parents, the three siblings agreed that they would like to have several family sessions. During these sessions the children shared their narratives with each other, Matthew, and their parents; this was a very emotional and healing experience for the family. The parents and children agreed that the earlier individual TF-CBT sessions were critical to the success of the conjoint family sessions.

Understanding Unique Needs of Reserve and National Guard Families

Unlike active duty families, Reserve and National Guard families typically live in largely civilian settings, often isolated from other military families.

These children may not know or attend school with any other military children, and their nondeployed parents may lack military friends to provide support throughout the deployment cycle, potentially putting National Guard and Reserve families at risk for increased distress or mental health problems during deployment.

CASE EXAMPLE

Ron was 10 years old when his father's Reserve unit was deployed to Iraq. His family lived in a suburban area where he didn't know other military children. Although he admired his father's military service and he was accustomed to brief absences during his father's Reserve training, Ron was upset when told that his father would be gone for a much more extended period. He was especially angry that his father would miss coaching his Little League baseball team, saying "Why do you always have to leave? Why can't one of the other dads do it this time?" Ron's older sister tried to help out at home but she was busy with her friends and annoyed at Ron's negative attitude, and as time went on she increasingly stayed out with friends and avoided being at home. As his father's duty was extended to a second and then a third deployment, Ron's mother became increasingly depressed over her husband's absence and grew ever more anxious about his safety. In response to his mother's difficulties, Ron's behavior became more problematic, especially at school, where he was not paying attention and he was fighting with peers. Ron was also worried about his father's safety, compounded by the fact that his father was communicating less and less and seemed to be withdrawing from the family. Ron's mother finally brought him for an evaluation at his pediatrician's suggestion. During the evaluation Ron told the therapist that he was mad because "no one at school knows what it's like. They talk about their dads all the time, they get to go hunting and fishing and play ball with their dads, and I don't even get to talk to my dad anymore. I hate everyone." Upon further assessment, Ron endorsed significant worries, anxieties, and some PTSD symptoms (intrusive thoughts about war-related media coverage, trying not to think about what might have happened when his father failed to call, and hyperarousal symptoms) related to the father's deployment.

A successful prevention program to prepare military children and families for deployment such as Project FOCUS (Families Overcoming under Stress, *www.focusproject.org*) could have prevented Ron's problems. However, Project FOCUS is not available in all areas, and for children who have developed deployment-related traumatic responses and/or who cannot access this type of military-specific resilience-building program, TF-CBT may be appropriate or can be used adjunctively to address trauma-specific symptoms.

Ron and his mother participated in TF-CBT to address his anxiety and behavioral problems and to support his mother's understanding and inform her parental responses. The therapist actively engaged Ron's father through several e-mail exchanges so he would understand the importance of his continued communication and involvement with his family during his deployment in relieving unnecessary anxiety. As TF-CBT progressed, Ron's father participated in some sessions via Skype, which was extremely meaningful to Ron and his mother. Even when Ron's father could participate for only a few minutes, it was enormously beneficial to the family and made them feel very united and supported. The shared sessions also provided opportunities for Ron to show his father newly acquired skills or for Ron's mother to discuss possible parenting strategies. The therapist also linked Ron and his mother to online resources through which Ron could connect with other Reserve and National Guard children in his area as well as in other parts of the country, thereby decreasing his sense of isolation.

Understanding the Changing Nature of Modern Military Wounds

As described previously, the types and severity of military injury are changing. The military is attempting to optimize communication to families after injury occurs (e.g., whenever possible, the wounded service member him- or herself is the one to contact the family), but therapists must be aware that the trauma of the service member's injury may be further complicated by any of the following: (1) children may receive inaccurate or age-inappropriate information about what happened to wounded parents, siblings, or other family members, or they may witness frightening emotional reactions of adult family members; (2) the service member may require extended care at a trauma center far from the family's home, leading to extended separations from children; (3) the nondeployed parent may join the wounded parent or family member, leading to children's separation from both caregivers; and (4) children may travel to visit wounded parents, siblings, or other family members, resulting in frightening exposures to disfiguring wounds, medical procedures, or equipment without age-appropriate explanation or preparation. Any of these experiences may contribute to children's distress or traumatic symptoms (Cozza & Guimond 2011).

CASE EXAMPLE

Mother brought 3-year-old Carlos for treatment shortly after his father returned to the family's home following a near-fatal combat injury in Afghanistan. The father's injuries required a double leg amputation, and left him with only partial use of his dominant arm. He was hospitalized for several months far from the family's home. Carlos stayed with his maternal grandmother for several weeks so his mother could be with his father. During the hospitalization, Carlos visited his father just after he had received his leg prostheses. The mother tried to prepare Carlos, telling him that "Daddy lost his legs but now he has new ones." However, Carlos started crying when he saw the metal prostheses, and screamed, "No monster legs!" For weeks after this visit, Carlos had nightmares about monsters chasing him, began wetting the bed, and became very clingy. At the initial assessment, Carlos's father told the therapist, "What's the point of therapy? I know my son's real feelings. I'll never be a real man to him again."

The therapist began TF-CBT by educating the parents about the impact of unexpected visual images on young children. Specifically, she told the parents that any confusing or frightening vivid image could be scary to a 3-year-old. She gave the example of her own 3-year-old son who had developed a phobia of ghosts one night when he mistook a bathrobe hanging in his closet for a ghost, thereafter refusing to go to bed until his mother (the therapist) checked the closet and under the bed to be sure there were no ghosts. Carlos's parents laughed in recognition and recalled a time when they had to do something similar the previous year when Carlos had become afraid of monsters. In fact, the parents recalled that the father had to reassure Carlos over the phone from Afghanistan that there were no monsters in the house. This helped the father understand that Carlos's fears of monsters was a normal 3-year-old fear, and not specifically related to his prosthetic legs. Carlos's father said that this made him feel better about the episode in the hospital. The therapist continued to provide TF-CBT to Carlos and his parents, emphasizing the importance of Carlos and his father spending quality time together doing things they both enjoyed. The family also benefited from the Sesame Workshop Talk, Listen, Connect resources at *www.sesameworkshop.org*. Over time Carlos accommodated to his father's physical condition. In addition, his father became increasingly comfortable lifting Carlos, playing games, and doing light household chores, even with the limited use of his dominant arm. Through his drawings and his transcribed words, Carlos's narrative described how he felt both scared and sad when "Daddy got hurt" and "Mommy went to the hospital without me," and later how he became "happy when Daddy came back." His wish for the future was for "Daddy to go to school and show my friends his new legs." When the therapist shared this with his parents, Carlos's father became emotional, saying that his son's narrative helped him realize that Carlos still looked up to him as a role model. During the conjoint session, the therapist read Carlos's story as Carlos sat on his father's lap. Father told Carlos that he would come to school with him and let the other kids see how his legs worked.

Understanding the Unique Military Rituals Surrounding Death

Therapists working with bereaved military families must understand the military rituals related to service members' deaths and how these rituals may contribute to trauma and loss reminders. Children and families may have difficulty recalling these details long after the death, making it exceedingly difficult for therapists to make connections and to identify ritual-related trauma cues.

Case Example

Laura was 15 when her father, a member of the National Guard, died during his second deployment to Iraq. Laura was called home from band practice when her mother received the death notification. She didn't tell her friends what happened because she was "in shock," but ran all the way home. When she got there, her mother was crying hysterically with two uniformed officers trying to comfort her. Laura told them to leave. Immediately following notification, local news reporters started calling and Laura stopped answering the phone. The mother agreed to her husband's parents' request for a military funeral (Laura's paternal grandfather was a retired service member). Although her paternal grandparents and younger brothers seemed to appreciate the military rituals at the funeral, Laura was angered by the presence of so many uniformed military members, who reminded her of the death notification officers, and worried that these uniforms would upset her mother, who was still crying much of the time. Indeed, Laura's mother did cry when she was handed the folded flag and when "Taps" was played. Laura wanted to leave, but her paternal grandparents insisted that the family stay and speak to all of the guests. When they were leaving, Laura saw protesters with signs reading "The only good soldier is a dead soldier." Her mother started sobbing when she saw these protesters, and Laura was so furious that she vowed to never return to the cemetery to visit her father's grave. Later, Laura became irritable and left the room whenever anyone mentioned her father, and she refused to talk about his death to her friends. Laura's maternal grandmother insisted that her daughter bring Laura for an evaluation.

During the evaluation, the therapist confirmed that Laura met criteria for military child traumatic grief. TF-CBT for Laura included skills for coping with military-specific trauma and loss reminders. For example, media coverage of combat activities that included political opinions against the war, which previously would have been only of minor interest to Laura, aroused extreme anger because it triggered trauma and loss reminders. During the affective modulation component, Laura acknowledged that it was hard not being able to talk to her friends about how she felt because they didn't get what it was like to be partly military, partly civilian. Her therapist suggested that Laura attend a regional Tragedy Assistance Program for Survivors (TAPS) Camp (*www.taps.org*), and Laura and her mother did so. This was a turning point for Laura, who met other bereaved National Guard and Reserve teens who felt similarly as her. Laura's mother also met several women at the TAPS Camp to whom she related well. Laura and her mother worked through the trauma narrative and bereavement-focused components of TF-CBT with positive results.

CLINICAL CASE DESCRIPTION

Ann was 9 years old when her father, an Army officer, returned from combat deployment to his home Army installation. Ann had experienced minor anxiety problems during her father's absence but was excitedly looking forward to his return. Family reintegration went smoothly, with the family quickly accommodating to new routines with the father's return, getting together with other close friends and families that had also reunited, and comforting a few families that had experienced loss, including one close friend of Ann's whose father had died. Initially, all seemed to be going well, but a few months later Ann developed sleep problems, nightmares, and school refusal behaviors, insisting that she was sick on school mornings and often returning home from school with a terrible stomachache. She was also throwing tantrums and refusing to follow rules at home, playing one parent against the other, and fighting with her younger sister. With the family's agreement, the school decided not to send Ann home when she complained of stomachaches, but to instead send her to the nurse's office. One day the school nurse noticed that Ann, while lying on a cot with a stomachache, was shaking under the blanket. When the nurse asked Ann to sit up so that she could check her temperature, Ann started sobbing. Asked what was wrong, Ann showed the nurse her blood-stained underpants. The nurse asked Ann whether someone had hurt her and Ann nodded her head yes. The nurse called Ann's mother and reported this incident to the FAP on post. Ann was examined by a military pediatrician and at the FAP later that day.

At the FAP Ann reported that her father's friend "Uncle Joe," a very well-liked member of her father's unit, had been sexually abusing her since shortly after the family's arrival at the current installation 2 years prior. The abuse had stopped when father and Uncle Joe were deployed to Iraq, but had restarted when the men had returned. About a month ago, Uncle Joe had begun forcibly raping Ann. Uncle Joe told Ann that if she told anyone about this he would not be able to help soldiers like her daddy win the war, and it would be her fault. Ann was scared that her disclosure would make her country lose the war, or that Uncle Joe would no longer help her father or be their family friend. She tearfully said, "I'm sorry but I had to tell." Physical findings confirmed Ann's report and charges against Joe were prepared.

Ann's parents were devastated and furious when they heard about what Ann had reported. Ann and her parents were referred for TF-CBT treatment, and the parents were eager to participate. Her parents were preoccupied about how to proceed in terms of the criminal charges, and at the initial evaluation were very focused on questions such as, "Will it be helpful or harmful for Ann to testify against Joe?" and "Should we try to get transferred so she doesn't run into people who know about this?" Ann endorsed significant symptoms of PTSD and anxiety about what her disclosure would do to her father and her family as well as how her friends and other parents in the community would respond to her allegation. Her UCLA PTSD Reaction Index score was 57, in the severe range.

Ann's parents were very supportive and determined to do whatever was in Ann's best interests. The therapist began TF-CBT by providing useful information to the family, emphasizing, for example, how important the parents' support was to Ann's positive recovery (Cohen & Mannarino, 1998, 2000). The therapist also normalized Ann's experience by informing parents that rates of sexual abuse among military girls appear to be similar to those in civilian communities (McCarroll et al., 2004); one out of four girls experience sexual abuse. Although shocked, the parents were also relieved that their daughter was not alone in this regard. The therapist also emphasized that Ann disclosed the abuse soon after it occurred, and that this was a credit to Ann's trust in her parents despite the huge guilt that the perpetrator had attempted to instill in her. The parents asked, "If this was the case, why didn't she tell us instead of the nurse?" The therapist helped the parents understand common responses and concerns of children who have experienced sexual abuse, including the desire to protect the people they love most (i.e., their parents). In Ann's case, feelings of loyalty, concerns about military mission, and Joe's popularity in his unit and the community likely made these feelings even stronger. Her parents understood and seemed comforted by this explanation.

The therapist then provided TF-CBT skills components to Ann and her parents. For relaxation, the therapist started by asking Ann what activities she really liked. Ann said she liked to sing, dance, collect butterfly stickers, and play with her friends. Using this information, the therapist and Ann designed several relaxation strategies for different settings. For example, for falling asleep, Ann would imagine a butterfly gently fluttering its wings until it slowly, slowly landed in a bed of grass. Ann practiced this with the therapist and then with her mother, and later reported that this visual image helped her fall asleep. In order to improve school attendance, Ann imagined herself dancing across a beach while relaxing each part of her body. When she had intrusive and scary thoughts about the sexual abuse, Ann agreed to sing her favorite song in her head or out loud (depending on the situation) in order to calm herself down. Her parents practiced this with her in session and agreed to reinforce this with her at home. They also spoke with the school nurse and Ann's homeroom teacher about how to reinforce these skills in school.

The therapist also taught Ann's mother and father important skills to optimize their parenting. For example, both parents were tempted to overindulge Ann following the sexual abuse disclosure because they felt guilty for not knowing what was happening, and the father, in particular, felt personally responsible for exposing Ann to the perpetrator. The therapist helped the parents understand that Ann needed to know that her parents did not see her as "damaged" and that all children need reasonable limits and rules in order to develop appropriate behavioral regulation. This was reassuring to parents and consistent with their military respect for predictable structure and rules. They were further reassured when Ann's behavior problems improved. The parents worked with the school to institute an *in vivo* plan to get Ann back to school (described shortly).

Ann could express a range of feelings (e.g., mad, sad, happy, frustrated, annoyed, excited), but she believed it was her job to help her mother when her father was deployed, and had mistakenly assumed that she should not talk about or need help with negative feelings. The therapist asked her, "What are you supposed to do with bad feelings?" Ann replied, "Just make them go away." The therapist clarified that "sometimes this doesn't work, making feelings too big to handle on our own and that it might be better to ask our parents for help." Ann said, "But then Mommy will have too much to handle." The therapist said, "When Mommy and Daddy say they want you to help out, they mean like helping with the dishes or helping your sister get dressed in the morning. They don't mean by ignoring big problems or worries. Mommies' and daddies' jobs are to help kids with their problems. If you don't believe me, let's go and ask them, OK?" Ann was reticent to ask her parents, but the therapist insisted. Ann's parents very clearly told Ann that they did not want her to keep worries or problems to herself. They explained that they were her parents, and while they appreciated all of her help, they wanted her to be a child, not another grown-up. Ann hugged her mother and said, "OK, Mommy." Together, the parents, Ann, and the therapist designed several affective modulation strategies for Ann, including seeking support from parents, spending time with peers, distraction through enjoyable activities such as dance and music, and self-soothing activities such as crafts and physical activities. The mother particularly reinforced these when Ann had intrusive reminders about the sexual abuse, such as when she was in places or situations where Joe abused her.

Cognitive coping was a very important component for this family, since many people on the base learned about the allegations. Joe was a well-known, well-liked member of the community, and the family encountered gossip about Ann's abuse allegations. People "took sides" and many did not believe Ann's disclosure. The parents felt ostracized by many of their former friends, leading Ann to feel like she "caused a lot of trouble for my family." At one point Ann told her mother that "I don't know if it really happened. Maybe I just dreamed it." The mother called the therapist, crying: "How could she say that, after all we're going through?" The therapist responded, "That may be exactly why she said it. Your daughter loves you so much she would try to do anything to keep you from pain." Ann's parents decided that her father should request a transfer. The father even considered leaving the military service since he felt disillusioned that some of his colleagues disbelieved what had happened. The therapist helped the parents reexamine this by asking "Before, when you were so close to Joe, if another child had accused him of sexual abuse and you didn't know all of the information you now know from Ann's perspective, would you have automatically believed it?" Parents were able to see that other people had heard a lot of inaccurate gossip (some of it distorted information spread by Joe and his friends). Ann's family had been instructed not to talk about her situation since she might have to testify in court proceedings in the future, so they had not been able to defend themselves with their version of the events. Ann's parents were able to change their thoughts from "Some of our military friends have deserted us" to "They don't know the facts," and this helped them to feel even more supported by the friends who had stuck by them even without knowing all of the details of the situation.

In Ann's trauma narrative, she included the additional information that Uncle Joe had threatened to sexually abuse her 3-year-old sister Emma if she ever disclosed the abuse. Ann said, "After he did that (the rape) the first time, I tried not to go to school so he couldn't hurt Emma (who did not yet attend school). When the nurse wouldn't let me go home, I knew I had to tell. He might go to my house when I was at school and do it to her." When the therapist shared this part of Ann's narrative with the parents during their parallel individual sessions, they both became tearful as they realized that Ann's school refusal and her disclosure had been attempts to protect her younger sister.

The therapist had been instituting *in vivo* mastery to help Ann return to school. However, this had only been moderately successful as a result of Ann's unexpressed worries about Joe abusing Emma. Once Joe was arrested (a process that took several weeks), Ann was more confident about returning to school and her school refusal diminished.

During the conjoint child–parent sessions, Ann shared her narrative. Her father was extremely helpful by reinforcing Ann's new cognitions. For example, he told Ann during this session, "Joe's job was to take care of his soldiers. Instead of doing that he abused one of our children. He hurt our soldiers. By telling the truth about him you helped every soldier in the Army. You made our Army stronger." The family worked together to develop a safety plan, and Ann asked if Emma could also be included. The parents, Ann, and Emma used the What Do You Know? game (Deblinger, Neubauer, Runyon, & Baker, 2006) and age-appropriate healthy sexuality education. At the end of treatment, Ann's UCLA PTSD Reaction Index score was 12 (in the normal range).

CONCLUSION

Military children and families face many challenges resulting from the duties of their military service member parents, siblings, and other family members. Since the start of combat operations in the Mideast in 2001, military families have been faced with multiple combat deployments that have resulted increased levels of distress in children and adults. In circumstances of complicated deployment, combat exposure may lead to the development of combat-related stress disorders (PTSD, depression, anxiety, and substance use disorders), combat injuries (including TBI), and, in the most severe circumstances, death. Military children and families are typically healthy, and they face these deployment-related challenges with strength and resilience. However, mitigating distress is an important goal of community, family, and individual prevention and intervention strategies. TF-CBT provides useful skills and strategies that can help military families manage successfully. When stresses are of a traumatic level, TF-CBT should be a critical component of the care of military children and families, given the evidence of its success in treating traumatic disorders. Clinicians who are unfamiliar with military communities can benefit from a further understanding of military children and families, their unique strengths, and the unique challenges that they face in order to more successfully implement treatments.

REFERENCES

Bates, M. J., Brim, W. L., Lunasco, T. K., & Rhodes, J. E. (in press). Military culture and warrior ethos. In M. N. Goldenberg, S. J. Cozza, & R. J. Ursano (Eds.), *Clinical manual for the treatment of military service members, veterans and their families*. Arlington, VA: American Psychiatric Publishing.

Brown, J., Cohen, P., Johnson, J. G., & Salzinger, S. (1998). A longitudinal analysis of risk factors for child maltreatment: Findings of a 17–year prospective study of officially recorded and self-reported child abuse and neglect. *Child Abuse and Neglect, 22*, 1065–1078.

Chandra, A., Lara-Cinisomo, S., Jaycox, L. H., Tanielian, T., Burns, R. M., Rider, T., et al. (2010). Children on the homefront: The experience of children from military families. *Pediatrics, 125*, 16–25.

Cohen, J. A., & Mannarino, A. P. (1998). Factors that mediate treatment outcome in sexually abused preschoolers: Six and twelve month follow-ups. *Journal of the American Academy of Child and Adolescent Psychiatry, 37*, 44–51.

Cohen, J. A., & Mannarino, A. P. (2000). Predictors of treatment outcome in sexually abused children. *Child Abuse and Neglect, 24*, 983–994.

Cohen, J. A., & Mannarino, A. P. (2004). Treatment of childhood traumatic grief. *Journal of Clinical Child and Adolescent Psychology, 33*, 820–832.

Cohen, J. A., & Mannarino, A. P. (2011). Trauma-focused CBT for traumatic grief in military children. *Journal of Contemporary Psychotherapy 41*(4), 219–227.

Cohen, J. A., Mannarino, A. P., & Deblinger, E. (2006). *Treating trauma and traumatic grief in children and adolescents.* New York: Guilford Press.

Cozza, S. J., Chun, R. S., & Polo, J. A. (2005). Military families and children during operation Iraqi Freedom. *Psychiatric Quarterly, 76,* 371–378.

Cozza, S. J., & Guimond, J. M. (2011). Working with combat-injured families through the recovery trajectory. In S. M. Wadsworth & D. Riggs (Eds.), *Risk and resilience in U.S. military families* (pp. 260–277). New York: Springer.

Cozza, S. J., Ortiz, C. D., Fullerton, C. S., Schmidt, J. S., & Ursano, R. J. (2011, November). *Responses of children to parental death: A report and comparison of military and civilian caregivers.* Poster session at the annual meeting of the International Society for Traumatic Stress Studies, Baltimore.

Deblinger, E., Neubauer, F., Runyon, M., & Baker, D. (2006). *What do you know?* Stratford, NJ: CARES Institute.

Flake, E. M., Davis, B. E., Johnson, P. L., & Middleton, L. S. (2009). The psychosocial effects of deployment on military children. *Journal of Developmental and Behavioral Pediatrics, 30,* 271–278.

Gibbs, D. A., Martin, S. L., Kupper, L. L., & Johnson, R. E. (2007). Child maltreatment in enlisted soldiers' families during combat-related deployments. *Journal of the American Medical Association, 298,* 528–535.

Greene-Sortrig, T. M., Britt, T. W., & Castro, C. A.(2007). The stigma of mental health problems in the military. *Military Medicine, 172,* 157–161.

Jensen, P. S., Grogan , D., Xenakis, S. N. & Bain, M. W. (1989). Father absence: Effects on child and maternal psychopathology. *Journal of the American Academy of Child and Adolescent Psychiatry, 28,* 171–175.

Jensen, P. S., Martin, D. & Watanabe, H. (1996). Children's response to parental separation during operation Desert Storm. *Journal of the American Academy of Child and Adolescent Psychiatry, 35,* 433–441.

Jordan, B. K., Marmar, C. R., Fairbank, J. A., Schlenger, W. E., Kulka, R. A., Hough, R. L. et al. (1992). Problems in families of male Vietnam veterans with posttraumatic stress disorder. *Journal of Consulting and Clinical Psychology, 60,* 916–926.

Lester, P., Peterson, K., Reeves, J., Knauss, L., Glover, D., Mogil, C., et al. (2010). The long war and parental combat deployment: Effects on military children and at-home spouses. *Journal of the American Academy of Child and Adolescent Psychiatry, 49,* 310–320.

Mansfield, A. J., Kaufman, J. S., Engel, C. C., & Gaynes, B. N. (in press). Deployment and mental health diagnoses among children of US Army personnel. *Archives of Pediatrics and Adolescent Medicine.*

McCarroll, J. E., Fan, Z., Newby, J. H., & Ursano, R. J. (2008). Trends in U.S. Army child maltreatment reports: 1990–2004. *Child Abuse Review, 17,* 108–118.

McCarroll, J. E., Ursano, R. J., Fan, Z., & Newby, J. H. (2004). Comparison of US Army and civilian substantiated reports of child maltreatment. *Child Maltreatment, 9,* 103–110.

Milliken, C. S., Auchterlonie, J. L., & Hoge, C. W. (2007). Longitudinal assessment of mental health problems among active and reserve component soldiers returning from the Iraq war. *Journal of the American Medical Association, 298,* 2141–2148.

Pine, D. S., & Cohen, J. A. (2002). Trauma in children and adolescents: Risk and treatment of psychiatric sequelae. *Biological Psychiatry, 51,* 519–531.

Rentz, E. D., Marshall, S. W., Loomis, D., Casteel, C., Martin, S. L., & Gibbs, D. A. (2007). Effect of deployment on the occurrence of child maltreatment in military and nonmilitary families. *American Journal of Epidemiol, 165,* 1199–1206.

Rosenheck, R., & Fontana, A. (1998). Transgenerational effects of abusive violence on the children of Vietnam combat veterans. *Journal of Traumatic Stress, 11,* 731–742.

Ruscio, A. M., Weathers, F. W., King, L. A. & King, D. W. (2002). Male war-zone veterans' perceived relationships with their children: The importance of emotional numbing. *Journal of Traumatic Stress, 15,* 351–357.

Steinberg, A. M., Brymer, M. J., Decker, K. B., & Pynoos, R. S. (2004) The University of California at Los Angeles Post-traumatic Stress Disorder Reaction Index. *Current Psychiatry Report, 6,* 96–100.

U.S. Department of Defense. (2009). *Demographics 2009: Profile of the military community.* Washington, DC: Office of the Deputy Under Secrtary of Defense.

Warner, C. H., Appenzeller, G. N., Mullen, K., Warner, C. M., & Greiger, T. (2008). Soldier attitudes toward mental health screening and seeking care upon return from combat. *Military Medicine, 173,* 563–569.

9

International Settings

LAURA K. MURRAY
STEPHANIE A. SKAVENSKI

OVERVIEW OF TF-CBT APPLICATIONS IN INTERNATIONAL SETTINGS

Trauma-focused cognitive-behavioral therapy (TF-CBT) has recently been employed and evaluated in a number of international settings, including western European countries (Germany, Norway, Sweden, Italy, and the Netherlands), Africa (Zambia, Tanzania, and the Democratic Republic of Congo [DRC]), and southeast Asia (Cambodia). TF-CBT training is also occurring in Japan and China. Other countries may be using TF-CBT as well. In this chapter we discuss characteristics of various populations and settings in which TF-CBT is being used, unique assessment and engagement strategies for each, training and supervision considerations, and an explanation of how the TF-CBT PRACTICE components have been applied with some modifications. We bring the use of TF-CBT to life through vivid case presentations from international low-resource settings.

Western Europe

At the first international TF-CBT conference, held in Italy, researchers from Norway, Italy, Sweden, Germany, and the Netherlands met to discuss ongoing TF-CBT studies and implementation methods. Collectively, western European sites reported few modifications beyond the obvious language differences in applying TF-CBT. Directors of the respective research studies stated that all TF-CBT components were relevant and could be implemented with no major cultural modifications in their settings. One minor modification noted by European sites is "toning down" the use of parental praise to fit with their cultures. However, they emphasized that the use of praise is a very important and effective intervention. In Germany, a pilot study demonstrated the feasibility of including foster parents or professional caregivers from group homes in the treatment (Kirsch, Fegert, Seitz, & Goldbeck, 2011). Some modifications reported included the additional collaboration with child welfare workers and biological (nonabusive) parents at the same time, with agreement on the different roles of adult caregivers with shared responsibility for the child (see Chapter 2, "Children in Foster Care," this volume). Given the limited modifications across these western European sites, the remainder of the chapter focuses on low-resource *settings*.

Low–Resource Settings

Countries considered "low resource" or "developing" are characterized by common challenges such as poverty, weak economy (World Bank, 2011), unrest of some kind, and limited organized health systems (i.e., little accessibility to effective treatments). TF-CBT has been used in at least four developing countries: Zambia, Tanzania, the DRC, and Cambodia. Examples here focus primarily on Zambia and Cambodia, where studies have been completed, with occasional reference to the ongoing studies in Tanzania and the DRC.

Zambia

Zambia is a landlocked country in sub-Saharan Africa with a population of 13,881,000 (Central Intelligence Agency [CIA], n.d.-c). It is the site of one of the world's most devastating HIV and AIDS epidemics. More than one in every seven adults in the country is living with HIV, and in 2009 nearly 76,000 adults were newly infected. HIV is most prevalent in urban areas rather than in poorer rural populations. The "feminization" of the HIV/AIDS epidemic is striking: Among those aged 15–24, HIV prevalence is nearly four times among females compared with males. Children have been significantly affected by the AIDS epidemic in Zambia: 120,000 children are estimated to be infected with HIV. In 2009, there were 690,000 AIDS orphans in the country. Orphans and other vulnerable children experience multiple traumatic experiences and stressors, including HIV-related stigma, abuse, poor health care, abbreviated childhoods and education, poverty, and reduced social support. Of particular relevance to TF-CBT, there is a belief that increasing numbers of child rape cases were being fueled by the "virgin cure" myth, which wrongly claims that sex with a virgin can cure AIDS. In a qualitative study, Murray and colleagues (2006) found that child "defilement" (i.e., sexual abuse) was identified as a major problem by the local Zambian community themselves.

The TF-CBT applications described later in this chapter were taken from two separate studies conducted in Zambia. The first study examined the feasibility of training, adapting, and implementing TF-CBT in Zambia with local lay workers. This study was conducted in Lusaka, Zambia, with 20 Zambian counselors. The second study was based in both Lusaka (urban) and Kabwe (peri-urban), and examined the ability to infuse evidence-based assessments and treatments into existing HIV health care systems. In both studies, outcomes included quantitative (validated assessment tools) and qualitative (perspectives of local counselors and families receiving TF-CBT) outcomes.

Tanzania

Tanzania, in east Africa, has a population of nearly 43 million, 42% of whom are younger than 14 years (CIA, n.d.-b). Tanzania was targeted for TF-CBT given its high rates of HIV and children orphaned by AIDS. In 2008 it was estimated that 1.3 million people were living with HIV in mainland Tanzania, 10% of whom were children. Currently, the area has an HIV prevalence rate of 6%. In 2009 an estimated 1.3 million children were orphaned from AIDS in Tanzania and 3 million orphaned for all reasons, including AIDS. The ongoing TF-CBT project in Tanzania focuses on group administration of TF-CBT for childhood traumatic grief with orphans who are living in a family environment (Murray et al., 2010).

Cambodia

Cambodia, in southeastern Asia, has a population of 14,701,717 (CIA, n.d.-d). In contrast to Africa, Cambodia has an adult HIV prevalence rate of 0.8%. Many of the issues related to TF-CBT for this population result from unrest and other social problems. In April 1975, after a 5-year struggle, Communist Khmer Rouge forcefully captured Phnom Penh and evacuated all cities and towns. At least 1.5 million Cambodians died from execution, forced hardships, or starvation during the Khmer Rouge regime under Pol Pot. Additionally, Cambodia is identified as a source of sexual trafficking for commercial exploitation and forced labor. As reported by Amnesty International (2010), the National Police Force statistics recorded 468 cases of rape, attempted rape, and sexual harassment in the 12 months preceeding November 2009, but noted that these figures are "extremely low and unreliable." The applications of TF-CBT and case presentations for Cambodia were taken from a joint project with World Vision on the feasibility of TF-CBT (Bass, Bearup, Bolton, Murray, & Skavenski, 2011). The different phases of the project were conducted in Phnom Penh (urban) across two different shelters for sexually trafficked female and male youth.

The Democratic Republic of Congo

The DRC is located in central Africa. Its current population is estimated at approximately 71,712,867 (CIA, n.d.-a). Since independence, the DRC has been in constant conflict with multiple rebel groups. Throughout these conflicts, large populations of children have been affected either as direct victims of violence, death, and sexual assault or as child soldiers. The project here has recently been undertaken by two graduate students from Belfast as part of their dissertation studies. TF-CBT is being conducted in groups, in collaboration with World Vision. All children included in this project are characterized as former child soldiers (P. O'Callaghan, personal communication, June 24, 2011).

UNIQUE ASSESSMENT STRATEGIES
IN INTERNATIONAL SETTINGS

In most developing countries, neither validated child mental health assessment tools nor trained personnel to administer them are readily available. Although some researchers may appreciate the importance of adapting and validating instruments to the local cross-cultural context, it is still common practice to assume local validity while allowing for some variation in the translation of more idiomatic symptoms. Although increasing, research investigating the psychometric properties of instruments across different ethnic and cultural groups is sparse (Iwata & Buka, 2002). While there is awareness and some evidence (e.g., Alami & Kadri, 2004; Ruchkin et al., 2005; Seedat, Nyamai, Njenga, Vythilingum, & Stein, 2004) that mental health syndromes defined in Western terms may exist in different forms in other cultures, operationalizing this variation in order to create valid and reliable instruments is a special skill in low-resource countries. Many of the relevant issues have been addressed by Bolton using a combined qualitative and quantitative methodology to develop or adapt and validate locally appropriate instruments in resource-poor countries (Bolton, 2001; Bolton & Tang, 2002). Briefly, this methodology includes beginning with a qualitative study to understand the local perception of problems, symptoms, causes, and solutions and to ensure cross-cultural sensitivity (e.g., Murray et al., 2006). Once the local symptoms and problems are understood, an assessment instrument can be developed and/or adapted. For example, the qualitative study in Zambia showed that the community considered defilement (sexual abuse), domestic violence, and physical abuse as children's major mental-health related problems; the most common symptoms included "crying," "thinking too much," "alone and withdrawn," "fearful that it will happen again," "feeling used," "looking confused," "damaged psychologically," "feeling rejected," "shy," "difficulty concentrating," "feeling uneasy and surprised," and "having an unsettled mind—thinking about what has happened." A review of diverse child mental health standardized instruments ensued to determine how closely symptoms included in each instrument corresponded with those described by the local informants in the preliminary qualitative study. Since PTSD symptoms from standardized instruments closely overlapped with prominent problems in the qualitative study for Zambia, the UCLA PTSD Reaction Index (Steinberg, Brymer, Decker, & Pynoos, 2004) was chosen as an instrument to adapt and validate using Bolton's (2001) methodology. This consists of reviewing the existing measure for the problems listed by the local population in the qualitative study. Local symptoms not represented in the measure are added. In Zambia the original items from the measure were maintained, and 18 additional signs and symptoms identified as locally relevant from the qualitative study were added (Murray, Bass, et al., 2011). Establishing local validity of a mental health assessment tool is critical to understanding the effectiveness of any treatment, including TF-CBT.

UNIQUE ENGAGEMENT STRATEGIES IN INTERNATIONAL SETTINGS

Particularly in light of trauma avoidance, engaging children and parents or other caretakers in TF-CBT is a critical component of treatment. In the United States, research has specifically focused on how to engage high-stress families (McKay & Bannon, 2004). One of the largest differences therapists encounter in engaging families in TF-CBT in developing countries is an overall unfamiliarity with structured mental health treatment. Specifically, the idea of seeing a therapist once a week for 12–16 sessions to address specific mental health problems in a structured manner is still a new concept in many developing countries. Most "counseling" in Zambia and Tanzania consists of one to two short (15- to 20-minute) sessions of advice giving. In contrast, counseling in Cambodian shelters typically consists of regular case management (e.g., legal support, court preparation, medical service) and general supportive counseling for the duration of the child's stay at the shelter (e.g., from a few months to 5+ years).

In Zambia and Tanzania, a unique engagement strategy was to spend time explaining the difference between TF-CBT and their current understanding of services (i.e., either monetary help or short "counseling", i.e., advice giving). In some cases, counselors also explained that TF-CBT was not a form of witchcraft or satanic ritual (other practices that are sometimes offered for suffering individuals in these cultures). In Tanzania, the study offers tea and biscuits for 30 minutes before the TF-CBT group begins as a method of engaging families to come to treatment and to come on time.

CASE EXAMPLE

Ms. P, the biological mother of Charity, brought her daughter in for the first TF-CBT treatment session. The counselor began to explain the components of TF-CBT and the number of times they would meet. The mother immediately said this was not what she was expecting, and she didn't understand why they had to come more than once or twice. The counselor explained that TF-CBT is a program that spends different weeks building different skills in the child, such as relaxation, and then spends time helping the child to talk about the trauma experienced. She used the analogy of attending school—talking about how skills are learned over time in the classroom. The counselor explained how she had been trained by professors from a university in the United States, and studies showed that this was a very effective way to help her child heal and no longer suffer from her "staying alone," "being closed," "sadness," and "sleeping problems" (symptoms that the child and mother indicated on the initial assessment). The mother said she did want to help Charity with these things as she seemed to be suffering so much, but she did not know how she could come so many times. The counselor encouraged her (a softer version of praise felt to be more appropriate to the Zambian culture) for being such a supportive mother to Charity and for bringing her in. The counselor asked the mother to tell about her week, her other children, and who else in her family helped her (as it was customary for nonbiological or extended family to help care for children). As the mother explained her situation, the counselor was empathetic to the challenge of her taking time (1 hour for the treatment and another hour for transport) each week for only Charity when she was caring for six other children, and had "more important" tasks like preparing food and selling at the market in order to support the family. They decided together that the grandmother and the "auntie" (a close neighbor) would bring Charity to treatment. The mother agreed to attend two sessions near the end—one in which she would hear the child's story and one when the child would share the story. The counselor also arranged for the project to help with the transport costs to and from TF-CBT (approximately $2.50 each way on a minibus).

CASE EXAMPLE

Goddfrey was a 14-year-old who resided with his grandmother in an overpopulated compound where there was a lot of violence. Goddfrey presented for his first session with his grandmother. During this initial meeting, Goddfrey's grandmother asked the counselor, "Is this just another way to use our children to get money from donors?" The grandmother then stated her suspicions about meeting at a hospice, that she was concerned they may try "to sacrifice the child to have money for the hospice." The counselor asked open-ended questions as a way to encourage the grandmother to tell her more about her concerns. The grandmother thought that since a lot of people who went to the hospice for treatment died, having the child come to the hospice would kill him (hospices are where many adults and children go for end-of-life care, and at one time a vast majority would die). The counselor understood and validated the grandmother's concern because many community members avoid hospices as a result of similar concerns. The counselor explained that the treatment was free, and its purpose was to help children who are having problems to face their fears. The counselor stated that the program has nothing do with the hospice, and that it was selected as a location for the treatment only because it is a central place in the community that is easily accessible and because it is near the compounds. The counselor also believed that it was necessary to directly address the grandmother's fears about satanism, since this was a known concern in the community. Rumors that the program is involved with satanism could quickly spread, preventing others from coming. After the counselor finished, the grandmother asked, "If this is true, then how come people who come to the hospice come out dead and not alive? Are you sure you aren't turning my nephew into a satanist?" The counselor normalized this concern, and suggested that it may help to explain more about what exactly she would be doing with her grandson. The counselor provided details about the eight components of the TF-CBT treatment and included step-by-step descriptions of the activities that would be involved, making sure to point out that none of the activities or topics involved satanism. The counselor also explained that, if possible, the grandmother would also be joining the treatment as often as possible and she could raise these questions or concerns again if she thought they were doing anything bad. The grandmother thanked the counselor for taking the time to explain and said that the program did not look religious at all, and that she was happy that the counselor would include her in the program going forward so that grandmother could make sure of this.

HOW TF-CBT IS APPLIED DIFFERENTLY IN INTERNATIONAL SETTINGS

Personnel, Training, and Supervision in Low-Resource Countries

Given the limited number of mental health professionals in low-resource countries, one of the most significant modifications is in the type of providers who deliver TF-CBT. In contrast to the United States, where TF-CBT is provided only by licensed master's-level mental health professionals, in all the TF-CBT studies discussed in this chapter, lay community members (usually with a high school education but no specific mental health training) have been trained to provide TF-CBT. This represents the current model within global mental health, wherein the task of providing therapy has been shifted away from the very limited number of mental health professionals to lay workers (Patel, 2009; Patel et al, 2010). The authors and others in the field of global mental health have tested and are using an apprenticeship model of training and ongoing supervision (Murray, Dorsey, et al., 2011). This model mimics other apprenticeship-style trainings, including (1) selection of apprentices who demonstrate interest and aptitude for the profession; (2) coursework/training; (3) application of knowledge "on the job" under direct supervision and coaching; (4) ongoing expansion of knowledge and skills under supervision; and (5) mutual problem solving by "master" or expert trainer and apprentice. Inherent in the apprenticeship model is the ability for local counselors themselves to make cultural modifications and actively guide the implementation process and the development of a local, sustainable supervision structure. This is accomplished through extended, intensive live trainings (10 days), specific live supervision training for local supervisors, ongoing Skype calls (2 hours/week), and experience with practice cases (minimum of one practice case per counselor). Research suggests that when the apprenticeship model is employed, mental health interventions delivered by lay counselors can have a positive impact on a range of important domains, including mental health, health, and functioning (Bolton et al., 2003; Patel et al., 2010; Rahman, Malik, Sikander, Roberts, & Creed, 2008). This model is obviously different from a one-time training, which is not recommended even for trained mental health professionals.

Particularly relevant to this chapter is the process of modification in low-resource and/or cross-cultural settings. Treatment outcome and implementation research from the West links fidelity of evidence-based practices to positive outcomes (Barber, Crits-Christoph, & Luborsky, 1996; Schoenwald, Carter, Chapman, & Sheidow, 2008), yet there is also a need to examine cultural modifications that may be important to mental health outcomes (Hwang, 2009; Rousseau & Kirmayer, 2009; Verdeli et al., 2003, 2008). Consistent with TF-CBT generally, training in low-resource countries attempts to maintain "flexibility within fidelity" (Kendall & Beidas, 2007), the critical line that balances room for creativity and adaptation to fit the population, including cross-cultural modifications, while maintaining fidelity (delivery of essential components) to the TF-CBT model. National counselors and leaders are critical in working with the trainers to make decisions about this balance. To operationalize this, concrete goals are created for each component of TF-CBT (e.g., for affective modulation: obtain a list of feelings from clients in their words, link these feelings to situations, where they feel them in the body, and the intensity of these feelings in these situations). These concrete goals define fidelity to the treatment model. The way in which these goals are reached, or how they are implemented, represents the flexibility built into TF-CBT and allows for cultural modifications or applications. Across the four sites where active TF-CBT research has occurred (Zambia, Cambodia) or is occurring (Tanzania, the DRC), the cross-cultural applications have been conceptualized as differences in *how* the components are implemented rather than changes required to the components themselves. In other words, we have been able to maintain fidelity while allowing for flexibility. The remainder of the chapter focuses on these cultural applications.

Logistical Modifications

Session length was modified in Zambia, with sessions ranging from 30 minutes to 2 hours. National counselors explained that punctuality is not critical in the Zambian culture, so families would often show up 30 minutes to 2 hours late for a counseling appointment, and this was culturally acceptable. This modification was also made to accommodate families who often have to travel long distances (or had to use local transportation, which can be unreliable) to their appointment and, therefore, would often rather stay for longer periods of time. If a longer session was held, the national counselor would complete more goals and/or components within one longer period of time and shorten the overall number of sessions (i.e., fidelity to the time frame of the intervention). In both Tanzania and the DRC, TF-CBT is being provided in group format for the first four components (psychoeducation and parenting, relaxation, affective expression and modulation, and cognitive coping and processing), and then each child's trauma narrative is created in individual sessions. The group resumes after the trauma narrative component. These groups are still split by age and gender, as is normally the case.

Psychoeducation

In both Zambia and Tanzania, one of their main differences from Western populations was families' unfamiliarity with counseling. Most families are familiar only with HIV-related voluntary counseling and testing, which is typically one meeting lasting 10–20 minutes to receive information about HIV. In addition, although caregivers were invested in helping their children, they often had other duties to attend to that were directly related to their livelihood (e.g., selling at the market, getting water for the family). Time was often spent carefully explaining the importance of involving caregivers in TF-CBT, if and when possible, and negotiating a plan for this.

CASE EXAMPLE

Loveness arrived with her aunt at the center for their joint psychoeducation session. The counselor began by greeting the family, explaining his role as counselor, the rationale for TF-CBT treatment and the length and duration of sessions. Loveness's aunt was very reluctant and questioned why she should be coming more often if it was her niece who needed help and not herself. The aunt explained that the program was long and time consuming and she had other important issues to attend to, such as walking a long distance to obtain clean water for the extended family. She stated that her other counseling, voluntary counseling and testing (VCT), for HIV had only been one session. The counselor praised Loveness's aunt for accepting this first invitation and accompanying the child to start her treatment. The counselor also acknowledged the difficulties many guardians and caregivers encounter in looking after children from extended families.

The counselor opened a discussion about how TF-CBT is different from VCT by asking the aunt to tell him about VCT. He thanked the aunt for sharing her understanding of VCT and then explained that TF-CBT is very new in Zambia and that in TF-CBT their goal is to work with the child and family to make sure the child is helped. The counselor explained that in TF-CBT they do not draw blood or do any other medical procedures. The aunt asked the counselor, "If you do not do medical tests, then what do you do? How will it help this child?" The counselor explained that TF-CBT is a special program for children who have been through very bad things in their life, as Loveness had: sexual abuse and witnessing two children drown in the river (two traumas she reported experiencing during the initial assessment). He stated that as a result of experiencing these bad things some children have bad behavior or problems in the home or at school. The counselor then asked the aunt what types of problems she has observed in Loveness. The aunt reported that Loveness was always distracted in school and now had bad grades, often woke in the night, was crying all the time, and was not helping around the home. The counselor explained that these are exactly the kinds of problems they work on in TF-CBT. He told the aunt that she was the expert on Loveness and that he needed her help in order to work through the program. The counselor explained that TF-CBT is different than VCT in that they will talk about the bad things that happened to the child, learn how to relax their bodies, and talk about how feelings and thoughts affect what we do, and that they will also talk directly about the bad things that happened and then about how to keep the child safe in the future. The caregiver said she understood much more now that this was something very different from VCT.

Parenting Skills

In Zambia, national counselors explained that Zambian parents use a wide range of techniques to discipline their children, including shouting, spanking, or punishing by withdrawing something important to the child. The parenting skills presented in TF-CBT were well liked by the counselors; however, they noted that they needed to use caution with these skills to ensure a fit within each family's current disciplinary approach and openness to change. In Cambodia, we worked with a population of youth living at shelters, many of whom had been sold by their parents to brothels. Unfortunately, there was no caregiver involvement in these cases.

CASE EXAMPLE

Mrs. N attended her second TF-CBT session with her daughter, 8-year-old Rose. As the counselor already had obtained buy-in from the mother the previous week, she explained that they would be working together over the next few sessions to learn and practice some skills Mrs. N could use at home to help with Rose's behavior as well as that of other children in the home. The counselor started by first explaining praise (this was the favorite parenting skill among her other clients' parents). The counselor explained that praising the child for specific behaviors is easy to do and can have a huge impact on increasing positive behaviors. The counselor then gave an example: "For instance, if the child never used to sweep the surroundings but suddenly she starts doing that, how would you react?" Mrs. N said that she would be very pleased (but would not say anything). The counselor suggested that she could encourage Rose and her other children to do this more often by praising them each time they sweep the surroundings. Mrs. N appeared hesitant and stated that she was not sure that would work because if she praised her, then Rose would just expect to get praise for doing something she is supposed to do anyway and "it would spoil her." The counselor normalized Mrs. N's thoughts and stated: "Yes, many of the parents with whom I work feel this way before they try using the technique. Let me ask you a question—is cooking nshima and relish something that you normally do?" Mrs. N replied that, of course, it is, and she does not expect to be praised for this. The counselor asked Mrs. N to imagine a situation where, after a long day of work, she spent time carefully preparing chicken, nshima, and relish for her family for dinner, and then her husband comes home, sits down to dinner with the family, and after only one bite of food declares that the meal was wonderful, the best he has had in a long time. The counselor then asked Mrs. N how that would make her feel and whether she would be more or less likely to cook that meal again. Mrs. N smiled and stated that she would feel very good and would try to do the same again and feel more encouraged to carefully prepare the meal in the future (she added that her husband has not done this in some time). The counselor related this back to Rose, and Mrs. N agreed to try to praise the child. Since this was a new skill for Mrs. N, the counselor did some role plays with her so she could practice using specific phrases such as "That is a very good job," "You swept the floor very nicely," "You worked very hard sweeping the floor today. Thank you."

During their next session together, Mrs. N and the counselor met individually to continue with parenting skills. The counselor checked in with Ms. N to see how the praising went over the course of the week. Mrs. N said that it went okay but she has not noticed any changes. The counselor asked Mrs. N how she praised the child. Mrs. N said that Rose had swept the surroundings three times that week, and each time when the child was finished she said to her, "That was good sweeping. I don't know why you are so lazy and don't always do it like that." The counselor returned to the situation of Mrs. N cooking dinner and asked her how she would feel if her husband said something like "That meal was wonderful. Why are you so lazy and don't cook like this all the time?" Mrs. N reported that she would be upset and would not want to cook at all. Again, the counselor related this to the situation with Rose and asked Mrs. N how she thinks Rose felt when she said that to her. Mrs. N admitted that Rose also probably felt bad. The counselor explained that when Mrs. N praises Rose she should only say the good and leave out the bad because the bad makes the praise meaningless. The counselor had Mrs. N roll-play again on how to praise using just positive phrases. Over the next few sessions, the counselor worked to help Mrs. N use positive feedback consistently and to model this behavior for her in session. In just a few weeks, Mrs. N reported back to the counselor that she began to see results and that the child began sweeping the floor without even being asked.

Relaxation

In international use of TF-CBT, we have found varying levels of relaxation practices. In Africa, the reception from local counselors was very positive, with minor modifications. For example, in the United States progressive muscle relaxation can be taught to young children using the analogy of a "cooked and uncooked noodle" or a "tin soldier and rag doll." In Zambia and Tanzania, national counselors chose to use analogies such as "cooked and uncooked okra." In Cambodia, national counselors indicated that adults and children use relaxation on a much more regular basis, including visual imagery and meditation. In fact, in the very first training, a local counselor ran a meditation exercise that the counselors continued to use for treatment of children. Counselors in Cambodia believed relaxation was such an important part of their culture that they often spent 1.5–2 sessions on this component.

CASE EXAMPLE

Sixteen-year-old Nary from Cambodia was starting relaxation during her third TF-CBT session. The counselor introduced the relaxation component using cooked and uncooked noodles. Since Nary had very limited experience in school, the counselor wanted to teach her by doing rather than talking. The counselor took Nary to the kitchenette at the shelter and pulled out a packet of noodles. She asked Nary to hold the noodles and describe what they felt like. Together, they cooked the noodles, and the counselor took one noodle out of the pot and asked Nary what it felt like. Nary was able to notice the difference between the stiff, hard, uncooked noodle and the soft, squishy, cooked noodle. After eating the noodles together, the counselor related this activity to relaxation and the feelings of stress in Nary's body, especially when she remembers the bad things that happened to her while she was in the brothel.

During their next session, the counselor introduced guided imagery—or "a walk in the mind," as often referred to by Cambodian counselors. The counselor started by asking Nary if she could tell her about a favorite place where she had been before and that she wishes to visit again. Nary replied that she would like to visit the riverside—her favorite place in Phnom Penh. The counselor then asked whether Nary had a preference for how she wants to get there. The client said that she wanted to take a *tuk tuk* (common form of transport in Cambodia). The counselor told Nary that in a few minutes they will go to visit the riverside by just sitting in this counseling room and doing "a walk in the mind." Before beginning this "walk," Nary rated her level of stress as 9 out of 10. The counselor then pulled out a picture they had drawn previously—of Nary's hand, and on each of the five fingers was written a question: What do you see? What do you hear about? What do you smell? What do you touch? What do you taste? The counselor explained that when they take a walk in the mind she wants Nary to remember and think about these questions. The counselor asked Nary to get in a comfortable position and begin the "breathe in and out" exercise they had practiced last session and to either close her eyes or to concentrate on a space on the floor in front of her. The counselor spoke softly, asking the five questions one by one. Following the activity, the counselor asked Nary what she saw, heard, smelled, touched, and tasted. The client reported that she traveled on a *tuk tuk* from the shelter to the main road and saw a lot of big houses and a green garden. And when she got to the riverside she saw a lot of people sitting on the long chairs and facing to the river. She felt happy to see a lot of young children running and eating their snack. She also smelled the roast beef and chicken and bought some to eat; it tasted so good and salty. She also smelled the air that was so pure and when it touched her skin it felt cool. When asked to rate her stress again, Nary reported her stress level as only 5 (out of 10). The counselor noted the difference between Nary's feelings before and after the activity and assigned her homework to practice this technique in the shelter every day, and especially when she feels stressed.

Affective Modulation

In Zambia, the goals of affective modulation were often accomplished by minor modifications such as using sticks to measure intensity of feelings, drawing on Styrofoam cups to show inside and outside feelings, and using fables about animals to describe feeling words. Creating a feeling list was the most difficult task in Zambia, since talking about feelings was a new skill and the tribal languages used for treatment often have one word that represents a number of different feelings (e.g., *ububi* can mean bad, angry, or frustrated). In Cambodia children were also not used to discussing their feelings openly. Activities used in Cambodia included using face feelings cards, a matching game where the child matches the face with the feeling, and reading a storybook and identifying feeling words and guessing the feeling ("play with karma").

Case Example

Sipho, a 7-year-old boy living in Lusaka, had just started affective modulation with the counselor. During the session the counselor asked the child to come up with a list of as many feeling and emotion words as he could in Nyanja (the local language he was most comfortable using). The child listed only two words: *bweno* (happy) and *sad* (the child spoke this word in English because he did not know the Nyanja word for sad). The counselor, also a Nyanja speaker, understood that often there were not direct translations for some feeling words (i.e., *sad*) and that some words for feelings, like *bweno*, could have multiple meanings (e.g., *bweno* can mean happy, joy, good). The counselor decided that she would need to be creative in order to help Sipho express additional feeling words. Toward this end, she introduced feeling exercises using different fruits and pictures of feeling faces. For example, the counselor handed Sipho a lemon and asked how he felt when he ate it. Sipho replied, "Bitter and sour." Then the counselor showed him pictures of feeling faces she had drawn herself, and asked Sipho to describe what that face looked like. Since there were still many words that seemed to represent a number of feelings (and different faces), the counselor asked Sipho to describe a situation when he felt "bweno." Sipho gave an example of when he passed his quiz in school and said that he felt good. The counselor asked what he looked like when he felt "bweno" for passing the quiz. The child said he was smiling and ran home. When asked about other situations that made him feel "bweno," Sipho was able to describe a range of times when "bweno" sometimes meant good or meant wonderful or joyful. For example, before she died his mother bought him a pair of shoes. Sipho reported he had lost the shoes, but later, after his mother died, he found them and this made him feel "bweno"—but not jump-up-and-down or smiling "bweno," but more like a warm-inside feeling. For each different feeling, they rated the intensity by marking different levels on a Coca-Cola bottle. The counselor continued using these techniques in order to reach all of the goals of the affective modulation component.

Cognitive Coping

Counselors in all four countries expressed that this component made sense to children and had cultural relevance, and many of them used cognitive coping frequently in their own lives. In all sites many children did not know how to read and/or write, so this component was implemented using pictures. While teaching cognitive coping in Zambia, children and caregivers often talked about religion or spirituality. In Cambodia, thoughts were often explained in reference to meditation (a very familiar activity for most).

CASE EXAMPLE

Thirteen-year-old Sin had been living at a shelter for trafficked girls for 2 years. Prior to living in the shelter, Sin had been living in a brothel and was not allowed to go to school (common among children in Cambodia who are forced to work in brothels). As a result, Sin had limited ability to read and write, and the counselor often used visual aids throughout TF-CBT to reach the goals of each component. At the beginning of session, the counselor asked Sin what she recalled from their last session, to which Sin replied that they had used animals to represent feelings. The counselor then introduced the concepts of thoughts and behaviors. The counselor stated that thoughts were "things that we say to ourselves like when we meditate or pray—sometimes we say the words out loud but sometimes we just say them in our head." The counselor then described behaviors as things that people do "like when we start a session we always do nail painting—your behavior then is painting your nails." To further help Sin distinguish among thoughts, feelings, and behaviors, the counselor drew a triangle and asked, "What picture would you draw to represent a thought—something that represents what we say to ourselves in our head when we meditate?" Sin drew a picture of a head for thoughts. With the counselor's guidance, Sin went on to draw a heart for feelings and a person dancing for behaviors. When the drawings were completed, the counselor provided several examples of situations in which two young people had different feelings and behaviors depending on their thoughts about the situation. For example, if the situation was that a handsome man passed a girl on the street and did not look at her, one girl might think, "He thinks I am worthless because I used to live in a brothel and that is why he does not look at me." She feels sad and angry, and her behavior is to stay in bed and not talk to anyone. Another girl might think, "He must be a very busy man; maybe he is thinking about taking good care of his mother or his little children." This girl feels happy thinking that the man is taking good care of his family, and she continues to go to school and to therapy. After discussing several of these examples, Sin said she understood how different thoughts affect how girls may feel and behave. The therapist photocopied the paper for Sin to take with her to help Sin remember thoughts, feelings, and behaviors.

CASE EXAMPLE

Nomsa was the mother of an 8-year-old girl who was seeing a TF-CBT counselor in Zambia. Nomsa and the counselor met for the first 15 minutes of session alone to review what the counselor was going to work on with her daughter that day while the mother ran to the market. The counselor introduced the idea of the cognitive triangle, saying "This is a way we show kids how thoughts, feelings, and behaviors are all connected." The counselor brought up a situation that she knew Nomsa had experienced many times—a minibus being very late and then arriving completely full with no room. The counselor helped her answer the questions "When this happens, what goes through your mind?"; "How do you feel?"; and What do you do?" Nomsa filled in the triangle as follows:

Situation: Minibus is late and when it arrives it is full.
Thought: I hate the minibus. There is no way I will be able to prepare dinner in time for my husband.

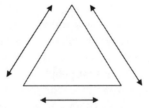

Feeling: Angry, frustrated   *Behavior:* Yelling, shouting

The counselor explained that they were now going to try to look at the same situation in a different way. "What are some other thoughts you could have in this same situation?" Nomsa responded that she could think it was the driver's fault. The counselor asked if there are any more helpful ways to look at the situation that would help her to feel a little better and maybe even change her behavior of yelling and shouting. Nomsa replied, "Well, sometimes I ask what the Bible would guide me to do. If I think about that, then I might think that this is unfortunate but that there are many worse things that could happen." The counselor suggested they could create a new triangle with this thought:

Thought: This is unfortunate but there are worse things that could happen. It is no one's fault.

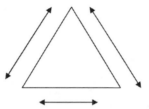

Feeling: Still a little frustrated   *Behavior:* Sigh, look around for a car going in that direction

Trauma Narrative

Children and caregivers often reported that this component was initially difficult but in the end very positive. Many parents and caregivers talked about how the trauma narrative allowed the child to "open up." Most cases in Zambia and Cambodia involved multiple traumas, so timelines or lists of traumatic events were often used. Both sites used different analogies to help explain the purpose of this component. For example, in Zambia counselors used riding a bicycle or cooking beans to explain the purpose of gradual exposure and the analogy of cooking nshima to help acquire the details (*nshima* is a staple food in Zambia made of a cornmeal product referred to as mielie meal). Zambian and Cambodian counselors used many drawings and sometimes dolls or figures to help children create their narratives. In Zambia counselors spent multiple sessions gradually exposing the caregiver to the child's story as most had their own similar traumatic experiences (e.g., raped when they were young; HIV infection). At times, counselors had to spend one session with the caregivers hearing their own trauma story so that the caregivers could be supportive in hearing the child's story. In Cambodia, it was not possible to share the narrative with caregivers because all of the youth were living in a shelter away from their families. These counselors added a session where the children would launch a balloon into the air to "let go" of the trauma. This activity fit with the cultural beliefs often described as "letting go" of bad things.

CASE EXAMPLE

Nine-year-old Elly had been living in an institutional care setting for street youth in Zambia for 4 years. When working with children in an institutional care setting, the TF-CBT counselors tried to work closely and collaboratively with the shelter staff, who often played the role of guardian. The counselor first met with the caregiver closest to Elly and explained that they would be starting to talk this week about the times she was sexually abused repeatedly by her grandfather. He used the analogy of cooking beans to explain the rationale again to the caregiver (which had already been done at the start of treatment): "I know you cook beans often for the children here. Tell me about that process again." The caregiver explained that it was a long and difficult process, but that she did it because the kids loved them so much. The counselor said, "In a similar way, the trauma narrative can be challenging and take some time, but once this is done it helps the child to feel better." The counselor was aware that talking about sexual body parts and sex was not something that most families did openly and that he also needed to prepare the caregiver ahead of time as to prevent any misinterpretations. The counselor explained this component to the caregiver to be sure she approved of it and knew the purpose. He told the caregiver that one of the most important parts of TF-CBT is when the child talks in detail about the bad things that happened, including, in Elly's case, the details of the rape. The counselor explained that in order to do this sometimes they needed to talk openly about sexual body parts and sex in order to get the details of the sexual abuse and provide accurate information. The counselor clarified that they do not do this in order to promote sexual activity or be disrespectful in any way. The caregiver agreed that the child could attend the sessions each week and the counselor would share the narrative with the caregiver each week as she was available.

The counselor met with Elly and introduced the rationale for the narrative in the same way he did at the beginning of TF-CBT, using an analogy of riding a bike since Elly had just recently learned how to ride a bike. He asked Elly to remember what that experience had been like. Elly talked about how it was hard, and sometimes she fell and hurt herself and even cried. She added proudly that now she has mastered it and could ride like the older kids. The counselor said, "The story we are going to start today is very similar to that. At the beginning, it may seem like you can't talk about the times your grandfather touched your private parts. But, as we practice more together, you will master this also and be able to talk about this without fear. This will help you feel better, be less sad, and want to be with friends more like you used to." After two sessions of working on the worst sexual abuse incident, Elly was still unable to mention the private sexual body parts using any words and thus was not talking about the "hot spot" or "worst moment." Through supervision the counselor and supervisor decided to try using dolls so the child could show the counselor what happened. They also thought it may be helpful for the caregiver to "give permission" to Elly to talk about sexual things with the counselor. The counselor also used another analogy to try to explain the amount of detail they needed. With the caregiver present for the first 10 minutes, the counselor asked if Elly had ever watched or helped someone cook nshima. The counselor, the caregiver, and Elly talked about all the little (and many) stages of cooking nshima and how each stage is very important. The counselor explained that Elly's story was similar in that each minute was very important to talk about, just like the steps of cooking nshima. The caregiver also explained to Elly that this was a "safe" and "OK" place to talk about sex. With just Elly in the room, the counselor introduced the dolls and named all the body parts of the dolls for both sexes. The child used the dolls to show what her grandfather did to her, even talking about the first time and then the "worst" time (which included vaginal and anal rape).

Cognitive Processing of the Trauma Narrative

In Zambia, counselors often used analogies to help explain the purpose of cognitive processing. For example, when trying to help children process the thought "I should have known he was a bad man," they might use the analogy of groundnuts (e.g., peanuts): "If you bought groundnuts in the shell, can you tell precisely whether or not they are all rotten inside?" or "Can you tell the shape of the groundnut inside a shell before you open it?" Counselors also used religion in restructuring, as described previously in the case example for cognitive coping, asking questions such as "What would the Bible guide us to do?" A culturally specific challenge of using cognitive restructuring was related to certain beliefs regarding witchcraft, which is common in some parts of Zambia. For example, a child might believe that her uncle raped her because she was possessed. Local counselors worked on the children to consider alternatives to the unhelpful thought, while being careful not to challenge any major beliefs (e.g., not insisting that children cannot be possessed). They were successful in reframing these to thoughts such as "If I am possessed, there are other ways to help me besides rape." Finally, a distinct thought in almost all the sex-trafficked youth within Cambodia was "My parents sold me." In many instances, this was true but unhelpful. Counselors addressed this as illustrated next.

CASE EXAMPLE

In his previous session, Savy, a 14-year-old who had been sold to a brothel by his parents, had included the thought "My mother is a bad mother because she sold me to the brothel," which resulted in strong feelings of depression and thoughts of suicide. His counselor, Minat, and Minat's supervisor agreed that he should work on processing this unhelpful thought in the next session. However, Minat was nervous because this was an accurate thought—the mother did, in fact, sell the child to a brothel.

At their next session, Minat started by praising Savy for being so brave and doing such a good job writing his story even though it was difficult. Minat told Savy that she had read through his trauma story and noticed he frequently mentioned the thought "My mother is a bad mother because she sold me to the brothel." Savy agreed that he thought about this a lot and that even now he thinks "My mother is bad." When asked how frequently he thinks about this, Savy replied, "Many times a day." Next, Minat asked Savy how he felt when he thought about this and Savy rated his feeling sad as 10/10 and angry 10/10. Minat told Savy that many children she works with who have been sold to a brothel also think and feel sad this way but that she does not want Savy to continue feeling this bad. She then asked Savy if he would be willing to do an activity to try and change this thought so that he could feel better; Savy agreed to try. Minat gave Savy a piece of paper and a pen, and said they were going to pretend they were the police or a lawyer investigating a case and Savy had to collect some information. Minat suggested they investigate what a good mother was by questoning other youth in the shelter. Savy liked the idea of being a "professional," and together they came up with questions to ask, such as "What do you believe the characteristics of a good mother are?" and "If you were a mother, what would you do for your children?" Together, they interviewed various staff and children at the shelter. Savy compiled a long list of responses, including (1) taking care of her children when they are sick, (2) providing them with food, (3) giving good advice, (4) allowing them to go to school, (5) helping children with their problems and homework, (6) protecting children from bad things, and (7) playing and laughing with their children. Many youth at the shelter also commented that their mothers were bad and had sold them to brothels. Minat then told Savy that she would read back the list to Savy, and every time she read a point that he thinks is true for his mom he should put a check mark next to it. Savy was able to validate that his mother took good care of him when he was sick, provided good food when she could, and helped him with problems. The counselor asked, "After doing this activity, what thoughts do you have about your mom that may be more helpful?" Savy replied, "My mom is bad for selling me but she also had some good points, and I guess a lot of moms sell their children so I'm not the only one." Minat drew a second triangle and had Savy write this new thought. The new thought still led to feelings of sadness and anger but to a lesser degree. Savy reported a helpful behavior as talking more with other children in the shelter. Minat asked Savy to practice saying this new thought to himself and to remember this activity every time he started thinking that his mom was bad and feeling sad and angry.

Conjoint Child–Parent Sessions

Conjoint sessions conducted in Zambia were often with multiple caregivers but at different times. Thus, a child may have two to three conjoint sessions—one with a grandmother, one with the mother, and one with an aunt. Conjoint sessions could not be used in Cambodia or the DRC since these children were not living with caregivers.

In Vivo Mastery of Trauma Reminders

In vivo mastery was rarely used in either Cambodia or Zambia given the nature of the traumas (e.g., it was not safe for a child to visit a brothel they feared and avoided; the perpetrator was often remained in the home, so trauma reminders were often still dangerous).

Enhancing Safety

Safety skills are an important part of TF-CBT and were introduced in all low-resource settings as important to use immediately when a safety issue arose. In most low-resource settings, mental health system "safety nets" that many of us are used to do not exist (e.g., child protection services, child legal services). In Cambodia, all the girls were relatively safe at a shelter, so counselors often discussed safety planning at the end of treatment, focusing on how to be safe in the future (i.e., healthy relationships as adults, safety issues when returning home). In Zambia, safety issues were often raised very early in treatment, making safety a necessary component throughout each week of TF-CBT.

CASE EXAMPLE

Ten-year-old Nkuka was referred for TF-CBT treatment after she disclosed to her aunt that her grandfather, whom the aunt was also looking after, had sexually molested and raped her. The counselor began the first session by meeting with the aunt alone because in this context it is seen as disrespectful to meet with the child first. The counselor began by asking what types of problems Nkuka was showing at home. The aunt replied that she has been acting disrespectfully and often running away, sometimes for the entire night. The aunt disclosed to the counselor that the grandfather who raped Nkuka was still in the home, as it was her responsibility to take care of him (there were no other family members living). The TF-CBT counselor flagged this as a safety concern and explained this to the aunt, calmly stating that they should work on this together because the very first task is to ensure that Nkuka is safe and to prevent her from running away. The counselor told the caregiver that she would like to call her supervisor, as was the standard first action when there was a safety concern. She explained that her supervisor, Violet, could help them decide on a good safety plan. During the call, the supervisor helped the counselor form a clear set of questions to ask the aunt while she made her way to the session to join the counselor and the aunt.

The counselor asked the aunt if there were any other placement options for the child or the grandfather. The aunt reported that the child had just lost her mother and she did not want to move her again but she also did not have anywhere to place her father. When asked if she had gone to the police to report the rape—after informing the aunt about the laws in Zambia against child sexual abuse and her obligation to report it—the aunt responded that she did but later dropped the case fearing that the police would imprison her father; she felt that he would not be able to handle prison and might die there. The counselor and aunt decided that for the short term Nkuka had to be able to stay somewhere else anytime the aunt wasn't home, particularly at night. The aunt thought of a neighbor who might help out and called her during the session. The neighbor agreed that Nkuka could spend the night at her house at least for the next few weeks while the aunt worked on an alternative plan.

The counselor and aunt then met conjointly with Nkuka to develop a detailed safety plan on what to do if the grandfather tried to approach her at the house, at the neighbor's house, in the street, or elsewhere. If Nkuka came home and did not find the aunt there, she was to go straight to the neighbor's house. Even though the grandfather was not to know where Nkuka was sleeping at night, the family agreed that Nkuka would sleep in the same room as the neighbor so that if he found her there he could not harm her. If the grandfather ever approached Nkuka in the neighborhood, she was to run to the neighbor's house and say "I have to go to the market," their code phrase for "I'm in trouble—my grandfather is near." Finally, Nkuka and the aunt signed a detailed list of safety steps to implement within the house. For example, when Nkuka took a shower, the aunt would stand directly outside the entire time and sing to Nkuka—a favorite childhood song that her mother used to sing—to let Nkuka know she was being protected. The entire daily schedule was also laid out so they could make sure that Nkuka was never alone with the grandfather. Although not a definitive solution, Nkuka expressed that she felt much better knowing all of these safety measures were in place, and she never ran away from home again. Over the next few weeks, Nkuka remained at the neighbor's home at night, and the aunt and Nkuka continued to attend TF-CBT sessions. At the beginning of each session, the counselor did a safety check-in and reviewed the safety plan with the child. After 3 weeks the aunt was able to locate some relatives of the grandfather in a distant village who agreed to take care of him in light of the current situation.

OTHER SPECIAL CONSIDERATIONS

When working in developing countries, daily stressors often have an impact on the individual and family as well as TF-CBT application. These may include poverty, HIV, limited mental health systems (e.g., child protection services), and limited law enforcement (e.g., police). We present an example where these multiple factors were present and how they were addressed in the context of TF-CBT.

CLINICAL CASE DESCRIPTION

Overview

Lubi, a 12-year-old girl who was diagnosed with HIV and, eventually, epilepsy, lived in a compound known for its violence and illicit drug distribution. Lubi lived down the street from a minibus driver who operated the bus route in her neighborhood and often took her mother, Mrs. K, to work. Because the minibus driver saw Lubi's mother every day, he came to know her fairly well and would often stop to talk and joke with her. He then began coming over when Mrs. K was at work and engaging Lubi in one-on-one conversation: "You know me," "We are familiar. I know your mother well, and she says it is OK to talk to me," and eventually "You are going to be my wife. Just wait and see." After a few weeks, he started bringing Lubi alcoholic drinks. After one of these visits he took Lubi to his bus and raped her; the sexual abuse continued over the next year, until her mother found out (through a neighbor). Mrs. K took Lubi to the police to report the multiple rapes.

Mrs. K brought Lubi to TF-CBT to address her posttrauma behavior. In an initial parent session, Mrs. K reported to the counselor that Lubi would often go out at night while Mrs. K was at work in order to find alcohol. Mrs. K told the counselor that on these occasions the minibus driver would follow Lubi, and there was concern that he would or had already managed to rape her again. Mrs. K reported concern about the "fits" the child had, which were getting worse as a result of the drinking.

Providing Safety Component First

Given the case presentation, the counselor had serious concerns for Lubi's physical safety as well as her health. Specifically, Mrs. K did not know the source of the child's "fits," and although Mrs. K had informed the counselor that Lubi was HIV positive, the child herself was not aware of her diagnosis (it is common for adults not to tell children). As a result, Lubi was noncompliant in taking her medicine because she did not understand why she needed it. The counselor asked Mrs. K's permission to contact his supervisor so that together they could develop a safety plan. In this discussion all parties decided that it was important to file another police report, as the minibus driver had not been detained following the initial report of the repeated rapes. Mrs. K agreed to a 24-hour watch over the child (with the help of a neighbor) to make sure she was safe in the interim while they waited for the police to take action, and the family would return later that week to the counseling center. This first session thus provided a combination of the psychoeducation and safety components. As part of the safety plan, the counselor helped to arrange an appointment at the University Teaching Hospital to evaluate Lubi's "fits" and also for the mother to see an HIV counselor.

Crisis between Sessions 1 and 2

Prior to their second visit, Mrs. K phoned the counselor when relatives of the minibus driver began threatening Lubi's life if the family did not withdraw the police report. Mrs. K reported that she was currently at the police station because Lubi went missing the night before, having been forced into the bus by the relatives, severely beaten, and then thrown out and abandoned in another compound. The police found Lubi late that night and called Mrs. K in the morning to pick her up. The counselor continued with the safety component, and instructed Mrs. K to first take Lubi to the medical clinic to make sure she was not seriously injured and then to come to the office. While waiting for Mrs. K to arrive, the counselor contacted his supervisor and the consulting psychologist from the University of Zambia, who had been assisting the counselors with high-risk cases. The team met before Lubi and her mother arrived and decided that for the client's own safety she needed to be moved out of the area, to a hospice for 24-hour observation and then to a confidential location where the minibus driver and his family could not find her. The team agreed that there were multiple issues involved, including (1) HIV disclosure and noncompliance with medication, (2) "fits" that needed a proper evaluation and likely medications, (3) imminent physical safety risks, and (4) severe trauma-related symptoms from the repeated sexual abuse. A local hospice agreed to admit Lubi for at least 1 month because of the HIV issues and also arranged for a doctor to consult on the "fits."

TF-CBT Components

Given that her health issues were being addressed, the counselor and team believed that it was important to continue with TF-CBT and focus on the trauma-related symptoms, which were believed to be contributing to Lubi's risky behaviors (drinking, going out at night). While Lubi was in the hospice, the counselor visited her twice a week. Lubi was very stable in the hospice as she was not allowed to go off grounds. Lubi learned the PRAC skills and used these often when she woke up from nightmares about the family of the minibus driver or when she missed her family and neighborhood. Because of Lubi's limited schooling and developmental delays, the counselor often had to work with her in a manner that was similar to that for a 7- or 8-year-old. All components were provided experientially through activities (rather than verbal). The trauma narrative resulted in detailed accounts of the sexual abuse, and Lubi also provided many unhelpful thoughts about the sexual abuse, HIV (which she had by now been informed of), and her recent diagnosis of epilepsy. Cognitive processing successfully addressed thoughts such as "No one loves me," "It was my fault he raped me," and "I am dirty now so I might as well go out and sleep with people." Her final chapter included statements that the rape was not her fault, and that she is able to do things to help protect herself from bad people in the community. She also wrote a letter to other children who find out they are HIV positive. She talked about how everyone kept it a secret from her, how initially she thought her life was over, and how she now takes medicines and understands that she can live a long life even with HIV. Lubi was still sad at times and felt "used," but her symptoms were greatly reduced. One of her new thoughts was "Even if I want to, it is not good to have sex with others who I am not in a relationship with because they probably don't love me." This led to her reporting feeling "stronger" and not engaging in such risky sexual behavior on her new triangle.

Wrapping Up

At the end of TF-CBT, the hospice team and Mrs. K agreed that it would not be a good or safe option for Lubi to return home given that the minibus driver's relatives were still living in the area and were still causing significant problems for Mrs. K. The hospice staff was able to identify a local boarding school that was only a short bus ride away so that Mrs. K could continue to see Lubi weekly while she worked on finding a new home in a different compound.

SUMMARY AND RECOMMENDATIONS

A growing number of studies are evaluating the effectiveness of TF-CBT for various international populations. In European sites, minimal if any modifications are being implemented. In low-resource settings, however, differences in culture and context require modifications in how TF-CBT is provided. Researchers and clinicians are repeatedly finding that such modifications do not interfere with the fidelity of TF-CBT and are generally minor alterations in how the components are implemented. This evidence is strengthened by the fact that the needed modifications have been determined by local counselors themselves, who are part of the respective cultures, rather than by Western TF-CBT trainers or developers. Results to date suggest that TF-

CBT is feasible, acceptable, and applicable for low-resource settings and can be implemented by lay persons. Even more exciting, preliminary research shows that TF-CBT is highly effective for the children and their families, as determined using both quantitative outcome data (Murray, Dorsey, et al., 2010; Murray, Skavenski, et al., 2010) and qualitative interviews with the families themselves (Murray, Skavenski, et al., 2011). These findings support the belief that both trauma impact and effective trauma treatments transcend cultural boundaries.

REFERENCES

Alami, K. M., & Kadri, N. (2004). Moroccan women with a history of child sexual abuse and its long-term repercussions: A population-based epidemiological study. *Archives of Women's Mental Health, 7*(4), 237–242.

Amnesty International. (2010). *Breaking the silence: Sexual violence in Cambodia*. London: Author. Retrieved May 25, 2011, from *www.amnesty.org/en/ library/asset/ASA23/001/2010/en/17ebf558-95f0-4cf8-98c1-3f052ffb9603/ asa230012010en.pdf*.

Barber, J. P., Crits-Christoph, P., & Luborsky, L. (1996). Effects of therapist adherence and competence on patient outcome in brief dynamic therapy. *Journal of Consulting and Clinical Psychology, 64,* 619–622.

Bass, J., Bearup, L., Bolton, P., Murray, L., & Skavenski, S. (2011). *Implementing trauma focused cognitive behavioral therapy (TF-CBT) among formerly trafficked-sexually abused girls in Cambodia: A feasibility study.* Baltimore: World Vision Cambodia & Johns Hopkins Bloomberg School of Public Health.

Bolton, P. (2001). Cross-cultural validity and reliability testing of a standard psychiatric assessment instrument without a gold standard. *Journal of Nervous and Mental Disease, 189,* 238–242.

Bolton, P., Bass, J., Neugebauer, R., Clougherty, K., Verdeli, H., Ndogoni, L., et al. (2003). Results of a clinical trial of a group intervention for depression in rural Uganda. *Journal of the American Medical Association, 279,* 3117–3124.

Bolton, P. A., & Tang, A. (2002). An alternative approach to cross-cultural function assessment. *Social Psychiatry and Psychiatric Epidemiology, 37*(11), 537–543.

Central Intelligence Agency. (n.d.-a). Africa: Democratic Republic of Congo. In *The World Fact Book.* Retrieved June 26, 2011, from *https://www.cia.gov/library/ publications/the-world-factbook/geos/cg.html*.

Central Intelligence Agency. (n.d.-b). Africa: Tanzania. *The World Fact Book.* Retrieved May 20, 2011, from *https://www.cia.gov/library/publications/the-world-factbook/geos/tz.html*.

Central Intelligence Agency. (n.d.-c). Africa: Zambia. In *The World Fact Book.* Retrieved May 20, 2011, from *https://www.cia.gov/library/publications/the-world-factbook/geos/za.html*.

Central Intelligence Agency. (n.d.-d). East and Southeast Asia: Cambodia. In *The World Fact Book.* Retrieved May 20, 2011, from *https://www.cia.gov/library/ publications/the-world-factbook/geos/cb.html*.

Hwang, W. (2009). The formative method for adapting psychotherapy (FMAP): A community-based developmental approach to culturally adapting therapy. *Professional Psychology: Research and Practice, 40*(4), 369–377.

Iwata, N., & Buka, S. (2002). Race/ethnicity and depressive symptoms: A cross-cultural/ethnic comparison among university students in East Asia, North and South America. *Social Science and Medicine, 55*(12), 2243–2252.

Juma, M., Askew, I., & Ferguson, A. (2007). *Situation analysis of the sexual and reproductive health and HIV risks and prevention needs of older orphaned and vulnerable children in Nyanza Province, Kenya.* Population Council.

Kandala, N., Ji, C., Cappuccio, P., & Stones, R. (2008). The epidemiology of HIV infection in Zambia. *AIDS Care, 20*(7), 812–819.

Kendall, P. C., & Beidas, R. S. (2007). Smoothing the trail for dissemination of evidence-based practices for youth: Flexibility within fidelity. *Professional Psychology: Research and Practice, 38,* 13–20.

Kirsch, V., Fegert, J. M., Seitz, D. C. M., & Goldbeck, L. (2011). Traumafokussierte kognitive Verhaltenstherapie (Tf-KVT) bei Kindern und Jugendlichen nach Missbrauch und Misshandlung: Ergebnisse einer Pilotstudie [Trauma-focused cognitive-behavioral therapy (TF-CBT) for children and adolescents after abuse and maltreatment. Results of a pilot study]. *Kindheit und Entwicklung, 20,* 95–102.

McKay, M. M., & Bannon, W. M. (2004). Engaging families in child mental health services. *Child and Adolescent Psychiatric Clinics of North America, 13,* 905–921.

Murray, L. K., Bass, J., Chomba, E., Imasiku, M., Thea, D., Semrau, K., et al. (2011). *Validation of the Child Post Traumatic Stress Disorder—Reaction Index in Zambia.* Manuscript submitted for publication.

Murray, L. K., Dorsey, S., Bolton, P., Jordans, M. J. D., Rahman, A., Bass, J., et al. (2011). *Building capacity in mental health interventions in low resource countries: An apprenticeship model for training local providers.* Manuscript submitted for publication.

Murray, L. K., Dorsey, S., Imasiku, M., Skavenski, S., Cohen, J. A., & Bolton, P. A. (2010, November). *TF-CBT internationally: Zambia and Tanzania.* Paper presented at the annual meeting of the Association for Behavioral and Cognitive Therapies, San Francisco.

Murray, L. K., Haworth, A., Semrau, K., Aldrovandi, G. M., Singh, M., Sinkala, M., et al. (2006). Violence and abuse among HIV-infected women and their children in Zambia: A qualitative study. *Journal of Nervous and Mental Disease, 194*(8), 610–615.

Murray, L. K., Skavenski, S., Familiar, I., Bass, J., Bolton, P., & Jere, E. (2010). *Catholic Relief Services, SUCCESS Return to Life, Zambia TF-CBT pilot project report to USAID.* Washington, DC: USAID.

Murray, L. K., Skavenski, S., Michalopoulos, L., Bolton, P., Bass, J., & Cohen, J. (2011). *Youth, family and counselor perspectives on the implementation of TF-CBT in Zambia.* Manuscript submitted for publication.

Patel, V. (2009). The future of psychiatry in low- and middle-income countries. *Psychological Medicine, 39,* 1759–1762.

Patel, V., Weiss, H., Chowdhary, N., Naik, S., Pednekar, S., Chatterjee, S., et al.(2010). Effectiveness of an intervention led by lay health counsellors for depressive and anxiety disorders in primary care in Goa, India (MANAS): A cluster randomised controlled trial. *Lancet, 376,* 2086–2095.

Rahman, A., Malik, A., Sikander, S., Roberts, C., & Creed, F. (2008). Cognitive behaviour therapy-based intervention by community health workers for mothers with depression and their infants in rural Pakistan: A cluster-randomised controlled trial. *Lancet, 372,* 902–909.

Rousseau, C., & Kirmayer, L. (2009). Cultural adaptation of psychological trauma treatment for children. *Journal of the American Academy of Child and Adolescent Psychiatry, 48*(9), 954–955.

Ruchkin, V., Schwab-Stone, M., Jones, S., Cicchetti, D., Koposov, R., & Vermeiren, R. (2005). Is posttraumatic stress in youth a culture-bound phenomenon?: A comparison of symptom trends in selected US and Russian communities. *American Journal of Psychiatry, 162*(3), 538–544.

Schoenwald, S., Carter, R. E., Chapman, J. E., & Sheidow, A. J. (2008). Therapist adherence and organizational effects on change in youth behavior problems one year after multisystemic therapy. *Administration and Policy in Mental Health, 35,* 379–394.

Seedat, S., Nyamai, C., Njenga, F., Vythilingum, B., & Stein, D. J. (2004). Trauma exposure and post-traumatic stress symptoms in urban African schools. *British Journal of Psychiatry, 184*(2), 169–175.

Steinberg, A. M., Brymer, M. J., Decker, K. B., & Pynoos, R. S. (2004). The University of California at Los Angeles Post-traumatic stress disorder Reaction Index. *Current Psychiatry Report, 6,* 96–100.

Verdeli, H., Clougherty, K., Bolton, P., Speelman, L., Lincoln, N., Bass, J., et al. (2003). Adapting group interpersonal psychotherapy for a developing country: Experience in rural Uganda. *World Psychiatry, 2*(2), 114–120.

Verdeli, H., Clougherty, K., Onyango, G., Lewandowski, E., Speelman, L., Betancourt, T. S., et al. (2008). Group interpersonal psychotherapy for depressed youth in IDP camps in northern Uganda: Adaptation and training. *Child and Adolescent Psychiatric Clinics of North America, 17*(3), 605–624.

World Bank. (2011). *How we classify countries* [country classifications data]. Retrieved May 20, 2011, from *http://data.worldbank.org/about/country-classifications.*

10

Children of Latino Descent
Culturally Modified TF-CBT

Michael Andrew de Arellano
Carla Kmett Danielson
Julia W. Felton

OVERVIEW AND DESCRIPTION OF POPULATION

Culturally competent assessment and treatment of ethnic minority populations has become a significant area of research and clinical work, including in the domain of trauma-informed treatment. Several published guidelines emphasize the importance of culturally competent treatment (e.g., American Psychological Association, 2002; Bernal, Bonilla, & Bellido, 1995; de Arellano, Ko, Danielson, & Sprague, 2008; Lopez, Kopelowicz, & Canive, 2002). These guidelines cite the need for considering the cultural context within which the family exists and adapting the approach to treatment accordingly. Consistent with these guidelines, the goal of this chapter is to describe cultural considerations and applications of trauma-focused cognitive-behavioral therapy (TF-CBT) for use with Latino populations. In this section, we address the need for cultural modifications of TF-CBT for these families.

The most recent U.S. census data indicate that Latinos (defined as any person who identifies his or her familial origins as Mexico, Puerto Rico, Cuba, Spanish-speaking Central and South American countries, or other Spanish cultures; U.S. Census Bureau, 2011) constitute 16% of the population, making them the largest minority group in the country. In the decade spanning 2000 to 2010, the Latino population grew by 43%, and in 2010, Latinos comprised 23% of the U.S. population under 18 years of age.

The term *Latino* encompasses people from a variety of nations, the largest being Mexico, Puerto Rico, and Cuba (Lopez & Dockterman, 2011). These minority groups are unequally distributed across geographic regions. For instance, Americans of Cuban decent constitute the largest minority in Miami, while Puerto Ricans are the largest Latino group in New York City. Furthermore, Latino subgroups encompass a range of socioeconomic status levels. Census data suggest that the occupational status of Mexicans and Puerto Ricans lags furthest from whites, while Cubans and non-Latino whites did not differ (Kochhar, 2005). There is also a great deal of heterogeneity found within cultural beliefs, practices, and contextual factors, including immigration history, language, education, socioeconomic status, exposure to stressors, racism, and discrimination as well as beliefs regarding mental health and treatment utilization practices, which should be considered when treating trauma-exposed Latino children.

Latino youth are often found to experience higher rates of trauma than other ethnic groups. In a nationally representative study, Finkelhor and Dzuiba-Leatherman (1994) found that Latino youth endorsed greater total numbers of victimization experiences than non-Latino white youth. A later study found that Latino youth had greater rates of sexual assault, sexual harassment, and family abduction only (Finkelhor, Ormrod, Turner & Hamby, 2005). In a community sample of adolescents, Latinos were significantly more likely to experience child sexual abuse (CSA) compared with non-Latino whites, and Latinas had the highest prevalence of CSA of all racial groups (Newcomb, Muñoz, & Carmona, 2009). In addition, data from the National Survey of Adolescents (Kilpatrick & Saunders, 1996) indicated that Latino adolescents experienced significantly more physical assault and sexual assault and witnessed more domestic violence than non-Latino white adolescents.

Trauma exposure is linked to a host of negative psychological sequelae, among them posttraumatic stress disorder (PTSD) and other anxiety disorders, depression, suicide attempts, substance abuse, and externalized behavior problems, including sexualized behaviors. Psychological trauma responses may be moderated by ethnic factors. For instance, Kilpatrick and colleagues (2003) found that trauma-exposed Hispanic adolescents were four times more likely to meet criteria for PTSD than white adolescents.

Differences in these rates may be due, in part, to environmental factors. Latino children specifically may face additional stressors, including poverty, limited access to community resources, and acculturation issues (e.g., legal status, English language proficiency). Immigration status may play a particularly important role in determining the psychological impact of trauma among Latino populations. A study of first-generation Latino youth found that almost 7% of the sample had symptoms of depression and 29% endorsed symptoms of anxiety (Potochnick & Perriera, 2010). Another study found that the number of years living in the United States is negatively correlated with psychopathology and fewer years in the United States was associated with experiencing greater numbers of traumas (Kaltman, Green, Mete, Shara, & Miranda, 2010). In addition, Jaycox and colleagues (2002) found that 32% of recent immigrant youth reported PTSD symptoms in the clinical range and 16% endorsed clinical levels of depression.

Minority groups in general are less likely to seek treatment following trauma than non-Latino whites, and of those with PTSD, less than half seek out services (Roberts, Gilman, Breslau, Breslau, & Koenen, 2011). Again, immigration status appears to be a moderating factor. For example, a recent study of service utilization among Latino adolescents found that foreign-born children utilize health services at a significantly lower rate than U.S.-born Latinos (Bridges, de Arellano, Rheingold, Danielson, & Silcott, 2010). One hypothesis is that treatment providers may be perceived as culturally insensitive, affecting both engagement in and response to treatment. For example, Yeh and colleagues (2002) found that between 10 and 15% of Latino families reported that the inability to find a provider who met their needs and incorporated their beliefs into therapy was a barrier to treatment. This lack of culturally competent service providers has been identified as a significant impediment to accessing treatment and receiving high-quality care, especially for Latino individuals with mental health problems (e.g., Hispanic Federation, 2005).

Improving cultural competence (e.g., incorporating important cultural values into treatment) has been shown to influence client–clinician communication and trust, the development of a successful therapeutic alliance, and the retention of culturally diverse clients in treatment (Bernal, Bonilla, Padillo-Cotto, & Perez-Prado, 1998). For example, premature termination is likely to be high when a therapist is experienced as cold or distant by a Latino client (Paniagua, 1994) or when treatment does not incorporate important cultural beliefs (Sonkin, 1995). Providing culturally competent mental health care can lead to increased patient satisfaction with care and reduce the likelihood of long-term economic costs resulting from untreated mental health problems (e.g., McCabe, Yeh, Garland, Lau, & Chavez, 2005). This relation between provider cultural competence and successful therapeutic outcome highlights the importance of culture in trauma and treatment utilization and outcomes. Even if a treatment has been shown to be efficacious with a minority population, it may have less than optimal efficacy if it has not incorporated cultural factors and culture-related processes (Santisteban, Muir-Malcolm, Mitrani, & Szapocznik, 2002).

Despite an overt promotion of culturally modifying empirically supported therapies, the mental health field has grappled with both defining cultural modification and delineating a process by which evidence-based therapies can be applied (Griner & Smith, 2006). Bernal, Jiménez-Chafey, and Domenech Rodríguez (2009, p. 362) defined cultural adaptation as "the systematic modification of an evidence-based treatment (EBT) or intervention protocol to consider language, culture, and context in such a way that it is compatible with the client's cultural patterns, meanings, and values." A recent synthesis of current thinking regarding cultural modifications of EBTs identified seven overarching guidelines: (1) flexibly administering EBTs by therapists; (2) enhancing meaning of therapies within the cultural context; (3) increasing assessment of client needs (before administering treatments); (4) openness to understanding and exploring client variables specific to therapy; (5) avoiding outright dismissal of traditional therapies, and incorporating these therapies as appropriate; (6) demonstrating client-focused empathy in a manner appropriate to the cultural context; and (7) avoiding categorizing cultural differences as weaknesses (Draguns, 2008). Although a recent meta-analysis (Huey & Polo, 2008) found that TF-CBT was "probably efficacious" for ethnic minority youth, in light of these guidelines we modified TF-CBT culturally to address the specific needs of children of Latino descent. The creation and components of culturally modified TF-CBT (CM-TF-CBT) are described next.

TF–CBT MODIFICATION PROCESS

TF-CBT was culturally modified for Latino children and families utilizing the theoretical and research literature on treatment with Latino populations, our qualitative and quantitative research with trauma-exposed Latino populations, and more than 15 years of clinical work providing TF-CBT with Latino children and their families. Common themes often arose in treatment with Latino populations, including the importance of spirituality/religion, traditional gender roles (e.g., *machismo/marianismo*), involvement of extended family in treatment, conservative beliefs about sex and the importance of virginity, and traditional childrearing practices. These constructs were integrated throughout treatment while serving this population, as dictated by the child and caregiver's endorsement of these beliefs.

CM-TF-CBT was further developed utilizing focus group methodology to determine the acceptability of the treatment and to solicit additional feedback to increase its cultural relevance and effectiveness. Focus groups (Davidson, de Arellano, Rheingold, Danielson, & Silcott, 2011) were conducted with Latino caregivers and providers serving Latino families in different geographic regions of the United States (e.g., south Florida, Texas, southern California, New York City), representing different nationalities, levels of socioeconomic status, and immigration/citizen statuses (e.g., recent immigrant, born in the United States).

While collecting qualitative data during the focus groups, particular attention was focused on beliefs regarding mental health and mental health treatment, views on trauma exposure and its effects, and reactions to each of the PRACTICE components of TF-CBT. After each component was presented, Latino parents participating in the focus groups discussed whether they felt the treatment component was consistent with their belief system. They also provided suggestions for making the interventions more culturally acceptable or culturally relevant. In general, the Latino parents recognized the importance of mental health treatment, especially for trauma-exposed children. However, they reported that the lack of knowledge about mental health services (e.g., What happens in therapy? Who needs therapy? Is it just for "crazy people"?) was a significant barrier to recent immigrant Latino families seeking services. They recommended providing more extensive psychoeducation to parents and children about mental health problems and treatment, including the "basics" (e.g., What is a therapist? What is therapy? What role do parents play in therapy?). They emphasized the importance of providing the psychoeducation to fathers as well as involving them in treatment. The Latino parents felt that each of the PRACTICE components of TF-CBT seemed to be acceptable culturally, if the rationale and clinical examples provided for each component were clearly culturally appropriate and relevant. They emphasized the necessity of providing a thorough rationale for the treatment component while continuing to focus on fundamentals (e.g., why feelings identification is important). Parents reported that engagement in treatment would likely be affected by the therapist's ability to incorporate spirituality and address other clinically relevant issues, such as general parenting practices, conflicts between parents, and difficulties associated with immigration, leaving families in their country of origin, and adjusting to a new culture.

IMPORTANT CULTURAL CONSTRUCTS

CM-TF-CBT is a tailored treatment that can be adapted to incorporate cultural beliefs as necessary depending on the beliefs of children and families and on their levels of acculturation. Numerous resources exist on cultural considerations in mental health and mental health treatment, including trauma-focused assessment and treatment (e.g., Abney, 1996; de Arellano & Danielson, 2008; de Arellano et al., 2008; Fontes 1995, 2005). Table 10.1 briefly reviews some of the primary cultural factors that were incorporated into CM-TF-CBT.

TABLE 10.1. Potential Cultural Constructs to Integrate in CM-TF-CBT

Cultural value or belief	Definition	Examples of application to and/or implications for CM-TF-CBT
Familismo	A preference for maintaining a close connection to the family. Stems from a collectivist worldview implying a willingness to sacrifice for the welfare of the family or group (Marin & Triandis, 1985) and is exhibited in a shared sense of responsibility among family members and close friends to care for children, provide financial and emotional support, and participate in group decision making (e.g., Falicov, 1998; Marin & Marin, 1991; Moore & Pachon, 1985).	• Includes all applicable family members in treatment (e.g., extended family members involved with caregiving). • Focus of treatment is on family as much as it is on the individual and thus stronger emphasis on building family-related skills (e.g., communication).
Personalismo	Valuing and building interpersonal relationships. Once a relationship has been established with a Latino who upholds personalismo, he or she is likely to pursue/desire a warm and personal relationship (Cuéllar, Arnold, & González, 1995).	• While establishing rapport, the goal for the clinician is to be perceived as warm and friendly immediately. • Potential challenges to traditional mental health boundaries (e.g., invitations for the therapist to attend important family functions, such as a birthday party or baptism).
Respeto and simpatia	Cultural values that dictate appropriate communication and social behavior both within and outside the family. Respeto implies setting clear boundaries in human relationships and is central in socialization (Santiago-Rivera et al., 2002). Simpatia is the need for social behaviors that promote pleasant social situations (Triandis, Marin, Lisansky, & Betancourt, 1984).	• *Respeto* and related deference to authority may mean that the therapist will be viewed in a more hierarchical relationship orientation (Santiago-Rivera et al., 2002). • *Simpatia* has clinical implications for teaching a child about discussing negative feelings. • Both *respeto* and *simpatia* can affect problem solving with family members and teaching revictimization risk reduction strategies, as this involves assertiveness, often with adults.
Marianismo	Tendency to try to attain the image of the ideal woman using the Virgin Mary as a role model. Women are expected to be spiritually strong, morally superior, and self-sacrificing (Lopez-Baez,	• May prevent females from wanting to alleviate suffering and get better because of a "suffer-and-endure attitude" (i.e., "This is a cross that I have to bear"; Garcia-Preto, 1990).

(continued)

TABLE 10.1. (*continued*)

	1999). Females must remain virgins until married.	• Feelings of shame and concerns about virginity may contribute to reluctance to disclose or discuss the abuse.
Machismo	Refers to a man's responsibility to provide for, protect, and defend his family. There has been some debate regarding some of the negative connotations surrounding the concept of *machismo*, including arrogance and sexual aggressiveness; however, it is argued that this is an anglicized interpretation of this concept (Morales, 1996).	• Efforts can be made to include the father in treatment or, at the very least, to receive the father's "blessing" with regard to therapy and therapy recommendations. • Reluctance of boys to disclose or discuss their victimization, particularly if the perpetrator was a male. • Difficulty for boys to discuss feelings of fear, sadness, and other emotions that may make them seem weak.
Espiritualismo, fatalismo, and folk beliefs	The interrelationship among religion, faith, and spirituality is fundamental to many Latinos (Flores & Carey, 2000). Roman Catholicism is the predominant religion of Latinos (Falicov, 1998). Many Latinos' traditional Catholicism places value on enduring human suffering and on self-denial. Fatalismo is the tendency to take life as it comes with a "resigned" mindset (Casas & Pytluk, 1995). Such beliefs may prevent some Latinos from seeking psychological help (Acosta, Yamamoto, & Evans, 1982). Some Latinos may adhere to folk beliefs about mental health problems and healing, and prefer treatment from *curanderos* or other forms of alternative medicine.	• *Espiritualismo* may contribute to feelings of shame experienced by Latino CSA victims. • *Fatalismo* and folk beliefs have implications for how mental health problems, therapists, and treatment are viewed and, therefore, should be assessed and addressed early in therapy. • Integrate alternative or traditional therapies as appropriate.
Dichos and cuentos	*Dichos* are short phrases that depict Spanish proverbs or sayings and are often used to communicate values and standards of behavior in daily conversation. *Cuento* therapy (Constantino, Malgady, & Regler, 1986) is an empirically tested, culture-specific therapeutic modality that utilizes folklore and storytelling with Latino children to teach therapeutic skills.	• Both *dichos* and *cuentos* can be utilized in therapy to teach new skills and improve client participation (Zuniga, 1992). • For religious families, *dichos* that are related to their religious beliefs can be included.

ASSESSMENT CONSIDERATIONS
FOR LATINO YOUTH

As noted earlier, there is great heterogeneity among families of Latino descent in their beliefs, practices, and other traditions. Especially when attempting to adapt EBTs to individuals from different cultural groups, it is crucial that cultural sensitivity not lead to individual insensitivity. In order to ensure that treatment will be individually tailored to meet the needs of the child and family, a careful assessment must be completed at the outset of treatment. Strategies for conducting a culturally informed assessment have been proposed, including techniques specifically for trauma-exposed Latino youth (de Arellano & Danielson, 2008). In general, a culturally informed assessment should include a broader range of traumatic events (e.g., immigration trauma, human trafficking, severe discrimination), a more tailored assessment of potential trauma-related symptoms, and an assessment of cultural beliefs and practices that may have a potential impact on treatment. In addition, the preferred language of the child and family members, social supports, current stressors (e.g., financial, legal), and family background (e.g., sociopolitical history of country of origin, immigration history) should be assessed (see de Arellano & Danielson, 2008, for a more detailed description).

During a culturally informed, trauma-focused assessment with Latino families, it is helpful to identify the various caregivers who are involved in the child's life and to attempt to collect assessment information from a broad range of caregivers (e.g., extended family members). This is related to a cultural construct, *familismo*, which is a preference for maintaining a close connection to the family, a common theme among many Latinos regardless of country of origin. *Familismo* stems from a collectivist worldview in that there is a willingness to sacrifice for the welfare of the family or group (Marin & Triandis, 1985). This worldview is exhibited in a shared sense of responsibility to care for children, provide financial and emotional support to family members, and participate in decision making that involves one or more family members (e.g., Falicov, 1998; Marin & Marin, 1991; Moore & Pachon, 1985). *Familismo* among Latinos includes valuing very close relationships, and stressing interdependence, cohesiveness, and cooperation among family members. *Familismo* extends to such relatives as grandparents, aunts, uncles, and cousins as well as close friends. If extended family members have significant involvement or influence over childrearing, their participation can be helpful in gaining a broader perspective on the child's level of functioning as well as in developing more effective intervention strategies. If it does not appear to be feasible to have extended family members involved in the assessment and/or treatment, contacts can be made over the telephone and/or periodically in person.

For bilingual children and families, language preference should also be assessed; however, this may not be as straightforward as simply asking what language is preferred. Often, children learn English faster than their caregivers, which can lead to a number of clinical considerations. When assessing for preference for treatment in English or Spanish, children who are learning English as a second language may be more likely to choose English in order to demonstrate their proficiency in the language, which is valued and rewarded in school. However, they may not be completely proficient and may have difficulty expressing themselves, especially when discussing more abstract concepts (e.g., thoughts and feelings). Therapists should encourage clients to express themselves in the language that best encapsulates how they think and feel throughout treatment. The children or caregivers may find it easier to talk about some topics in Spanish and some things in English. If a Spanish-speaking therapist is not available, an interpreter can help to facilitate integrating Spanish content into treatment. When using interpreters, it is ideal to use the same interpreter with each case whenever possible because of the relationship that the children and their caregivers develop with him or her. In addition, interpreters should also receive training in the treatment model so that there is an understanding of the overall process and goals of treatment and the purposeful use of language (e.g., using appropriate terminology for body parts, using behaviorally specific terms). For example, situations can arise when the interpreter, as a person from the same culture, might perceive that certain terminology is inappropriate or too "graphic" and as a result may temper the translation to the family out of *respeto*.

Of course, an accurate and thorough assessment of trauma exposure is critical to providing trauma-focused treatment. It may be helpful to broaden the range of traumatic events assessed to account for traumatic events commonly experienced by the Latino population being served. For example, Latino families who may have immigrated with the help of a coyote (e.g., human smuggler) may have witnessed physical or sexual assaults and other forms of violence during the immigration process. In addition, other events experienced by Latino families, including natural disasters (e.g., earthquakes, hurricanes), violence (e.g., drug-related shootings), human trafficking, and racism/discrimination can have serious mental health consequences and should be assessed (Kessler, Mickelson, & Williams, 1999). An effective trauma assessment for Latino children and families should also include a wider range of mental health problems than what is typically assessed in the general population (e.g., depression, PTSD, other anxiety disorders). For example, somatic complaints (e.g., headaches, stomachaches) may be a more acceptable manifestation of distress (Raguram, Weiss, Channabasavanna, & Devins, 1996) and should be assessed and monitored accordingly if present.

Level of acculturation among families presenting for trauma-focused treatment is an important factor to assess, particularly for those in which some or all members have immigrated to the United States. Marin (1992) defined acculturation as a process of attitudinal and behavioral change undergone by individuals who reside in multicultural societies or who come in contact with a new culture as a result of colonization, invasion, or other political changes. Acculturation is relevant to mental health treatment because it has been viewed as a stressful process, particularly among recent immigrants (Diez de Leon, 2000). Prolonged acculturative stress may produce negative psychological consequences (Saldana, 1994). In addition, children of immigrant families tend to acculturate at a faster rate than their caregivers. This acculturative gap can also be a source of significant distress among immigrant families (Szapocnik & Kurtines, 1993). Thus, it is important for the therapist to assess acculturation levels of family members and to be aware of the degree of acculturation each is experiencing. This will both provide information about distress and give some indication of the degree to which the family upholds specific cultural values and beliefs. The Acculturation Rating Scale for Mexican Americans–II (ARSMA-II; Cuéllar, Arnold, & Maldonado, 1995) is an example of a standardized scale that can be used to access acculturation in adolescents and adults of Mexican descent. It evaluates acculturation across three domains: language, ethnic identity, and ethnic interaction. In addition, two subscales measure orientation toward Mexican culture and Anglo culture. The ARSMA-II has been found to have good internal consistency, strong construct validity, and strong concurrent validity (Cuéllar, Arnold, & Maldonado, 1995). Similarly, a range of cultural constructs can be assessed with the Multiphasic Assessment of Cultural Constructs—Short Form (Cuéllar, Arnold, & González, 1995), which measures the following theoretical cultural constructs in Latino origin populations: *fatalismo*, *familismo*, folk beliefs, *machismo/marianismo*, and *personalismo*. Such standardized measures provide an efficient means of assessing important cultural constructs at the outset of treatment, allowing for immediate integration of these constructs and tailoring of treatment.

ENGAGEMENT STRATEGIES FOR LATINO FAMILIES

As with all TF–CBT treatment, the therapeutic relationship between the therapist and Latino clients in CM-TF-CBT is central. Establishing rapport and trust with recent immigrant children and families is essential but there may be any number of obstacles, such as lack of experience or negative experiences with mental health providers, shame related to the trauma exposure (e.g., child sexual abuse), fear and mistrust of agencies perceived to be linked with legal or government entities, and/or immigration concerns. Not only is the relationship with the child and family likely to have an impact on treatment progress, but it is also likely to affect the degree to which the family engages in therapy and whether or not the family terminates treatment prematurely. Thus, much effort should be put into establishing trust throughout treatment, but particularly in the first several sessions. In general, the less acculturated a family is, the more time the therapist will need to devote to educating them about what to expect in therapy.

It is helpful to understand cultural constructs that dictate interpersonal interactions, such as *personalismo* and *respeto*, to facilitate the development of a strong therapeutic relationship. *Personalismo* refers to valuing and building interpersonal relationships. Once a relationship has been established with a Latino who upholds *personalismo*, a warm, personal relationship is often pursued. Given that therapy involves a personal and supportive relationship, *personalismo* may translate into invitations for the therapist to attend important family functions (e.g., baptisms, *quinceañeras*). Again, this construct can be beneficial for therapy, as the valuing of warm, friendly, and personal relationships has important implications for how the family may respond to treatment. The therapist can contribute to *personalismo* by increasing the "warmth" of the mental health environment when the family comes in for services.

Just as the construct of *respeto* impacts the therapeutic alliance, it can also have an effect on communication among the child, family, and therapist. *Respeto* implies setting clear boundaries in human relationships and is central in socialization (Santiago-Rivera, Arredondo, & Gallardo-Cooper, 2002). It represents sensitivity to the individual's position and helps guide social interactions to avoid conflict. In building rapport with the family, the emphasis on *respeto* and deference to authority can lead to the therapist being viewed in a more hierarchical relationship orientation (Santiago-Rivera et al., 2002). The child and caregiver may subsequently come across as agreeable with the therapist and less likely to question new therapeutic concepts and skills, even when they are not well understood. For this reason, the therapist should assess the client's understanding of therapy content. A common strategy used by the CM-TF-CBT therapist includes asking the child and/or caregiver to reflect explanations of concepts back to the therapist in their own words rather than asking, "Do you understand?" or "Do you have any questions?" Because of the aforementioned construct of *respeto*, these types of questions are usually met with affirmation regardless of whether the target concept is, indeed, understood.

TF-CBT MODIFICATIONS FOR LATINO FAMILIES: INTEGRATION OF CULTURAL CONSTRUCTS

The core components of TF-CBT are summarized by the acronym PRACTICE: **P**sychoeducation and **P**arenting; **R**elaxation; **A**ffective expression and modulation; Cognitive coping and processing; Trauma narrative; *In vivo* mastery of trauma reminders; Conjoint parent–child sessions; and Enhancing future safety and development (Cohen, Mannarino, & Deblinger, 2006). In CM-TF-CBT, suggested cultural modifications can be made to each PRACTICE component. In addition to the suggestions and examples presented next, it is important to note that it is ideal to weave in cultural modifications—based on cultural constructs identified as valued by the family—throughout treatment (e.g., prayer as a relaxation strategy, religious *dichos* for cognitive coping, addressing the importance of virginity during cognitive processing of the narrative) rather than simply including these constructs and modifications once or twice.

During the *psychoeducation* component, it is important to have a thorough understanding of the child and family's perceptions of mental health and mental health treatment, which may include inaccurate and unhelpful beliefs (e.g., "Therapy is only for very mentally ill and impaired individuals"). This can be achieved by asking the child and family members Socratic-type questions (e.g., "Who typically receives mental health treatment?") and to provide corrective psychoeducational information based on their responses (e.g., treatment is for trauma-exposed youth experiencing difficulties as a result of the trauma exposure). Some important views to address may include causes of trauma and trauma-related problems (e.g., weakness, lack of faith, lack of respect, fate) and their previous/preferred strategies for addressing these problems (e.g., seeking help from a physician, priest, *curandero*/folk healer). Relatedly, a more detailed description of therapy and therapists can be helpful, including how long treatment lasts, what are the roles of the therapist, child, and parent in treatment (using analogies that the family understands), and what a typical trauma-focused therapy session looks like.

The psychoeducation component is also an opportunity to frame the treatment intervention approach in a manner that is culturally congruent. For example, some families for whom spirituality is important may believe in *fatalismo* and that, through their faith, "God will provide" (i.e., that therapy is not necessary). One way to help the concept of therapy fit into this belief is to talk about such intervention and mental health services as a possible way that God may, indeed, be providing for the family. Another similar strategy would be to frame the family's seeking services in the context of "God helps those who help themselves" (i.e., participating in treatment can be a way they can help themselves). It is also important to include psychoeducational information that is directly relevant to the child's and family's background. For example, in a case involving a child who had immigrated from Mexico and was referred for treatment secondary to sexual abuse, the therapist discussed stressors and potential traumatic events experienced by other families during the immigration process and while attempting to adapt to U.S. culture. This helped to validate and normalize the child's emotional reactions and subsequently led to further detailed disclosure of the violence she had witnessed while immigrating as well.

A useful strategy to teach skills during psychoeducation and other CM-TF-CBT components is the use of *dichos* (proverbs), which are short Spanish proverbs or sayings learned through language that are often used in daily conversation. *Dichos* can be used to create a comfortable environment, facilitate rapport, and communicate to Latino clients that their needs and identities will be respected (Aviera, 1996). *Dichos* have been found to "link the phenomenological world of the Latino immigrant with the symbols and metaphors available" to therapists in the process of addressing and reframing emotional struggles (de Rios, 2001, p. 5). *Dichos* are applicable to a variety of life events, and their use serves as an excellent example of a culturally informed strategy that can be implemented to teach new skills in therapy. The use of *dichos* in therapy has been shown to improve client participation, reframe problems, and increase motivation (Zuniga, 1992). An example of a *dicho* that may be used to give a child hope is "Despues de la tormenta, sale el sol entre las nubes" (literal translation: "After the storm, the sun shines through the clouds"), the English equivalent of which is "After the rain, comes the sun."

Some relevant resources for clients include:

- *Todos Tenemos Sentimientos* (Everybody Has Feelings) for adolescents (Avery, 1998).
- *Vegetal Como Eres: Alimentos con Sentimientos* (Vegetable as You Are: Food with Feelings) for preadolescent children (Freymann & Elffers, 1999).

As in traditional TF-CBT, in the *parenting* component of CM-TF-CBT it is important to gain a thorough understanding of the caregiver's approach to child rearing. While childrearing practices differ across families, certain common Latino cultural values may impact this aspect of treatment. A common goal is to help children become *bien educado* (well educated) and not *malcriado* (disrespectful, rude, spoiled). Becoming *bien educado* refers not to formal education but rather to the process of learning adequate social graces and skills (Nava, 2000). Specifically, obedience, *respeto* (respect), humility, and affectionate behaviors are encouraged in the socialization process in raising children in order to become *bien educado*. With this worldview, children are taught to be deferential to adults and maintain a hierarchical relationship with them. Understanding Latino beliefs about childrearing practices has implications for the manner in which such strategies are framed in therapy.

While developing a plan to address problematic behaviors, it is critical that the therapist assess childrearing styles and preferences (e.g., respect toward one's parents, preference for punishment vs. reward). The therapist should be attentive to existing childrearing styles and preferences and, to the extent possible, should adjust parenting interventions to be congruent with caregiver beliefs. For example, for families who prefer punishment and other "active parenting strategies," time-out can be framed as *la esquina de castigo* (the corner of punishment) or *la esquina de aburrimiento* (the corner of boredom). With regard to praise, it is recommended that parents be provided with a thorough rationale, including addressing concerns about reinforcing the child for doing things she or he is already supposed to be doing. If parents are not comfortable with the terminology of "praising," the therapist can describe it in an alternative way that is consistent within their framework (e.g., "Tell the child what she or he is doing that you like and provide reasons why you like it"). The therapist can help parents focus on the opposite of the problematic behaviors by explaining that the child is trying to gain their attention and that the caregivers should only give attention (i.e., the reward) for desired behaviors (McCabe et al., 2005). In addition, for caregivers who have strong beliefs regarding child obedience out of *respeto* rather than a system of rewards or punishments, behavioral interventions can be framed as a means to achieve greater *respeto* from the child (evidenced by increased behavioral compliance). For example, while working with a grandmother who was serving as primary caregiver for her 11-year-old granddaughter who had witnessed domestic violence, the grandmother indicated significant concern that her granddaughter would frequently not obey her (e.g., not pick up her room, not do required chores). The grandmother reported that this would make her very angry because it demonstrated a lack of respect. The therapist agreed that respect for caregivers is very important and made helping her granddaughter to be more respectful a treatment goal. The strategies that were implemented included having the grandmother "point out" the behaviors she wanted to see continue immediately after her granddaughter engaged in these behaviors (labeled praise). The granddaughter's compliance increased through the implementation of various behavioral strategies, and the grandmother was pleased to see that her granddaughter was being more respectful toward her.

The *relaxation* component consists of teaching the child and caregiver various relaxation skills to manage physiological symptoms of fear and anxiety that typically develop following exposure to traumatic events, especially since Latinos endorse more somatic complaints than other symptoms of distress. To capitalize on the strengths of the child and family and to tailor the relaxation component to be more culturally relevant for Latino families, care should be taken to assess for existing strategies that the family utilizes to reduce distress. Lists of relaxation strategies that the child and family identify as being effective can be created, and they can be reminded to utilize these techniques. The therapist can then work with the child and family to identify new relaxation strategies to incorporate into their repertoire, including culture-related strategies. For example, if spirituality is important to the child, the therapist can assess whether there are any aspects of the child's spiritual beliefs that help him or her to relax (e.g., prayer, meditation). These aspects can be integrated into treatment, along with other relaxation techniques.

Another important consideration for the relaxation component is ensuring that the examples used to teach the techniques are understandable and appropriate to the knowledge and experiences of the child and family. For example, imaginal scenes commonly used to teach and practice visual imagery (e.g., sitting on the beach watching the ocean) may not be as familiar to some children and could be difficult to visualize effectively (e.g., identifying multisensory details). Similarly, in progressive muscle relaxation exercises for young children that compare the body to objects in order to demonstrate tense muscles versus relaxed muscles (e.g., uncooked spaghetti vs. cooked spaghetti), the examples used should be culturally relevant and familiar to the child and family (e.g., uncooked fideos/noodles vs. cooked fideos/noodles; tortillas vs. duritos/tortilla chips). Even if children understand the examples, tailoring them to be more closely related to Latino culture can often help with engagement.

The *affective expression and modulation* component focuses on assisting children in identifying and labeling the full range of emotions that accompany exposure to traumatic events, including negative (e.g., shock, fear, anger, sadness, shame) and positive (e.g., love, curiosity, positive physical sensations) feelings as well as mixed or confusing emotions. As noted previously in the discussion of psychoeducation, one strategy to introduce the importance of being able to talk about a broad range of feelings within CM-TF-CBT is the use of *cuentos*, or stories, that present information within a culturally congruent context. Numerous such storybooks are available in English and Spanish, and some are available in both languages, which is sometimes preferable for bilingual children.

Language can be an important consideration when discussing feelings with Latino families, especially for bilingual families. Not all words in English and Spanish translate perfectly back and forth. If the children are bilingual and young, their vocabulary for emotions may be selectively different in English and Spanish. That is, they may be familiar with some emotion words in English and some in Spanish. Children who primarily have spoken Spanish in their home and did not learn English until they started school may have learned some basic language associated with emotion prior to entering school and may not have learned emotional language as well in English. It may be necessary to go through feeling exercises and games in both languages to ensure that the children understand the emotions discussed.

In addition to typical feeling identification games and exercises, therapists can culturally modify exercises, such as watching age-appropriate *novelas* (soap operas) or other television programs in session, and have the child pick out emotions the characters are displaying (e.g., What is that character feeling? How do you know? What would be a better way for him or her to demonstrate that emotion?).

Children's or family's beliefs about traditional gender roles can have an impact on the ways that the children express emotions, and should also be assessed. For example, traditional gender roles such as *machismo* may have some implications for how boys and men perceive they should "behave" (e.g., men should be "strong"). Boys who adhere to traditional gender roles, such as *machismo*, may believe that males should not express negative emotions such as fear or sadness, which can be interpreted as a sign of weakness. A potential strategy to address this challenge is to discuss how difficult it is to talk about sadness and fear, and how it is a demonstration of true strength and *machismo* to be able to express such emotions. The goal for the therapist in these situations is to help boys be able to express negative affect in a way that is healthy and culturally congruent.

Similarly, children may feel uncomfortable talking about negative feelings in general because of a desire to maintain *simpatia*, the need for social behaviors that promote pleasant social situations (Triandis et al., 1984). One strategy to assist in distinguishing this from trauma-related avoidance is to engage children in discussions about negative emotions that are not part of their traumatic event (e.g., school stressors, conflicts with peers). If the difficulty speaking about strong negative emotions is confined to trauma-related cues or reminders, then it is more likely due to traumatic avoidance rather than *simpatia*.

To overcome this reluctance to disclose emotions—whether related to machismo or *simpatia*—caregivers can assist by reassuring the child that talking about such negative emotions in therapy is acceptable. The therapist may first need to work with the caregivers independently to increase their own comfort with and acceptance of experiencing and expressing negative affect, especially in contexts where a male caregiver typically does not model expression of these feelings.

Finally, the feeling identification and expression skills developed in session can be used to set the stage for discussions about abuse-related emotions. At this point, the therapist should assess whether the child and parent feel that it is okay to talk about "family things" outside of the family. This will help in identifying areas in need of troubleshooting prior to developing the trauma narrative.

During the *cognitive coping and processing* component, the therapist teaches families to identify and share their innermost thoughts or internal dialogues first about everyday events and later in therapy, during the narrative process, in relation to the traumatic experiences. Using nontrauma examples, the therapist explains how thoughts are related to feelings and behaviors and teaches how to identify inaccurate or maladaptive thoughts and to challenge thinking mistakes by replacing them with more accurate, helpful, and adaptive thoughts. This is another CM-TF-CBT component in which *cuentos* can be introduced and utilized to help demonstrate the skill of changing thoughts to modify feelings and behavior. There are many *cuentos* to choose from that demonstrate situations in which changing thoughts to be more helpful can lead to more desirable behavioral and emotional outcomes. Two examples are Little Red Ant and Laughing Skull:

Cuento of the Little Red Ant

There once was an ant that was smaller than everyone else and thus believed she was weaker and different. One day she came across a piece of cake that she really wanted to bring home for her family to eat. She did not believe that she could carry this cake by herself and as she came across many other animals, she asked them to help her. However, no one could help her. In the end, she told herself to at least try to carry the cake before giving up and it ended up that she was able to carry the cake all by herself after all!

The message is that by changing her thoughts about being able to carry the cake the ant gained confidence and learned she was capable of a lot more than she thought.

Cuento of the Laughing Skull

A long time ago, next to the convent of Santo Domingo, there was a skull that sat in a niche in a wall. People would pass by this skull all the time, but no one seemed to notice it. One night, guards walking by heard noises and all of a sudden the skull was floating and shaking and screaming. This happened many nights in a row until finally one of the guards decided to look closer at the skull, despite being very scared. The skull fell to the ground as he approached and the guards quickly learned that it was mice, which had built their home under the skull that were causing all of the noise and movement.

The message is that challenging one's thoughts, or the meanings attached to certain situations, can help improve feelings (e.g., change fear to courage to relief) and behaviors. There are numerous variations of these stories across different Latin American countries, but the central point of the *cuentos* remains the same.

The therapist should discuss the advantages and disadvantages of different ways of coping, including avoidance. Avoidance coping in response to stressful events has been identified as a strategy that may be more common among Latinos. The therapist can assess whether the child or caregivers have been taking an approach of *no pensar* (trying not to think about the trauma, or avoidance) or trying to forget about it altogether and "just put it behind them" as a way of coping. The therapist can discuss how this approach may not make the problems go away. With the child's help (via Socratic questions), the therapist can generate examples of how avoidance has not resolved prior problems and where it has not worked to "leave the past in the past." For the child and family who report identifying strongly with avoidance coping, it will be particularly important to present a strong rationale for creating a trauma narrative. This can include sharing the research and clinical evidence for the use of TF-CBT, including with families of Latino descent, and how it has helped many trauma-exposed children with similar symptoms feel better. The therapist can also reiterate that avoidance coping is not likely working if there is evidence that the child is still having trauma-related symptoms.

As discussed earlier, beliefs about traditional gender roles can impact the application of TF-CBT components. Culturally specific beliefs about the female gender can present unique obstacles in cognitive coping. In some families with strong traditional spiritual beliefs and/or those with a strong endorsement of *marianismo* (using the Virgin Mary as a role model of one who is spiritually strong, morally superior, and self-sacrificing; Lopez-Baez, 1999), girls and/or their mothers may have been raised to believe that the suffering related to the trauma exposure is merely a "cross to bear" and/or that adverse problems are God's way of testing them. The use of Socratic questioning may help the client to view the notion of "It is my duty to suffer" as an unhelpful cognition. In this case, the therapist can discuss modeling and encourage the mother to set an example for her daughter with regard to challenging this belief. Reframing these culturally specific beliefs about gender roles could focus on participation in trauma-focused therapy as consistent with being a "strong woman," honoring her duty in the family by doing this important, challenging trauma-focused work.

If it has not yet been raised earlier in treatment, the therapist will want to begin eliciting parents' feelings and underlying thoughts related to their child's traumatic experiences. In addition to trauma-related thoughts offered by the parent, it is appropriate to specifically prompt parents for thoughts commonly associated with cultural beliefs (e.g., for caregivers with a strong sense of *fatalism* and/or spirituality: "This happened to him because it was part of God's plan"). In addition, for other families with strong spiritual beliefs, concerns regarding negative events being brought on as a result of committing a sin (i.e., a punishment) are not uncommon, and a belief in a just world may be present ("Good things happen to good people, and bad things happen to bad people"). These and similar unhelpful thoughts should be assessed and addressed if present.

Another manner to encourage cognitive coping strategies is the use of positive self-statements. Incorporating common Latin American *dichos/* proverbs, as noted earlier, can help make this strategy more culturally relevant. Some common *dichos* that may be useful in this component of CM-TF-CBT include:

- *Donde hay gana hay mana.* (Where there is a will there is a way.)
- *No hay mal que por bien no venga.* (There is no misfortune from which good does not come, or Every cloud has a silver lining.)
- *La esperanza no engorda pero mantiene.* (Hope does not make you gain weight, but it sustains you.)

The *trauma narrative* component directly addresses the child's responses to the traumatic event. During these sessions, the child creates a story, or narrative, of the traumatic events to recount the details of the incident and process negative thoughts and feelings associated with it. This serves as imaginal exposure to help the child experience the negative feelings related to the traumatic event, with the therapist's support in a safe and controlled environment while also helping the child to contextualize and process the traumatic experiences.

Presenting a strong rationale for creating the trauma narrative is very important, particularly for children and families who have culturally based concerns about talking about sexual abuse (e.g., religious concerns, belief that it is inappropriate for children to discuss sex) or those whose typical coping style is avoidance. Similar to addressing other culture-related challenges during this model, it can be extremely helpful to engage the caregivers in reassuring the children that it is appropriate for them to discuss the traumatic events while constructing the narrative. Often, caregiver concerns about discussing the trauma are fueled by their own distress about their children's trauma exposure. Working with caregivers in parallel sessions from the start of treatment can significantly reduce their distress by further developing their own coping skills and addressing avoidance behavior through gradual exposure. This process also encourages the development of stronger trust with the therapist.

Presenting a treatment rationale can be more effective using culturally familiar examples. For instance, to explain and review the concept of gradual exposure, the therapist uses the analogy of playing in cold water: "You wade deeper into the cold water a little at a time until your body gets used to it and it doesn't feel cold anymore." In this example, a river, stream, or the ocean may be more relevant to the clients than a swimming pool as the body of water. In addition, the use of *cuentos* can help convey the importance of completing the trauma narrative. The *cuento* of Tossing Eyes can be used to illustrate the point that sometimes we may be asked to do something that is painful initially for a brief time, but then it pays off in a significant way in the long run (i.e., as with gradual exposure).

Cuento of Tossing Eyes

There once was a jaguar that used to toss his eyes into the ocean for fun and they would be tossed right back to him. However, one day a shark came and ate his eyes. The jaguar was very frightened, because now he could not see and would not be able to hunt for food, which would mean that he would surely die. A large, magical bird known as "king condor" came and saw that the jaguar was in trouble. The jaguar said, "Please help me and I will hunt for you." So the bird gave him mud and told him to put it on his eyes. When he did this, the jaguar became very uncomfortable and began to run around, saying "This hurts!" The bird then told him to remove the mud and open his eyes. Magically, his eyes were now glowing and he could see even better than before.

Therapists can highlight that although it was initially painful, the short amount of discomfort brought about stronger eyesight in the jaguar.

A potential language consideration when constructing the trauma narrative for bilingual children is attempting to determine the language in which the memory was encoded. Some studies suggest that more complete memory recall occurs if the memory is elicited in the language in which it was encoded (Javier, Barroso, & Muñoz, 1993; Javier & Marcos, 1989). For example, for a child who was trauma exposed as a monolingual Spanish speaker (e.g., victimized prior to immigrating from a Latin American country or prior to leaning English in school), attempts should be made when possible to elicit details about the trauma narrative in Spanish.

During cognitive processing of the trauma narrative, in addition to common negative distortions such as self-blame, overestimating danger, and a changed worldview, potential culturally related maladaptive thoughts and beliefs should be assessed directly if they have not yet been identified. For example, depending on the degree to which children and families adhere to various cultural beliefs, thoughts associated with *marianismo* (e.g., "I am no longer a virgin"), religious beliefs (e.g., "God is punishing me for something I did"), and other culturally related beliefs should be assessed when processing the narrative. The therapist must be careful to not discount cultural values but rather focus on the healthy, helpful aspects of these cultural values though progressive logical questioning and reframing. For example, one strategy to address concerns about the loss of virginity is to discuss with the child and caregiver how virginity is not something that can be taken away; it can only be given. It can be framed as being less associated with physical actions and more associated with a spiritual gift that is given in a loving relationship when individuals are mature enough to do so. In the case of sexual abuse, a child is being victimized and is thus unable to give his or her virginity away. Therefore, the child is still a virgin.

In a case example in which Michael de Arellano applied CM-TF-CBT, a child's father was having significant concerns about his daughter's loss of virginity and did not seem to experience relief from the explanation that virginity cannot be taken away, only given. The father was deeply Catholic and the importance of virginity stemmed from his religious beliefs. In order to better address his unhelpful thoughts, an "expert" in his faith was brought into treatment—a Latino Catholic priest in the community who had already met with the therapist to discuss this challenge in treatment. When the priest presented the same rationale as the therapist for why the child was still a virgin, the father experienced significant relief, likely because the priest could address the father's unhelpful thoughts from a position of authority and *respeto* related to the father's cultural beliefs.

In vivo mastery is a TF-CBT treatment component utilized when children's avoidance behaviors interfere with important activities such as going to school, playing with friends, and/or sleeping in their own bed. *In vivo* mastery helps children to gradually face these "trauma reminders" with the assistance and support of the caregiver and/or therapist. This component can be even more challenging than the imaginal exposure utilized in the trauma narrative component for some caregivers, who may prefer avoidance coping themselves or who are experiencing significant distress related to the children's trauma exposure. As with the trauma narrative, in CM-TF-CBT it is important to present a strong, clear rationale for the component and to reassure the children and caregivers that the *in vivo* exposure is done in a gradual manner that is very manageable. The use of encouraging *dichos* noted earlier can also be helpful in accomplishing this component

Conjoint parent–child sessions occur throughout the duration of CM-TF-CBT treatment, in which the children, caregivers, and/or extended family members meet with the therapist for joint therapeutic activities to review information, learn new techniques or skills, and share the trauma narrative. The therapist helps to prepare the caregivers for these conjoint sessions and uses clinical judgment to determine when they are appropriate. When working with Latino families in particular, it is important to consider the possibility that caregivers also have their own trauma exposure and may not have received treatment, especially given the research that suggests Latinos are at greater risk for trauma exposure and less likely to access services (Bridges et al., 2010; Kilpatrick & Saunders, 1996; Newcomb et al., 2009). In preparation for and handling of conjoint sessions, the therapist should be sensitive to the possibility of increased caregiver distress, including triggering their own trauma-related symptoms. Fortunately, caregivers can greatly benefit from learning all the same coping strategies in the parallel caregiver treatment and experience symptom relief (see Stewart

& Chambless, 2009, for review). However, for caregivers who are overwhelmed by their distress and have great difficulty managing it in treatment, referrals should be considered focused on addressing the caregivers' trauma-related symptoms.

During the final component, *enhancing future safety and development*, the therapist addresses general and personal safety skills with the children and caregivers, and works with the family to develop a safety plan for dangerous situations. It is important for caregivers to be involved in this process given that they can assist in enhancing the safety of the children's environment. If multiple caregivers tend to be involved with the children, the therapist should consider including them to help make safety planning even more effective. In families where *respeto* and *simpatia* are emphasized, and the children are taught to always be respectful of adults, to never question adults, and to avoid conflict, it will be especially important for the therapist and the parents to work with the children in understanding the exceptions to these rules (e.g., not OK. Touching is never OK—whether it is coming from an adult or someone else you know).

At times, a caregiver's beliefs may pose potential challenges to safety planning, such as reluctance to talk about sex education with children or to discuss concerns about dangerous situations that may be sexual in nature. Given that the primary goal of this component is to increase safety, accommodations should be made to ensure that the safety plan that is developed with the child and caregiver is culturally congruent and realistic in order to make it more likely that it will actually be used upon completion of treatment. For example, if a male caregiver does not think it is appropriate to talk about sex education or sexual concerns with his daughter, the therapist can consider identifying other individuals who are readily accessible and supportive with whom the child could speak about this topic. Using strategies such as these can increase the likelihood that the child's safety will be enhanced and the risk for future victimization reduced. In addition, for many Latino families, there is a preference to keep discussions of personal matters within the home. This can be a motivator for the caregiver to have more of these difficult discussions (e.g., sex) with the child at home in order to avoid having the child seek out information outside the home (e.g., friends, media) from sources that may not share the same value system.

For Latinos, termination of CM-TF-CBT treatment can often be particularly difficult, as the therapist may have become part of the *personalismo* or even *familismo* of this family. Issues around termination and loss should be thoroughly discussed. Medical doctor analogies may be given if the family has difficulty understanding the termination of the therapeutic relationship (e.g., "After a doctor fixes a broken leg, you do not continue to see that doctor"). Celebrating the last session in a formal way, with a focus on the success of the family in treatment rather than solely on the termination, is helpful in setting a joyful tone to the session.

CONCLUSION

Research and clinical evidence suggest that modifying EBTs to be more culturally relevant can enhance the effectiveness of interventions for use with different cultural groups. A careful, culturally informed assessment of trauma exposure, trauma-related sequelae, and important cultural constructs is critical for optimizing culturally competent treatment. CM-TF-CBT allows TF-CBT to be more culturally congruent and individually tailored for the level of acculturation and cultural beliefs and practices of Latino children and families. The tailoring process used in CM-TF-CBT may be a model for tailoring trauma-informed interventions for other cultural groups.

REFERENCES

Abney, V. D. (1996). Cultural competency in the field of child maltreatment. In J. Briere, L. Berliner, J. A. Bulkley, C. Jenny, & T. Reid (Eds.), *The APSAC handbook on child maltreatment* (pp. 409–419). Thousand Oaks, CA: Sage.

Acosta, E., Yamamoto, J., & Evans, L. (1982). *Effective psychotherapy for low income and minority patients*. New York: Plenum Press.

American Psychological Association. (2002). *Guidelines on multicultural education, training, research, practice, and organizational change for psychologists*. Washington, DC: Author. Retrieved from *www.apa.org/pi/oema/resources/policy/multicultural-guidelines.aspx*.

Avery, C. E. (1998). *Everybody has feelings/Todos tenemos sentimientos: The moods of children*. Silver Spring, MD: Gryphon House.

Aviera, A. (1996). "Dichos" therapy group: A therapeutic use of Spanish language proverbs with hospitalized Spanish-speaking psychiatric patients. *Cultural Diversity and Mental Health, 2*(2), 73–87.

Bernal, G., Bonilla, J., & Bellido, C. (1995). Ecological validity and cultural sensitivity for outcome research: Issues for cultural adaptation and development of psychosocial treatments with Hispanics. *Journal of Abnormal Child Psychology, 23*, 67–82.

Bernal, G., Bonilla, J., Padillo-Cotto, L., & Perez-Prado, E. M. (1998). Factors associated to outcome therapy: An effectiveness study in Puerto Rico. *Journal of Clinical Psychology, 54*, 329–342.

Bernal, G., Jiménez-Chafey, M. I., & Domenech Rodríguez, M. M. (2009). Cultural adaptation of treatments: A resource for considering culture in evidence-based practice. *Professional Psychology: Research and Practice, 40*(4), 361–368.

Bridges, A. J., de Arellano, M. A., Rheingold, A. A., Danielson, C. K., & Silcott, L. (2010). Trauma exposure, mental health, and service utilization rates among immigrant and United States-born Hispanic youth: Results from the Hispanic family study. *Psychological Trauma: Theory, Research, Practice, and Policy*, 2(1), 40–48.

Casas, J. M., & Pytluk, S. D. (1995). Hispanic identity development: Implications for research and practice. In J. G. Ponterotto, J. M. Casas, L. A. Suzuki, & C. M. Alexander (Eds.), *Handbook of multicultural counseling* (pp. 1155–1180). Thousand Oaks, CA: Sage.

Cohen, J. A., Mannarino, A. P., & Deblinger, E. (2006). *Treating trauma and traumatic grief in children and adolescents*. New York: Guilford Press.

Constantino, G., Malgady, R. G., & Regler, L. H. (1986). Cuento therapy: A cultural sensitive modality in Puerto Rican children. *Journal of Consulting and Clinical Psychology, 54*, 639–645.

Cuéllar, I., Arnold, B., & González, G. (1995). Cognitive referents of acculturation: Assessment of cultural constructs in Mexican Americans. *Journal of Community Psychology, 23*(4), 339–356.

Cuéllar, I., Arnold, B., & Maldonado, R. (1995). Acculturation Rating Scale for Mexican Americans-II: A revision of the original ARSMA Scale. *Hispanic Journal of Behavioral Sciences, 17*(3), 275–304.

Davidson, T. M, de Arellano, M. N., Rheingold, A. A., Danielson, C. K., & Silcott, L. (2011, November). *Culturally-modified trauma-focused cognitive behavioral therapy for Latino children: Focus groups*. Paper presented at the annual conference of the National Latinao/Psychological Association, Los Angeles.

de Arellano, M. A., & Danielson, C. K. (2008). Assessment of trauma history and trauma-related problems in ethnic minority child populations: An informed approach. *Cognitive and Behavioral Practice, 15*(1), 53–66.

de Arellano, M. A., Ko, S. J., Danielson, C. K., & Sprague, C. M. (2008). *Trauma-informed interventions: Clinical and research evidence and culture-specific information project*. Los Angeles: National Center for Child Traumatic Stress.

de Rios, M. D. (2001). *Brief psychotherapy with the Latino immigrant client*. New York: Haworth Press.

Diez de Leon, C. (2000). Acculturation and family therapy with Hispanics. In M. T. Flores & G. Carey (Eds.), *Family therapy with Hispanics: Toward appreciating diversity* (pp. 283–297). Needham Heights, MA: Allyn & Bacon.

Draguns, J. G. (2008). What have we learned about the interplay of culture with counseling and psychotherapy. In U. P. Gielen, J. G. Draguns, & J. M. Fish (Eds.), *Principles of multicultural counseling and therapy* (pp. 393–417). New York: Routledge/Taylor & Francis.

Falicov, C. J. (1998). *Latino families in therapy: A guide to multicultural practice*. New York: Guilford Press.

Finkelhor, D., & Dzuiba-Leatherman, J. (1994). Victimization of children. *American Psychologist, 49*(3), 173–183.

Finkelhor, D., Ormrod, R., Turner, H., & Hamby, S. L. (2005). The victimization of children and youth: A comprehensive, national survey. *Child Maltreatment, 10*(1), 5–25.

Flores, M. T., & Carey, G. (2000). *Family therapy with Hispanics: Toward appreciating diversity*. Needham Heights, MA: Allyn & Bacon.

Fontes, L. A. (1995). Culturally informed interventions for sexual child abuse. In L. A. Fontes (Ed.), *Sexual abuse in nine North American cultures: Treatment and prevention* (pp. 259–266). Thousand Oaks, CA: Sage.

Fontes, L. A. (2005). *Child abuse and culture: Working with diverse families.* New York: Guilford Press.

Freymann, S., & Elffers, J. (1999). *Vegetal como eres: Alimentos con sentimientos* [Vegetable as you are: Food with feelings]. New York: Scholastic.

Garcia-Preto, N. (1990). Hispanic mothers. *Journal of Feminist Therapy, 2,* 15–21.

Griner, D., & Smith, T. B. (2006). Culturally adapted mental health intervention: A meta-analytic review. *Psychotherapy: Theory, Research, Practice, Training, 43*(4), 531–548.

Hispanic Federation. (2005). Las Olvidadas/The Forgotten Ones. Available at *www.hispanicfederation.org/images/pdf/publications/policy_brief/las_olvidadas-the_forgotten_ones_latinas_and_hivaids_epidemic.pdf.*

Huey, S. J., & Polo, A. J. (2008). Evidence-based psychosocial treatments for ethnic minority youth. *Journal of Clinical Child and Adolescent Psychology, 37*(1), 262–301.

Javier, R. A., Barroso, F. & Muñoz, M. A. (1993). Autobiographical memory in bilinguals. *Journal of Psycholinguistic Research, 22,* 319–338.

Javier, R. A., & Marcos, L. R. (1989). The role of stress on the language-independence and code-switching phenomena. *Journal of Psycholinguistic Research, 18*(5), 449–472.

Jaycox, L. H., Stein, B. D., Kataoka, S. H., Wong, M., Fink, A., Escudero, P., et al. (2002). Violence exposure, posttraumatic stress disorder, and depressive symptoms among recent immigrant schoolchildren. *Journal of the American Academy of Child and Adolescent Psychiatry, 41*(9), 1104–1110.

Kaltman, S., Green, B. L., Mete, M., Shara, N., & Miranda, J. (2010). Trauma, depression, and comorbid PTSD/depression in a community sample of Latina immigrants. *Psychological Trauma: Theory, Research, Practice, and Policy, 2*(1), 31–39.

Kessler, R. C., Mickelson, K. D., & Williams, D. R. (1999). The prevalence, distribution, and mental health correlates of perceived discrimination in the United States. *Journal of Health and Social Behavior, 40,* 208–230.

Kilpatrick, D. G., Ruggiero, K. J., Acierno, R., Saunders, B. E., Resnick, H. S., & Best, C. L. (2003). Violence and risk of PTSD, major depression, substance abuse/dependence, and comorbidity: Results from the National Survey of Adolescents. *Journal of Consulting and Clinical Psychology, 71*(4), 692–700.

Kilpatrick, D. G., & Saunders, B. E. (1996). *Prevalence and consequences of child victimization: Results from the National Survey of Adolescents.* Washington, DC: U.S. Department of Justice, Office of Justice Programs, National Institute of Justice.

Kochhar, R. (2005, December 15). *The occupational status and mobility of Hispanics.* Retrieved from *http://pewhispanic.org/reports/report.php?ReportID=59.*

Lopez, M. H., & Dockterman, D. (2011, May 26). *U.S. Hispanic country of origin counts for nation, top 30 metropolitan areas.* Retrieved from *http://pewhispanic.org/reports/report.php?ReportID=142.*

Lopez, S. R., Kopelowicz, A., & Canive, J. M. (2002). Strategies in developing culturally congruent family interventions for schizophrenia: The case of Hispanics. In H. P. Lefley & D. L. Johnson (Eds.), *Family interventions in mental illness: International perspectives* (pp. 2061–2090). Westport, CT: Praeger.

Lopez-Baez, S. (1999). Marianismo. In J. S. Mio, J. E. Trimble, P. Arredondo, H. E. Cheatham, & D. Sue (Eds.), *Key words in multicultural interventions: A dictionary* (p. 183). Westport, CT: Greenwood Press.

Marin, G. (1992). Issues in the measurement of acculturation among Hispanics. In K. F. Geisinger (Ed.), *Psychological testing of Hispanics* (pp. 1235–1251). Washington, DC: American Psychological Association.

Marin, G., & Marin, B. V. (1991). *Research with Hispanic populations*. Newbury Park, CA: Sage.

Marin, G., & Triandis, H. C. (1985). Allocentrism as an important characteristic of the behavior of Latin American and Hispanics. In R. Diaz (Ed.), *Cross-cultural and national studies in social psychology* (pp. 85–104). Amsterdam: Elsevier Science.

McCabe, K. M., Yeh, M., Garland, A. F., Lau, A. S., & Chavez, G. (2005). The GANA program: A tailoring approach to adapting parent child interaction therapy for Mexican Americans. *Education and Treatment of Children, 28*(2), 111–129.

Moore, J., & Pachon, H. (1985). *Hispanics in the United States*. Englewood Cliffs, NJ: Prentice Hall.

Morales, E. (1996). Gender roles among Latino gay and bisexual men: Implications for family and couple relationships. In J. Laird & R. J. Green (Eds.), *Lesbians and gays in couples and families: A handbook for therapists* (pp. 272–297). San Francisco: Jossey-Bass.

Nava, Y. (2000). *It's all in the frijoles: 100 famous Latinos share real-life stories, time tested dichos, favorite folklore, and inspiring words of wisdom*. New York: Simon & Schuster.

Newcomb, M. D., Muñoz, D. T., & Carmona, J. V. (2009). Child sexual abuse consequences in community samples of Latino and European American adolescents. *Child Abuse and Neglect, 33*(8), 533–544.

Paniagua, F. A. (1994). *Assessing and treating culturally diverse clients: A practical guide*. Thousand Oaks, CA: Sage.

Potochnick, S., & Perreira, K. (2010). Depression and anxiety among first-generation immigrant Latino youth: Key correlates and implications for future research. *Journal of Nervous and Mental Disease, 198*(7); 470–477.

Raguram, R., Weiss, M. G., Channabasavanna, S. M., & Devins, G. M. (1996). Stigma, depression, and somatization in south India. *American Journal of Psychiatry, 153*(8), 1043–1049.

Roberts, A. L., Gilman, S. E., Breslau, J., Breslau, N., & Koenen, K. C. (2011). Race/ethnic differences in exposure to traumatic events, development of post-traumatic stress disorder, and treatment-seeking for post-traumatic stress disorder in the United States. *Psychological Medicine, 41*(1), 71–83.

Saldana, D. H. (1994). Acculturative stress: Minority status and distress. *Hispanic Journal of Behavioral Sciences, 16*(2), 116–128.

Santiago-Rivera, A. L., Arredondo, P., & Gallardo-Cooper, M. (2002). *Counseling Latinos and la familia: A practical guide.* Thousand Oaks, CA: Sage.

Santisteban, D. A., Muir-Malcolm, J. A., Mitrani, V. B., & Szapocznik, J. (2002). Integrating the study of ethnic culture and family psychology intervention science. In H. A. Liddle, D. A. Santisteban, R. Levant, & J. H. Bray (Eds.), *Family psychology: Science-based interventions* (pp. 2331–2351). Washington, DC: American Psychological Association.

Sonkin, D. J. (1995). *The counselor's guide to learning to live without violence.* San Francisco: Volcano Press.

Stewart, R. E., & Chambless, D. L. (2009). Cognitive-behavioral therapy for adult anxiety disorders in clinical practice: A meta-analysis of effectiveness studies. *Journal of Consulting and Clinical Psychology, 77*(4), 595–606.

Szapocznik, J., & Kurtines, W. M. (1993). Family psychology and cultural diversity: Opportunities for theory, research, and application. *American Psychologist, 48*(4), 400–407.

Triandis, H. C., Marin, G., Lisansky, J., & Betancourt, H. (1984). Simpatico as a cultural script of Hispanics. *Journal of Personality and Social Psychology, 47*(6), 1363–1375.

U.S. Census Bureau. (2011). *The Hispanic Population: 2010.* Washington, DC: U.S. Department of Commerce, Economics and Statistics Administration.

Yeh, M., McCabe, K., Hurlburt, M., Hough, R., Hazen, A., Culver, S., et al. (2002). Referral sources, diagnoses, and service types of youth in public outpatient mental health care: A focus on ethnic minorities. *Journal of Behavioral Health Services and Research, 29*(1), 45–60.

Zuniga, M. E. (1992). Using metaphors in therapy: *Dichos* and Latino clients. *Social Work, 37*(1), 55–60.

11

~

American Indian
and Alaska Native Children
Honoring Children—Mending the Circle

Dolores Subia BigFoot
Susan R. Schmidt

OVERVIEW AND DESCRIPTION OF POPULATION

Commonly referred to as the Great Turtle Island, what is now known as the United States of America includes more than 650 federally recognized tribes and native villages, with the majority of American Indians and Alaska Natives living in the western states and in nonreservation areas (Bureau of Indian Affairs, 2008). Indian Country is legally defined to include American Indian reservations, select American Indian communities, Alaska Native villages, rancheros, and all American Indian allotments (BigFoot & Braden, 1999). Many extend this definition to include all Indigenous people served through tribal or Native organizations or service systems, including those living in rural or off-reservation sites, in urban areas surrounding or adjacent to reservation lands, and in communities with a substantial American Indian/Alaska Native population within the continental United States (BigFoot & Schmidt, 2009).

Historical events and federal policies have dramatically affected the lives of American Indians and Alaska Natives. The military action, missionary efforts, the Federal Indian Boarding School Movement, the Dawes Act, the Indian Self-Determination and Education Assistance Act, and the

Indian Child Welfare Act forever changed the economic, physical, and social lives of American Indian/Alaska Native people (BigFoot, 2000; Manson, 2004). Policies of the federal government forced once self-reliant and self-sufficient Tribes/Indigenous people toward removal, relocation, isolation, and in some cases termination and extinction, resulting in social, economic, and spiritual deprivations. Over the past 200 years, American Indian and Alaska Native people have suffered from a lack of education, unemployment and economic disadvantage, family disorganization, and personal despair (Manson, 2004). Approximately 26% of American Indian/Alaska Native live in poverty compared with 13% of the general population and 10% of European Americans (National Child Abuse and Neglect Data System [NCANDS], 2002). Single-parent American Indian/Alaska Native families have the highest poverty rates in the country.

Violence is an all too common occurrence in Indian Country. The yearly average rate of violent crimes among American Indians and Alaska Natives is 124 per 1,000, almost more than 2½ times greater than the national rate (Bureau of Justice, 2004). American Indian/Alaska Native women report more domestic violence than men or women of any other race (Centers for Disease Control and Prevention [CDC], 2004). One study found that American Indian/Alaska Native women were twice as likely to be physically or sexually abused by a partner as non-American Indian/Alaska Native women (CDC, 2004). The incidences of repeated exposure to family violence can create a reverberating effect with American Indian/Alaska Native children and youth, since they are at higher risk for subsequent victimization.

American Indian/Alaska Native children are victims of child abuse and neglect more frequently than other children. In 2002 (NCANDS, 2002), the American Indian/Alaska Native population was found to be the only group to experience an increase in the rate of abuse or neglect of children younger than 15. When comparing the rates of one substantiated report of child abuse or neglect for every 30 American Indian/Alaska Native children age 14 or younger (Perry, 2004) with the national rate of 12.3 per 1,000 (NCANDS, 2002), it is easy to understand that American Indian/Alaska Native children are at an increased vulnerability to trauma exposure. American Indian and Alaska Native children are also at heightened risk for experiencing other forms of trauma, including the premature loss of loved ones. This population leads the nation in death by alcohol-related motor vehicle accidents, chronic liver disease, and cirrhosis. They also lead the nation in deaths resulting from diabetes-related complications.

Given the multiple risks present in American Indian/Alaska Native communities, it is not surprising that the prevalence of posttraumatic stress disorder (PTSD) is substantially higher among American Indian/Alaska Native persons than in the general community (22% vs. 8%; Kessler, Sonnega, Bromet, Hughes, & Nelson, 1995). It is likely that higher rates of exposure to traumatic events coupled with the overarching cultural, historical, and intergenerational traumas make this population more vulnerable to PTSD and negative long-term health outcomes. The rates of depression among American Indian/Alaska Native children range from 10 to 30% (Satcher, 1999) while the level of substance abuse can be even higher, with illicit drug use highest among American Indian/Alaska Native youth, at a rate of 9.9%. Substance use may also be a signal for other mental health needs, as American Indian youth in treatment for substance abuse often have significant untreated psychiatric comorbidity (Novins, Beals, Shore, & Manson, 1996). In addition, children of substance-abusing parents are at increased risk for harm or injury as a result of car accidents, behavioral problems, parental neglect, suicide, and personal substance abusive behaviors.

Suicide has been a continuous concern for American Indian/Alaska Native children and youth. In their survey of American Indian/Alaska Native adolescents (n = 13,000), Blum, Harmon, Harris, Bergeisen, and Resnick (1992) reported that 22% of females and 12% of males indicated that they attempted suicide at some point. This rate is higher than that for other age ranges and ethnic groups. Among adults, American Indian/Alaska Native men are four times more likely and American Indian/Alaska Native women three times more likely to attempt suicide than their counterparts of other racial groups (CDC, 2004). The suicide rate is particularly high among young American Indian/Alaska Native males ages 15–24. Accounting for 64% of all suicides among the American Indian/Alaska Native population, the suicide rate among this age group is two to three times higher than the general U.S. rate (Kettle & Bixler, 1991; May, 1990; Mock, Grossman, Mulder, Stewart, & Koepsell, 1996).

SPECIAL APPLICATIONS OF TF-CBT ARE NEEDED FOR AMERICAN INDIAN/ ALASKA NATIVE YOUTH

Historically, government and social service organization use of non- or poorly suited mental health treatments with diverse populations has led to widespread distrust and reluctance among such populations to seek mental health services. Service providers, and even families themselves, may discount or fail to recognize American Indian/Alaska Native traditional practices that are instrumental to healing and well-being. Although mainstream and traditional American Indian/Alaska Native approaches may differ considerably (e.g., a support group compared with a traditional sweat ceremony), common principles of connection are embraced by both approaches. Traditional American Indian/Alaska Native healing practices such as sweat ceremonies may lack scientific evidence for their efficacy; however, their incorporation has been reported to improve client engagement and retention among both American Indian/Alaska Native adults and adolescents.

In 2003, as part of the National Child Traumatic Stress Initiative, the University of Oklahoma Health Sciences Center, Center on Child Abuse and Neglect, established the Indian Country Child Trauma Center (ICCTC) to develop trauma-focused treatments and outreach materials specifically designed for American Indian/Alaska Native children and their families. ICCTC identifies existing evidence-based treatments that share common elements with American Indian/Alaska Native cultural beliefs and practices. Its goal is to design culturally relevant approaches that respect shared and tribal-specific teachings, practices, and understandings while recognizing the substantial individual variability in cultural affiliation among American Indian/Alaska Native people. The interventions developed by ICCTC are designed to be useful for rural and/or isolated tribal communities where licensed professionals may be few.

Based on a review of research-supported child trauma treatments, trauma-focused cognitive-behavioral therapy (TF-CBT; Cohen, Mannarino, & Deblinger, 2006) was selected to serve as the foundation for the cultural enhancement Honoring Children–Mending the Circle (HC-MC). Originally described as a cultural "adaptation," we have shifted to the term cultural "enhancement" to emphasize that we are not presenting a new model, but rather broadening the focus of TF-CBT to encompass the foundational framework of Indigenous teachings that TF-CBT complements. The presentation of TF-CBT within an American Indian/Alaska Native well-being framework enhances healing through the blending of science and Indigenous culture understandings and practices. What makes cultural enhancement successful is the translation not just of language but of core principles and treatment concepts so that they become meaningful to the culturally targeted group while still maintaining fidelity. Much has been written regarding the complementarity of cognitive-behavioral theory (CBT) and American Indian/Alaska Native traditional teachings. The core construct in CBT—the connection between one's thoughts, feelings, and behaviors—is Old Wisdom evident throughout Indigenous teachings and traditions (LaFromboise, Trimble, & Mohatt, 1990). Moreover, TF-CBT is consistent with American Indian/Alaska Native traditional beliefs such as the centrality of family, the importance of attending to and listening to children, education through recounting experiences (e.g., storytelling, ceremony), and the importance of identifying and expressing emotions. The HC-MC adaptation seeks to honor what makes American Indians and Alaska Natives culturally unique through respecting the healing beliefs, practices, and traditions within their families, communities, and tribes and villages.

Partners in the HC-MC development process included stakeholders (tribal leadership, consumers, and traditional, ceremonial, warrior societies, helpers, and healers), programs (e.g., schools, tribal colleges, behavior health agencies), TF-CBT providers, and the TF-CBT developers, who provided ongoing consultation. There was consensus on traditional American Indian/Alaska Native concepts to be incorporated into the enhancement as they are common to most, if not all, tribal communities: extended family and relational connections, practices, and behaviors regarding respect, beliefs regarding the concept of the Circle, and the interconnectedness between spirituality and healing. Indigenous knowledge, or Old Wisdom, is also a foundational aspect of the cultural enhancement as generations of Indigenous people intuitively relied on teachings and behavioral principles prior to the labeling and description of such concepts through the written word (BigFoot, 2008).

The framework for HC-MC is the circle. For many Indigenous people, the Circle is a sacred symbol that has long been used to understand the world. The symbolism of the Circle is Old Wisdom transmitted in oral stories, carved into rock formations, sculpted in wood or clay, woven into reed baskets, and painted in colored sand. The most widely recognized American Indian/Alaska Native symbolic circle is the Medicine Wheel. The constructions of the Medicine Wheel and its teachings have been documented since 7000 B.C.E. (*http://solar-center.stanford.edu/AO/*). Other symbolic circles include the Sacred Hoop, Sacred Circle, children as the center, and cycle of life. The circle or hoop typically includes colors, directions, animals, symbols, teachings, developmental levels, dynamic movement, and connections or relational links between and among each element while providing Indigenous wisdom about life (BigFoot, 2008). The concept of the circle is incorporated into American Indian/Alaska Native lifestyles through practices, teachings, and ceremonies such as at the beginning of the grand entry for pow wows, the physical placement of participants during sweat lodge, the shape of the drum, ceremonial structures such as medicine lodges and many kivas, and dwellings such as grass or reed shelters and wattle or daubs.

The HC-MC circle bears similarities to the Medicine Wheel, but is conceptualized within this model as a model of well-being. The HC-MC circle is based on tribal teachings, but remains flexible to accommodate individuals of diverse cultures and spiritual and religious beliefs. It is an elaboration on the CBT core construct of the cognitive triangle—that our thoughts, feelings, and behaviors are interconnected. Core HC-MC constructs are based on American Indian/Alaska Native worldviews: (1) all things are interconnected, (2) all things have a spiritual nature, and (3) existence is dynamic. HC-MC defines well-being as balance and harmony both within and between one's spiritual, relational, emotional, mental, and physical dimensions. Figure 11.1 depicts the HC-MC circle, which is composed of the five well-being dimensions.

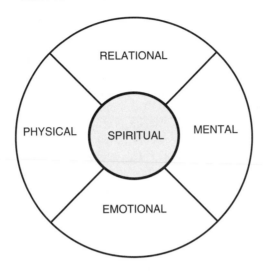

FIGURE 11.1. HC-MC well-being model. Copyright 2008 by Dolores Subia Big-Foot and Susan R. Schmidt. Reprinted by permission.

Spirituality serves as the core of the HC-MC circle. Central to wellness and healing is the American Indian/Alaska Native belief that all things—human and earth—have a spiritual nature. Spirituality has played and continues to play an important role in the individual and collective well-being of American Indians. American Indian/Alaska Native helpers and healers have been taught words, prayers, practices, rituals, and ceremonies that help connect the physical world with the spiritual to bring about wellness, balance, and harmony. The spiritual dimension is interwoven with the physical, mental, emotional, and relational well-being dimensions.

HC-MC defines personal imbalance as disharmony in one or more of the circle dimensions. Imbalance may manifest in such ways as spiritual disconnection, unhealthy behaviors, emotional instability, distorted beliefs, and poor relationships. Trauma exposure is one pathway with the potential to cause such imbalance. As a result, the goal of the healing process is to restore one's personal balance within the five dimensions, thus reestablishing personal well-being.

UNIQUE ASSESSMENT STRATEGIES FOR AMERICAN INDIAN/ALASKA NATIVE YOUTH

When and to what degree to blend HC-MC elements into the TF-CBT treatment model is dependent on the individual youth's and family's level of

American Indian/Alaska Native affiliation. Collaboration and exploration with the family to learn about each member's level of American Indian/Alaska Native cultural affiliation is necessary to determine the extent to which the incorporation of HC-MC enhancements into the treatment process will be beneficial. It is critical to recognize that cultural affiliation is an individual developmental process. Although some family members may possess a strong American Indian/Alaska Native identity, others may identify more strongly with different aspects of their personal identity such as their religious affiliation, professional role, or other racial or ethnic affiliation. Exploration of client cultural identity at both the individual and the familial level is critical not only during the initial assessment and early stages of therapy, but also throughout the therapeutic process as cultural affiliation is dynamic and multidimensional.

The American Indian/Alaska Native affiliation model, as depicted in Figure 11.2, is designed to assist therapists in understanding the level of affiliation that a particular American Indian or Native Alaskan has with their Indigenous culture. The chart illustrates the range of affiliation for American Indian/Alaska Native people: (1) individuals who have strong ties to their American Indian/Alaska Native culture, (2) individuals with limited ties to their American Indian/Alaska Native culture but a desire to

(1) High/Strong Cultural Affiliation—AI/AN	(2) Limited or No Affiliation—Insecure
• Identity as AI/AN is secure • Highly desirous to maintain high/strong affiliation • May have other cultural heritage(s) that are not assumed	• Identity as AI/AN is insecure • Highly desirous to acquire high/strong affiliation • May have other cultural heritage(s) that are not assumed or are not valued • Affiliation marginal
(3) Limited or No Affiliation—Secure	**(4) High/Strong Cultural Affiliation—Other**
• Identity as non-AI/AN is secure • Limited or no interest in affiliation with AI/AN or other cultural base • May or may not be expressive about limited interest in own AI/AN background/heritage • May or may not identify with other heritage(s) • Has found value in other aspects of self-identity	• Identity as non-AI/AN is secure • Has a high/strong affiliation with selected or elected heritage(s) • Highly values maintaining high/strong affiliations with selected or elected heritage(s)

FIGURE 11.2. American Indian/Alaska Native affiliation model. Copyright 2009 by Dolores Subia BigFoot. Reprinted by permission.

strength their affiliation, (3) individuals with limited ties to their American Indian/Alaska Native culture and more strongly identify with other aspects of their self-identity, and (4) individuals whose personal identities are strongly tied to other cultural heritages. Individuals and families with a strong American Indian/Alaska Native affiliation may benefit from incorporation of several elements from the HC-MC enhancement into TF-CBT treatment. HC-MC elements may serve to further facilitate the healing process and support the return to well-being through connection to one's American Indian/Alaska Native heritage. For individuals who have strong affiliations with other culture or heritages (e.g., limited or no American Indian/Alaska Native Affiliation—secure; high/strong cultural affiliation—other), the families may prefer to work within the original TF-CBT framework. For American Indian/Alaska Native individuals with limited or no American Indian/Alaska Native affiliation but who would like to grow in this identity, the incorporation of HC-MC enhancements may be beneficial to the therapeutic process. HC-MC therapists have shared the benefits of the model enhancements with American Indian/Alaska Native youth within this affiliation category who have come from abusive and neglectful home environments. These youth may have developed negative or inaccurate perceptions of American Indian/Alaska Native culture and have had few positive American Indian/Alaska Native role models. Therapists report that the HC-MC enhancement supports opportunities for corrective educational and emotional experiences, leading to a healthier personal identity and the development of positive relationships within the youth's tribe and community. Of key importance regardless of the individual youth's and family's cultural affiliation is their inclusion in determining what level of cultural integration into the treatment model best fits their needs.

ENGAGEMENT STRATEGIES FOR AMERICAN INDIAN/ALASKA NATIVE FAMILIES

Safety and trust are often key issues for traumatized American Indian/Alaska Native individuals entering therapy given the personal violations they may have endured. Intergenerational impacts from historical traumatic experiences may further compound youth's and families' ability and willingness to enter and commit to treatment. Clinicians in Indian Country have not had the luxury to expect that families will be committed to the multisession format of structured treatment approaches. Families who utilize therapeutic services tend to participate in only a few sessions before attendance becomes sporadic or stops. In fairness to families, their therapeutic experiences have often been less than ideal with few options for effective interventions. Most therapeutic encounters have focused on crisis intervention, therapeutic approaches of long-term duration with limited skill building, and practices without cultural foundations. Recent developments in culturally based interventions have begun to lead to more meaningful understandings of the impact of historical trauma as well as recent or current traumatic events on American Indian/Alaska Native individuals and families (BigFoot, 2010).

The TF-CBT model emphasizes the centrality of the therapeutic relationship in treatment (Cohen, Mannarino, & Deblinger, 2006). The establishment of a safe and effective therapeutic environment is dependent on such factors as therapist genuineness, warmth, empathy, and creativity. As stated by McDonald and Gonzalez (2006), the first session with American Indian/Alaska Native clients is the most significant because it is in this session that the client determines whether or not to trust the therapist and engage in the treatment process. This is especially true for children and families impacted by trauma. It is in the first session that therapists may begin to develop a broader understanding and appreciation of the family system, including their cultural affiliations, values, and experiences. It is important for therapists to convey in the first and subsequent sessions their respect for the family's steps toward healing and to begin joining the family as a helper in their healing process. Given the historical devaluation experienced by American Indian/Alaska Natives, the family should be provided with the opportunity to teach the therapist about their family, family history, and levels of cultural affiliation. Therapists should provide the information necessary to support families in making thoughtful decisions about their treatment experience, not only at the beginning of treatment but throughout the therapeutic relationship.

Opportunities exist throughout the TF-CBT model to incorporate HC-MC enhancements into the treatment process. Families may wish to incorporate such things as tribal-specific songs, names, words, or healing ceremonies into sessions. Tribal stories that incorporate familiar animals, birds, or locations may carry increased meaning for American Indian/Alaska Native children and families. It is important to recognize that the HC-MC enhancement of TF-CBT will likely look different for each individual and family because it is designed to be personalized by the therapist based on the family's needs, experiences, and understandings. Images, stories, and practices familiar and meaningful to individuals from one tribe or geographic area may have little meaning, or possibly an opposite meaning, for those from another. For example, ivory carvings are common to Native Alaskan culture but have no history with tribes in the Southeast. Whereas the Scissor-tailed Flycatcher is a revered bird with tribes in Oklahoma, the Raven has a more prominent place within Northwest Indigenous cultures. Therapists implementing the HC-MC enhancement are encouraged to appreciate and to learn more about the customs, traditions, stories, and symbols relevant to tribes within their geographic area.

The following section provides a sampling of HC-MC therapeutic considerations and enhancements that may be incorporated into a selection of TF-CBT PRACTICE components.

PRACTICE COMPONENT ENHANCEMENTS

Two tools have been designed to assist therapists in the implementation of HC-MC. Figure 11.3 displays a worksheet that may be used to guide therapeutic work within a specific PRACTICE component. The HC-MC component worksheet helps incorporate cultural considerations via tangible reminders to address the relational, emotional, mental, physical, and spiri-

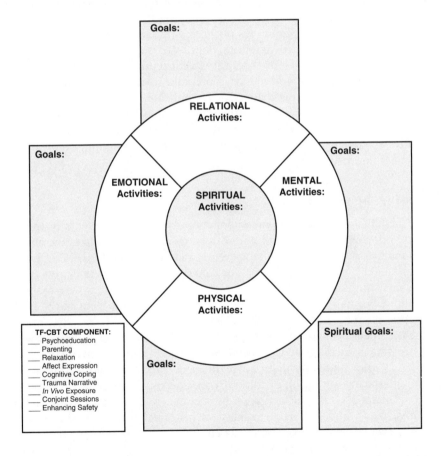

FIGURE 11.3. HC-MC component worksheet. Copyright 2008 by Dolores Subia BigFoot and Susan R. Schmidt. Reprinted by permission.

tual dimensions within each of the PRACTICE components. Some HC-MC therapists have expanded their use of the components worksheet to therapy sessions in order to facilitate psychoeducation about well-being and the impact of trauma on children and families. The worksheet has also been utilized for in-session treatment planning with families. Figure 11.4 depicts a linear representation of this worksheet designed to assist therapists further in treatment plan development and tracking. This worksheet provides an example of a personalized treatment plan specific to the psychoeducation TF-CBT component within the HC-MC well-being model.

The American Indian/Alaska Native healing practices worksheet was developed as a training tool to help therapists conceptualize how such practices fit within the wellness model and within TF-CBT. As shown in Figure 11.5, the form has three areas: (1) the healing practice, (2) the usefulness or purpose of that practice, and (3) the meaningfulness or value/belief surrounding that practice. Examples of three different practices are provided to demonstrate the range of activities, objects, or items that could be used in this manner. The intent is for therapists to conceptualize the family's Indigenous healing practices and identify outcomes from those practices. Feedback from therapists using the worksheet indicates this is effective in identifying activities, objects, or items the family sees as helpful; how the family would like to incorporate these into the therapeutic process; and what the family expects to achieve as a result of the integration of familiar Indigenous practices into treatment.

Psychoeducation

The TF-CBT psychoeducation component provides developmentally appropriate information about common trauma reactions, normalizes the child's and family's response to traumatic events, and introduces the TF-CBT treatment model (Cohen et al., 2006). For American Indian/Alaska Native families, this component is critical to treatment engagement. It is here that the therapist begins to learn about the family and join with them in the healing process. The establishment of a safe, accepting, and culturally responsive therapeutic environment is key to supporting the family's commitment to treatment participation. Depending on youth and caregiver American Indian/Alaska Native affiliation, treatment engagement may be enhanced through the incorporation of culturally specific and developmentally appropriate materials such as factsheets on trauma in American Indian/Alaska Native youth and families; readings on historical trauma when relevant to the family's experience; culturally congruent descriptions of well-being, trauma, and healing (previously described); and the use of familiar analogies and stories to explain the treatment process.

HC-MC therapists have found that the use of culturally based analogies can enhance treatment participation among clients wavering in their

PSYCHOEDUCATION
Goals and considerations specific to this family:
1. Help parents consider the impacts of intergenerational and historical trauma on their family.
2. Provide teen and parents with education on trauma in AI/AN youth and their families.
3. Enhance engagement through explanation of TF-CBT treatment process in culturally relevant terms.
4. Identify family's goals for treatment and the healing process.

Activity	Member(s) Involved		Domain(s) Involved				
	Child	Care-giver	Relational	Mental	Physical	Emotional	Spiritual
Review "What is trauma? A guide for parents" (Indian Country Child Trauma Center, n.d.)	√	√	√	√	√	√	√
Review intake assessment findings and discuss in context of current and intergeneration family trauma.	√	√	√	√	√	√	√
Use analogy of beading to describe TF-CBT model to family.	√	√	√	√			
Explore youth's and parents' American Indian affiliation and explore external helpers, healers, and activities the family may include in the healing process.	√	√	√				

FIGURE 11.4. HC-MC component treatment plan. Copyright 2011 by Dolores Subia BigFoot and Susan R. Schmidt. Reprinted by permission.

commitment to the comprehensive TF-CBT protocol. The following two analogies may be adapted specific to clients' understanding and developmental level to provide education on the TF-CBT model structure and process. Therapists may find similar protocols, ceremonies, or relevant activities that emphasize the importance of structure, patience, consistency, and commitment to the TF-CBT therapeutic process.

Activity/Object/Item	Use/Purpose	Meaningfulness/Value/Belief
Singing a good-bye song after a family member has passed away	• To help family members say good-bye to the deceased family member • To recognize that the family member's spirit is on a new journey	• Gives permission for the spirit to journey onward • To acknowledge that this is a transition period for everyone • To give permission to mourn • To provide a supportive structure for mourning • Serves as a reminder of the loved one when sung again in the future

FIGURE 11.5. American Indian/Alaska Native healing practices worksheet. Copyright 2009 by Dolores Subia BigFoot and Susan R. Schmidt. Reprinted by permission.

Grand Entry Procession

Since 1889, the Arlee Celebration (*www.arleepowwow.com*) has been held on the Flathead Reservation in Arlee, Montana, and is one of many spectacular pow wows held across Indian Country, especially during the summer months. A pow wow is a social and spiritual gathering of American Indian people that primarily involves music, dancing, and various customs depending on the location, tribal affiliation, and purpose. One common feature of all pow wow events is the beginning "grand entry" procession, consisting of a strict protocol of drummers, singers, and warriors (active, retired, or former military) who start the event. Dancers (e.g., traditional, fancy, straight, grass, chicken, buckskin, cloth) follow a strict line of placement depending on dancer type. Following pow wow protocol is expected and considered respectful to self and others. This protocol, which has been built around hundreds of years of tradition, addresses order, structure, pacing, and meaning. Whether it is the acknowledgment given to elders as they start a procession, the feast dinner to celebrate the first laughter of a baby, the chief song sung at the beginning of an event, or the single folded dollar laid at the feet of a dancer, protocol instructs Indigenous people in ways to respectfully honor each other.

Protocol is not new to American Indians or Alaska Natives; it provides instruction in how to conduct specific activities in order to achieve consistent good outcomes. Values reinforced through protocol include respectfulness, acknowledgment, order, purpose, expectations, and beginnings and endings. It brings an understanding of knowing what to expect next and that there is purpose to each activity. Similarly, there is a structured protocol within TF-CBT that is designed to support children and families in achieving good treatment outcomes and moving beyond their traumatic experiences.

Beading

Beadwork is a common but highly personalized skill among many American Indian and Alaska Native artists, with exquisite variety in design and application. However, certain features remain the same. Specific items are necessary for beading such as a needle, thread, backing, colored beads, cutting implements, wax, chosen design, required measurements, and buckskin or similar material for shape and form. The creativity and beauty of the beadwork are at the heart and hands of the gifted artist; however, the structure, form, and function come from the common elements that the artist uses to bring forth the exquisite piece. The TF-CBT therapeutic process is similar to beading in that the TF-CBT core components create the basic structure; the therapist and client then work together to add complementary features to make treatment most meaningful to the client.

Parenting

The TF-CBT model aims to increase parents' confidence and ability as caretakers of their children. Historical concepts of parenting may be utilized to introduce specific parenting skills. The following stories offer examples of how the HC-MC therapist may utilize descriptions of Indigenous practices and beliefs to introduce parenting concepts emphasized within the TF-CBT model:

THE IMPORTANCE OF ATTACHMENT AND RECOGNIZING CHILDREN'S POTENTIAL

Upon discovering that she was pregnant, an American Indian woman would actively engage in song and conversation with the unborn child to touch with words and intent. This was to ensure that the infant knew it was welcome, respected, and loved. This new life was viewed as being eager to learn and a willing seeker of those traits that would help in knowing and understanding self and others. The caregiver's responsibility was to nurture and expand the positive nature of the child, to touch the child with honor and respect. Because a child was considered a gift from the Creator, the caretakers had the responsibility to return to the Creator an individual who respected him- or herself and others.

THE IMPORTANCE OF ATTACHMENT AND POSITIVE ROLE MODELING

Within the family, children, parents, and grandparents were secure in their relationships with each other. Children respected their parents, but just as important was the parents' respect for children. Children knew they were the center of existence for all family members. They were honored by celebrations and feasts given by relatives that left no doubt as to their worth and value. Today some children continue to be honored by birthday celebrations, graduation dinners, first tribal dance, school or athletic achievement ceremonies, or other kinds of acknowledgment of accomplishment.

BEHAVIOR MANAGEMENT

Understanding and shaping human and animal behavior is old American Indian/ Alaska Native wisdom. There is a rich legacy of Indigenous people training birds of prey, domesticating dogs, and in the past 500 years becoming skilled horsemen. In the 1800s, many tribes became known for their exceptional skill in warfare because their horses were highly responsive to subtle commands and expert maneuvering. Teaching, instructing, shaping, modeling, coaching, training, tutoring, and rewarding are ways common to American Indian/Alaska Native people.

Relaxation

The relaxation TF-CBT component assists the youth in learning skills to reduce physiological manifestations of stress and PTSD. This often incorporates the teaching of deep breathing and progressive muscle relaxation as methods for stress reduction. In the HC-MC model, the therapist can reinforce the cultural application of relaxation by incorporating familiar soothing traditional images and activities. These may have the added benefit of reinforcing the youth's spiritual and relational connectedness.

Diaphragmatic breathing may be taught through pairing inhalations and exhalations with relaxing images such as the sway of windswept grasses or the movement of a woman's shawl during a ceremonial dance. Youth who engage in singing, chanting, or playing traditional instruments such as the flute or drum may learn to pace their breath to the beat and intensity of the music. Progressive muscle relation may be taught through such imagery such as the tensing and relaxing of a bowstring to explain the difference between relaxed and tense muscles. Muscle relaxation may also be supported through the reinforcement of activities that are naturally relaxing, such as canoeing, hiking, horseback riding, or other sports in which the youth participates.

The therapist may inquire as to the spiritual practices that the youth and family engage in that facilitate relaxation. This not only supports the family's own sense of spirituality and their engagement in naturally relaxing practices, but also reinforces the family's connectedness with one another and with other helpers and healers in their community. When considering the emotional and mental components to relaxation, the therapist may assist the child in understanding how one's thoughts and feelings can support physical relaxation. For example, with the trauma-exposed child, intrusive thoughts may create anxiety and an inability to relax. Common reactions to trauma include physical sensations of rapid heartbeat and breathing that result in distress or discomfort. Relevant traditional instructions during ceremonial or related activities such as the Sweat Lodge may include such words as "Know that this is a safe place for you. Leave bad or scared thoughts outside. Close your eyes and breathe in. Feel how you are sitting and think about who is sitting next to you." This instruction encourages the relaxation response through altering one's thoughts and emotions.

Affective Modulation

Historically, Indigenous cultures have highly valued emotional understanding and expression. Traditionally, direct verbal emotional expression is less favored over such creative forms as song, dance, and artistic symbolic representations. However, the emotional devastation of intergenerational trauma within many American Indian/Alaska Native cultural groups has led to high rates of depression, anxiety, and suicidal ideation among younger generations. Many youth have had poor role models for healthy emotion management, instead seeing older generations use harmful methods of coping such as drug and alcohol abuse.

For the HC-MC therapist, it is important to assess youth's family's norms, beliefs, and practices regarding emotional expression. American Indian/Alaska Native youth may be supported in the development of healthy emotional expression skills through a variety of traditional activities, such as the sharing of stories incorporating animals/elements/colors/directions; the development of physical emotional representations such as beading, painting, drawing, masks, totems, or shields; learning the words for feelings in their Native language; singing or playing traditional musical instruments; and dancing.

Cognitive Coping

Historically, Indigenous people have understood and recognized the interplay among thoughts, feelings, and behaviors. Certain ceremonial instructions guide participants to direct thoughts toward better behavior, decision making, coping, and the future. Counsel may be given to remind individuals that someone offered prayer for them, that they are thought of, that good things are wished for them, and that what they do is important to others. Additionally, how they treat themselves is as important as how they treat others.

As with previous components, the use of Indigenous stories can support skill development. Stories involving the coyote or trickster teach problem solving and decision making. Tribal creation stories have been retold for generations to help bring understanding and a way to manage life when life circumstances are overwhelming. Every tribe has a creation story that tells of their origin and what behaviors led them forward. Many tribal websites have posted their creation stories to share the wisdom of their history and important tribal teachings. In 2003, Cheyenne historian John L. Sipe wrote of the discovery of the Lost Cheyenne:

> This Cheyenne creation story describes a mighty migration that forced the Cheyenne to separate when a water monster broke the ice over which they were traveling. A portion of the Tribe was isolated from the main body when the ice broke and they never reconnected, leaving them to decide how to survive on their own and manage their new circumstances. It is told that they confronted many adversities before eventually settling in the far north country, where they built structures to house their families, tended the land, hunted game, and fished the many streams.

What can be learned from this and other creation stories is that when circumstances change and adversities occur, one must develop new understandings, make thoughtful decisions, and change behaviors to overcome these challenges.

Trauma Narrative; Conjoint Sessions

The trauma narrative is a key healing element of TF-CBT involving a structured and repetitive retelling of the traumatic event in gradually increasing detail in order to reduce the child's distress related to the memory. Within Indigenous cultures, stories are transmitted from generation to generation in order to remember and learn from the past, to carry wisdom forward, and to offer resolutions for present and future life difficulties. Indigenous stories capture understandings, explanations, solutions, acceptance, and compassion. The essence of a story is borne from the thoughts, feelings, and actions of the storyteller. Wisdom imparted through the story may reveal the pathway toward well-being. The act of storytelling may be as important as the end result because it is sometimes the process of the journey where one gains insight and wisdom.

For some American Indian/Alaska Native individuals, certain intergenerational beliefs may contribute to hesitancy to participate in the trauma narrative process, and these will subsequently need to be addressed before narrative work can begin. Some families believe that to discuss trauma invites it to recur or that talking about a deceased loved one may hinder his or her journey to the next world. With such families, it may be beneficial to support the family in seeking guidance from their spiritual leader regarding their participation in the trauma narrative component. For some, such beliefs may not be spiritually or culturally based but instead developed as a result of the family's intergenerational history of trauma. Cognitive processing techniques may help these families move forward into narrative work. Indigenous stories may also help reduce avoidance. The following story serves as an example:

> Millions of buffalo once roamed the Great Plains. As was common then, and still common today, tumultuous thunderstorms covered the landscape from early spring into the summer months. We are familiar today with those raging, darkening storms that typically form in the West and move toward the East, especially those that grow quite menacing with torna-does, strong forceful winds, pounding hail, and/or icy rain. Out in open prairie, the buffalo were intensely aware of approaching storms. How do you think they responded as a storm approached? Did the millions of buffalo run into the menacing storm force or did they run away from it? When watching buffalo out on the plains, the people saw that the buffalo ran into the storm. The buffalo instinctively knew that beyond the storm was calm, brightness, sunshine, and peaceful grazing.

The following story also incorporates animal imagery to introduce the trauma narrative:

> When animals get hurt, their natural instinct is to clean their wounds to promote healing. This is their way of taking care of themselves. The bear may find it painful to remove debris from an injury. But he does this knowing that this is necessary for his body to become well. Heal-ing must take place for the bear to be able to use his body to gather food and to protect himself. The bear must tend to the hurt until it is healed. Then he is ready to return to his path on the circle. (BigFoot & Schmidt, 2008)

When beginning trauma narrative work, the HC-MC therapist collaborates with the youth and family to determine in what format the narrative will be developed and with whom and how it will be shared. Protocols may be involved when inviting certain helpers or healers to participate. Families may also wish to coordinate healing ceremonies or practices with narrative completion. As some American Indian/Alaska Native children may be less comfortable with writing or telling their story, alternate methods grounded in American Indian/Alaska Native cultural practices may include such activ-ities as creating a journey stick, totem, song, carving, beading, mask, pot-tery, or traditional dance. Some families select to develop a family "narra-tive" after the child's individual narrative completion, such as the creation of a family totem or journey stick.

Families who have experienced intergenerational trauma may wish at this point in treatment to honor loved ones who did not have the opportunity to heal from their traumatic experiences. The therapist may work with the family to determine how they would like to address their family's trauma history. It will be important for the therapist to work with the caregivers to consider the needs of their child when determining the child's level of participation in such an endeavor. The therapist may support the family in seeking out helpers and healers within their community or tribe to symbolically and ceremonially help their ancestors to complete their healing journey.

SUMMARY

This chapter has provided an overview of HC-MC and an introduction to the methods utilized in the cultural enhancement. The HC-MC cultural enhancement does not change the basic tenets of TF-CBT; rather, the TF-CBT foundation is observed from a worldview that honors the teachings and practices that have been part of American Indian and Alaska Native understandings for untold generations. This model is designed to assist the therapist and family in recognizing and understanding how traditional cultural practices have value and application within TF-CBT.

The rich cultural teachings and practices of American Indians and Alaska Natives are much broader than presented here. Caution should be exercised when considering how to culturally enhance or modify any EBP not originally developed for this population. In fact, there may be great skepticism that cultural adaptation of any EBP is simply another strategy of oppression by the dominant culture. There is the need to understand how oppressive legacies are embedded (e.g., policies, institutions, and social systems) and perpetuated (e.g., practices, belief systems, and behaviors) today in the form of institutional and structural or systemic racism as well as its individual manifestations (*www.overcomingracism. org*).

The cultural enhancement of TF-CBT is mindful of the family's cultural context while maintaining the integrity of the original EBP through grounding in Old Wisdom. That is to say that the underlying premises of TF-CBT are consistent with core dimensions of American Indian/Alaska Native traditional teachings and beliefs about healing. The concept of the circle stress the importance of family; attending to and listening to children; telling about experiences (e.g., through storytelling or ceremony); the interrelationships among emotions, beliefs, and behaviors; the importance of emotional identification and expression; and movement toward self-healing and well-being.

The Indigenous people of today—and of the past—present a broad cultural picture. There is much diversity in the traditional concepts and tribal beliefs of American Indians and Alaska Natives. It is important not to assume that all tribal and native people have similar traditions. Especially critical is the respect for the process of healing and well-being that each child and family is capable of achieving through the thoughtful blending of cultural traditions and practices and scientifically based interventions. Through our work at the ICCTC, we seek to respect the unique traditions seen across American Indian and Alaska Native people while honoring the collective values, practices, and wisdom that provide them with support and strength.

REFERENCES

BigFoot, D. S. (2000). History of victimization. In D. S. BigFoot (Ed.), *Native American topic-specific monograph series*. Washington, DC: Office for Victims of Crime.

BigFoot, D. S. (2008). Cultural adaptations of evidence-based practices for American Indian and Alaska Native populations. In C. Newman, C. J. Liberton, K. Kutash, & R. M. Friedman (Eds.), *A system of care for children's mental health: Expanding the research base*. Tampa, FL: University of South Florida, Louis de la Parte Florida Mental Health Institute, Research and Training Center for Children's Mental Health.

BigFoot, D. S. (2010, February). *The effects of trauma on America Indian and Alaska Native children*. Paper presented at the 30th Annual Conference of the National Association of Social Workers, New Mexico Chapter, Albuquerque, NM.

BigFoot, D. S., & Braden, J. (1999). *Upon the back of a turtle: A training curriculum for criminal justice personnel working in Indian Country*. Oklahoma City: Center on Child Abuse and Neglect, University of Oklahoma Health Sciences Center.

BigFoot, D. S., & Schmidt, S. R. (2008). *Honoring Children, Mending the Circle training manual*. Oklahoma City: University of Oklahoma Health Sciences Center.

BigFoot, D. S., & Schmidt, S. R. (2009). Science-to practice: Adapting an evidence based child trauma treatment for American Indian and Alaska Native populations. *International Journal of Child Health and Human Development, 2*(1), 33–44.

Blum, R.W., Harmon, B., Harris, L., Bergeisen, L., & Resnick, M. D. (1992). American Indian/Alaska Native youth health. *Journal of the American Medical Association, 267*(12), 1637–1644.

Centers for Disease Control and Prevention. (n.d.). *Understanding suicide: factsheet*. Retrieved from *www.cdc.gov/violenceprevention/pdf/suicide-FactSheet-a.pdf*.

Cohen, J. A., Mannarino, A. P., & Deblinger, E. (2006). *Treating trauma and traumatic grief in children and adolescents*. New York: Guilford Press.

Kessler, R.C., Sonnega, A., Bromet, E., Hughes, M., & Nelson, C.B. (1995). Post-traumatic stress disorder in the National Comorbidity Survey. *Archives of General Psychiatry, 52*(12), 1048–1060.

Kettle, P. A., & Bixler, E. O. (1991). Suicide in Alaska Native, 1979–1984. *Psychiatry, 54,* 55–63.

LaFromboise, T. D., Trimble, J. E., & Mohatt, G. V. (1990). Counseling intervention and American Indian tradition: An integrative approach. *Counseling Psychologist, 18,* 628–654.

Manson, S. M. (2004). *Cultural diversity series: Meeting the mental health needs of American Indians and Alaska Natives.* Abstract retrieved November 12, 2007, from *www.azdhs.gov/bhs/ccna.pdf.*

May, P. A. (1990). Suicide and suicide attempts among American Indians and Alaska Natives: A bibliography. *Omega, 21*(3), 199–214.

McDonald, J. D., & Gonzalez, J. (2006). Cognitive-behavioral therapy with American Indians. In P. A. Hays & G. Y. Iwamasa (Eds.), *Culturally responsive cognitive-behavioral therapy: Assessment, practice and supervision* (pp. 23–46). Washington, DC: American Psychological Association.

Mock, C. N., Grossman, D. C., Mulder, D., Stewart, C., & Koepsell, T.S. (1996). Health care utilization as a marker for suicidal behavior on an American Indian reservation. *Journal of General Internal Medicine, 11*(9), 519–524.

National Child Abuse and Neglect Data System. (2002). *Child maltreatment 2002.* Washington, DC: Department of Health and Human Services, Administration on Children and Families.

Novins, D. K., Beals, J., Shore, J. H., & Manson, S. M. (1996). The substance abuse treatment of American Indian adolescents: Comorbid symptomatology, gender differences, and treatment patterns. *Journal of the American Academy of Adolescent and Child Psychology, 35*(12), 1593–1601.

Perry, S. W. (2004). *American Indians and crime: A BJS statistical profile, 1992–2002.* Washington, DC: U.S. Department of Justice. Retrieved November 8, 2005, from *www.justice.gov/otj/pdf/american_indians_and_crime.pdf.*

Satcher, D. (1999). *Mental health: A report of the surgeon general.* Paper presented at the 92nd Annual Convention of the National Association for the Advancement of Colored People, New Orleans, LA.

Sipe, J. L. (2003). The Lost Cheyennes. *Watonga Republican.*

Stanford Solar Center. (2008). *Ancient observatories, timeless knowledge.* Retrieved October 2, 2009, from *http://solar-center.stanford.edu/AO/.*

Index

Page numbers in *italic* refer to figures